W9-AZG-159

PHACODYNAMICS

Mastering the TOOLS AND TECHNIQUES of Phacoemulsification Surgery

Third Edition

Barry S. Seibel, MD

Clinical Assistant Professor of Ophthalmology

University of California

Los Angeles School of Medicine

SLACK Incorporated, 6900 Grove Road, Thorofare, NJ 08086-9447

Publisher: John H. Bond
Editorial Director: Amy E. Drummond
Senior Associate Editor: Jennifer J. Cahill
Illustrations by Barry S. Seibel, MD

Printed in the United States of America
Published by: SLACK Incorporated
6900 Grove Road
Thorofare, NJ 08086-9447 USA
Telephone: 609-848-1000
Fax: 609-853-5991
WWW: http://www.slackinc.com

Seibel, Barry S.
Phacodynamics: mastering the tools and techniques of phacoemulsification surgery/Barry S. Seibel.--3rd ed.
p. cm.
Includes bibliographic references and index.
ISBN 1-55642-388-8
1. Phacoemulsification. I. Title.
[DNLM: 1. Phacoemulsification--methods. 2. Phacoemulsification--instrumentation. WW 260S457p 1999]
RE451.S38 1999
617.7'42059--dc21
DNLM/DLC 98-29336
for Library of Congress

Contact SLACK Incorporated for more information about other books in this field or about the availability of our books from distributors outside the United States.

Last digit is print number: 10 9 8 7 6 5 4 3 2 1

Dedication

To my wife, Rhonda, for her patience, love, understanding, and inspiration.

Contents

Ultrasound

Section Two: Logic of Setting Machine Parameters

Section Three: Overview of Phacoemulsification Techniques

Section Four: Irrigation and Aspiration Techniques

Section Five: Physics of Capsulorhexis

Appendices

Acknowledgments

I would like to acknowledge first and foremost phaco's inventor, Dr. Charles Kelman, without whose persistent dedication the field of ophthalmology might still be limited to large incision extracapsular cataract surgery, and without whom this book would simply have no subject. This third edition of *Phacodynamics* also is indebted to John Bond, Amy Drummond, and, of course, Peter Slack of SLACK Incorporated for appreciating the need for a new edition in the face of advancing technology and techniques. As in previous editions, I am grateful for the feedback that I have received from engineers at various phaco companies, including Alcon's Gary Sorensen, Don Lobdell, and Mikhail Boukhny, as well as AMO's Mark Cole, Ken Kadziauskas, and, of course, Ed Zaleski. I am especially grateful to Bob Blankemeyer, Jim Tiffany, Chuck Hess, Bob Mosher, Ash Mahmood, Blake Michaels, and Dennis Casey of Bausch & Lomb Surgical/Storz Ophthalmics for the extensive allocation of their engineering resources and staff for wet lab research in fluidics and ultrasonics. Thanks also to the individual Storz engineers, including Jim Perkins and Rob Naslund. A very special thanks to Storz's Bill Neubert and senior engineer Tom Moore for their additional help in proofreading the book for technical accuracy. Alex Urich, president of Circuit Tree Medical, and Ed Terpilowski, president of MicroSurgical Technology, were instrumental in the development of the Flat-Head Phaco tip, and Rhein Medical's president, John Bee, was invaluable in bringing the Seibel Chopper to market.

I would also like to acknowledge the valuable role that lecturing has played in the development of this new edition; answering impromptu questions forces me to constantly analyze, update, and clarify my thoughts and explanations about fluidics and ultrasound. I am therefore grateful to the numerous physicians, medical societies, and groups that have invited me to lecture around the world in the past several years. Thanks also to Storz for including me in the excellent domestic and international phaco courses directed by Dr. William Maloney, as well as to Allergan for my inclusion in the domestic courses organized by Susan Zajfen. A very special thanks in this regard to the outstanding Australian Allergan team of Peter Abrahamson, Craig Stamp, and Jason McCabe, who organized a truly excellent series of educational programs in which I was honored to participate. Thanks also to Dr. Bill Fishkind, with whom I have instructed our AAO course "The Physics of Phaco" for the past 3 years. I also appreciate Dr. Kevin Miller for including me in various instructional courses at the Jules Stein Eye Institute.

Finally, besides Dr. Kelman, I would like to acknowledge some additional people whose work has inspired my own. I am always amazed at the energy of Dr. Lucio Buratto, a prolific author and originator of the live surgery VideoCataract courses. I further wish to acknowledge Drs. Sam Masket, Howard Fine, Bob Osher, and Doug Koch; although the field of ophthalmology has many fine teachers, I have found these friends and colleagues to be especially inspirational in that they help to establish the benchmark in ophthalmic education through their dedication to teaching, their intellectual honesty, and their energetic curiosity.

Preface to the Third Edition

During the 4 years since the second edition of *Phacodynamics* was written, two significant factors have evolved which prompted this new edition. First, significant new machine technologies and surgical techniques have been introduced. Dr. Nagahara's chop technique has continued to grow in popularity and variations as the benefits of this innovative method have become increasingly apparent clinically as well as from the perspective of ultrasonic and fluidic efficiency; correspondingly, the third edition has several new illustrations and text devoted just to these chop variations. My own fault-line phaco technique was developed as an exercise in the application of phacodynamic principles with regard to surgical methodology as well as instrumentation. Similar application of phacodynamic principles was applied to the design of the Seibel Chopper, as well as the Flat-Head Phaco tip, and the logic behind these particular tools and techniques is explained in this new edition. New pumps have been developed since the previous edition, including the rotary vane pump and the scroll pump. The larger number of pumps on the phaco market has prompted this new edition's categorization of all pumps into either a flow-based or vacuum-based classification with comparison and contrast between the two with regard to clinically relevant fluidics. This classification system will help the surgeon to more knowledgeably assess new phaco machines as well as better understand the logic behind setting parameters on his or her current machine. The section on ultrasonics has greatly expanded with emphasis on new tip designs and their effect on clinical utility as well as machine fluidics. Finally, a significant new control modality is described in the third edition, the Dual Linear foot pedal, which allows simultaneous linear control of two different parameters, such as vacuum and ultrasound.

Thc sccond factor that has prompted this new edition is my 4 additional years of lecturing, during which I have continued to refine my explanations of the physics of machine technology and microsurgical technique. I am grateful to the many intelligent questions which have resulted in what I feel are even better schematic graphics and descriptions than in previous editions; over half of the illustrations and accompanying text are either completely new or revised. Moreover, my abilities in graphic illustration have continued to develop in the past 4 years, as have my computer hardware and software used in this endeavor. Finally, additional cross-referencing and categorization has been included to further reinforce the multifactorial nature of phacodynamic principles. It is this multifaceted approach to understanding the logic behind machine technology and surgical techniques which I have endeavored to carry over from previous editions and significantly enhance in this third edition.

Preface to the Second Edition

The preface to the first edition is just as relevant to this second edition: understanding the underlying principles of the surgical equipment and techniques results in maximum safety, control, and adaptability. A working knowledge of these principles has become even more vital in the past couple of years, during which time the phaco equipment has evolved to allow even greater surgical finesse and control to the operator who fully understands the parameters involved. The second edition's new section on *Anterior Chamber Fluidics* analyzes the currents involved in phaco surgery so that you can understand when and how to adjust vacuum and aspiration flow rate to achieve maximum safety and efficacy at various stages of surgery. New material has been added to the *Machine Technology* section which explains the concepts of surge, compliance, venting, bottle height function, and fluidic resistance. Understanding these concepts will not only allow an educated evaluation of the many different phaco machines on the market, but they will also maximize your effectiveness with your current machine. All of the illustrations have been carefully scrutinized for fluidic accuracy and have been revised as necessary. For example, IA tips have been changed to phaco tips in the flow diagrams because recent lab measurements have demonstrated that the flow volume depicted would not be accurate for the high resistance IA port. Even the number of drops in the drip chambers of the flow diagrams has been revised to accurately reflect the results of recent fluidic experiments. Material on Dr. Nagahara's phaco chop method as well as Dr. Koch's stop and chop method have been included in Sections Two and Three. The *Physics of Capsulorhexis* section has doubled in size in order to include even more clinical options for different surgical situations. As in the first edition, however, the emphasis of *Phacodynamics* is not so much on individual methods or techniques as it is on the underlying principles which are common to all.

Preface to the First Edition

The fundamental goal of phacoemulsification is to remove a cataract with minimum disturbance to the eye. You should use the least number of surgical manipulations necessary to accomplish the surgery; random, superfluous movements must be actively avoided. Each maneuver should be performed with the minimum force required; maximum efficiency is attained by applying principles of physics and mechanical advantage. Physical manipulation of intraocular tissues can be decreased by taking full advantage of a phaco machine's capabilities by using principles of fluid dynamics. Minimum effort yields maximum safety.

Every phacoemulsification course teaches one or more step-by-step methods, including one-handed, two-handed, chip and flip, in-the-bag, divide and conquer, and others. Each method has its own attributes, and you should familiarize yourself with all of them. However, every step-by-step method shares the same disadvantage: not every operation will necessarily proceed in an orderly fashion to the next appropriate step. The goal of this book is to teach the fundamental principles of both the phaco machine and the microsurgical maneuvers shared by all of the step-by-step methods. By understanding these underlying principles, you will be able to transpose as necessary between methods, improvise your own methods, and adapt to virtually any surgical situation with confidence.

Foreword

In the late 1960s when I was in the process of developing the instrumentation and procedure we now know as phacoemulsification, I found myself at the limits of that era's technology. Even today with all the advances made in computers, metallurgy, and the like, the same can be said regarding improvements in the functionality of modern phaco machines.

It is certainly fair to say that the phacoemulsification procedure relies as heavily on the surgeon's skill as it does on the apparatus. With this in mind, I have always stressed the importance of the surgeon having ample knowledge regarding the technology behind the instrumentation he or she wields.

The procedure has, from its inception, evolved in lock step with advances in technology, the most significant of which has been the introduction of microprocessor control and feedback of machine function. This advancement allows the surgeon to customize the machine to his or her own requirements. But this also implies that the surgeon have a firm understanding of the principles involved.

Dr. Seibel, in his expanded third edition of *Phacodynamics,* brings the phaco surgeon up-to-date in this marriage of technology and surgical technique. The numerous illustrations and diagrams bring the technology behind the technique to the broader ophthalmic community in a manner that is logical and concise.

Charles D. Kelman, MD
The Eye Center
New York, New York

SECTION ONE

Machine Technology

Machine Overview

Phacoemulsification is comprised of two basic elements. First, ultrasound energy is used to emulsify the cataract so that a 10mm lens may be removed (aspirated) through a 3mm or smaller incision. Second, a fluidic circuit is employed to counteract the potential heat buildup and repulsive action of the ultrasonic needle, as well as to remove the emulsate via the aspiration port while maintaining the anterior chamber (Figure 1-1). This circuit is supplied via the irrigation ports by an elevated irrigating bottle which supplies both the fluid volume and pressure to maintain the chamber hydrodynamically and hydrostatically, respectively; anterior chamber pressure is directly proportional to the height of the bottle. The fluid circuit is regulated by a pump which not only clears the chamber of emulsate, but also provides significant clinical utility. When the phaco tip is unoccluded, the pump produces currents in the anterior chamber, measured in cc/min, which attract nuclear fragments. When a fragment completely occludes the tip, the pump provides holding power, measured in mm Hg vacuum, which grips the fragment. In order to fully exploit the potential of a phaco machine, the surgeon must understand the logic behind setting the parameters of bottle height, ultrasound power, vacuum, and flow.

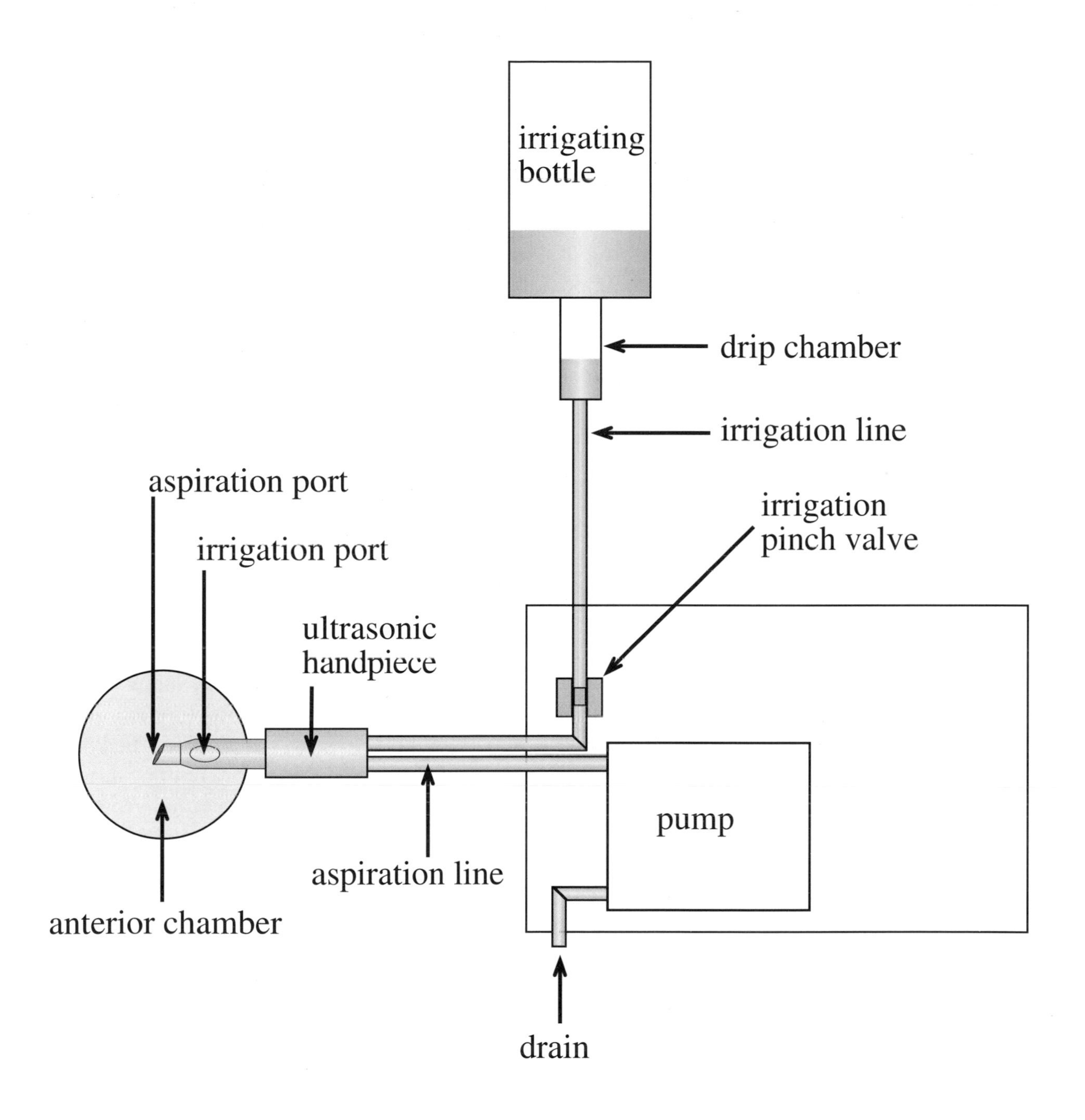
irrigating bottle
drip chamber
irrigation line
aspiration port
irrigation port
irrigation pinch valve
ultrasonic handpiece
pump
aspiration line
anterior chamber
drain

Figure 1-1

Foot Pedal

The phaco machine is controlled intraoperatively by the surgeon via the foot pedal. Note the four positions in phaco mode, designated 0, 1, 2, and 3 (Figure 1-2); the pump is inactive in positions 0 and 1. Note that **position 0** refers to the resting, fully upright **point** of foot pedal travel, whereas the other positions each refer to a particular **range** of foot pedal travel. The irrigation tubing passes through a fixture on the phaco machine in which a plunger pinches the tubing in position 0, thereby completely interrupting the fluidic circuit at this point. When the surgeon steps into **position 1**, the plunger snaps away from the tubing, completing the fluidic circuit and pressurizing the anterior chamber in proportion to the bottle height; no actual flow is present except for any possible incisional leakage. Some machines have a **continuous irrigation mode** that eliminates position 0 by keeping the pinch valve open throughout all pedal travel, thereby pressurizing the fluidic circuit even when the pedal is in the relaxed, fully upright baseline position. Position 1 is useful for many maneuvers that do not require vacuum, flow, or ultrasound yet benefit from a formed anterior chamber, including nuclear rotation and splitting.

As **position 2** is entered, the pump head begins to rotate in a flow pump; vacuum is created in the rigid drainage cassette of a vacuum pump. In either case, pump activity produces flow through the aspiration port when it is unoccluded, and vacuum just inside the aspiration port when it is occluded. In a vacuum pump machine with **linear control**, vacuum increases as the pedal is pushed further into position 2, thereby increasing both the aspiration flow rate (with an unoccluded tip), as well as the potential maximum vacuum (with an occluded tip) up to the maximum preset value, which is reached when the pedal is in the bottom of position 2 and continues at this level throughout position 3. In a flow pump machine with linear vacuum control, the maximum potential vacuum is also increased as the pedal is pushed further into position 2 up to the maximum vacuum level which is preset by the surgeon. However, flow rate (on most flow pump machines) stays constant throughout position 2 travel; the pump head can be observed to have a constant rotational speed throughout position 2 (and 3) travel. Some newer machines offer the option of linear control of either flow or vacuum (see Figure 4-7).

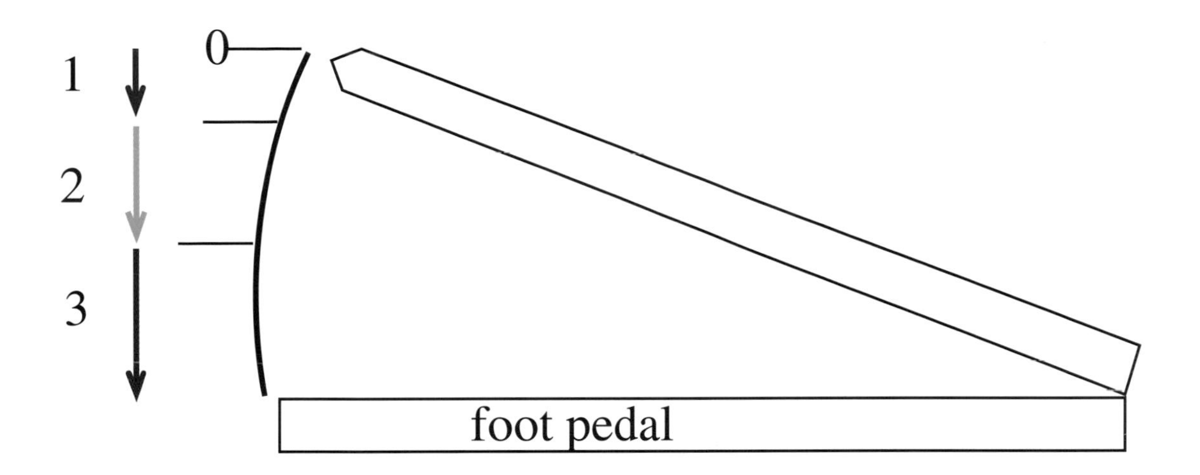

Figure 1-2

Foot Pedal (continued)

Position 3 represents the range in which ultrasound energy is active. A **linear control** machine will give progressively more ultrasound energy as the pedal is progressively depressed until the maximum amount (preset by the surgeon) is reached at the bottom of pedal travel; if the ultrasound mode is set to **fixed power panel control** (nonlinear), the full preset ultrasound power will be abruptly engaged as soon as position 3 is entered and will be maintained throughout position 3's travel.

Note that the irrigation (I) line pinch valve which opened in position 1 continues to be open throughout positions 2 and 3. Similarly, pump activity (A) which starts in position 2 continues throughout position 3 (Figure 1-3). Many machines also have a foot pedal **reflux** control which reverses flow so that fluid (and any capsule, iris, or other inadvertently aspirated tissue) will flow out of the aspiration port. Some machines have an identical pedal setup for both phaco and IA, although most combine the travel of positions 2 and 3 into a single longer excursion for position 2 in IA (see Figure 1-3).

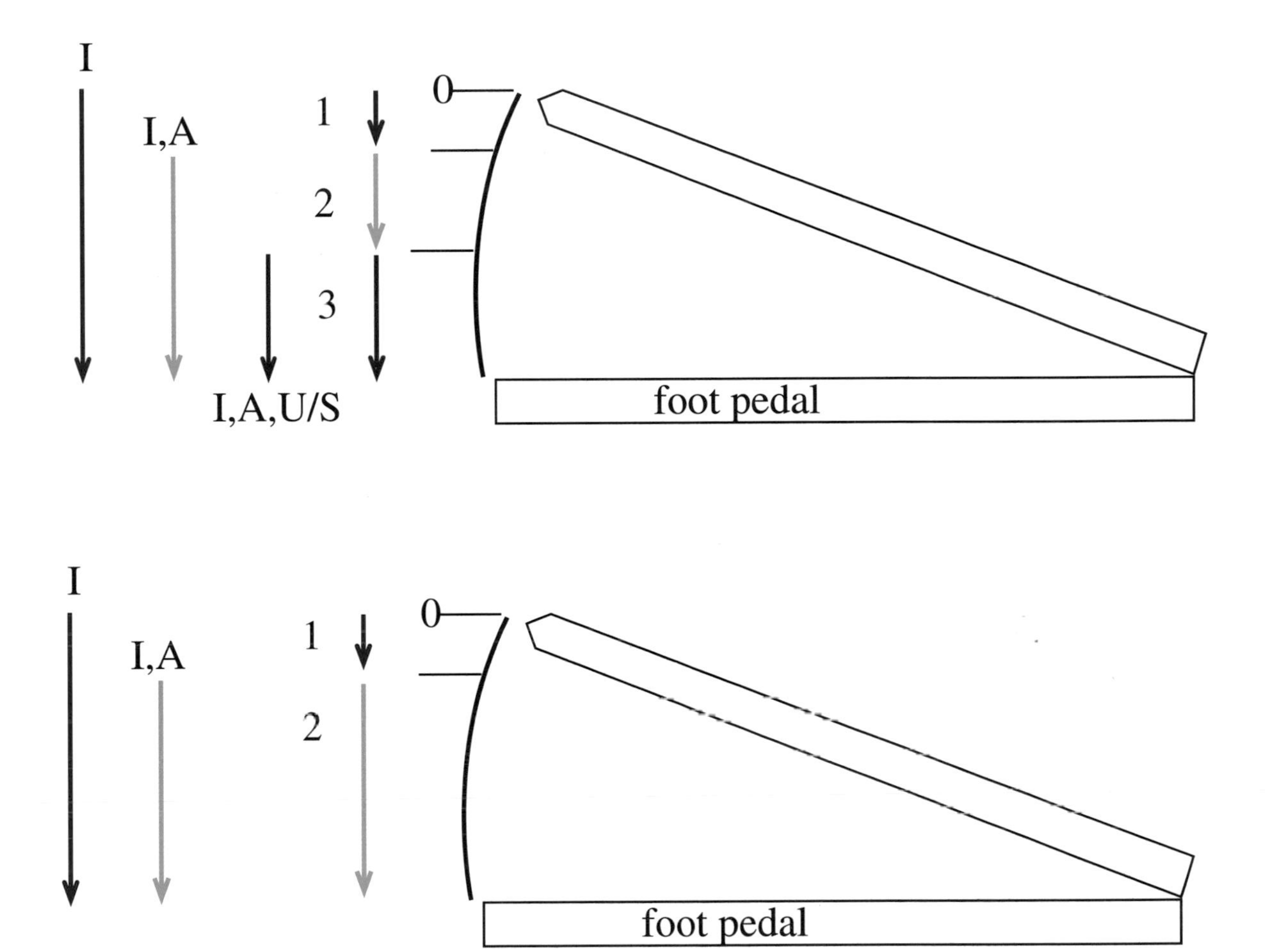

Figure 1-3

Foot Pedal (continued)

A new mode of pedal control has recently been introduced by Bausch & Lomb Surgical on the Storz Millennium platform. The **Dual Linear pedal** allows simultaneous linear control of both ultrasound and vacuum by separating these parameters into two different planes of pedal movement; a new lateral yaw movement has been added to the traditional pitch excursion of the pedal (Figure 1-4). This configuration has some significant advantages. First and foremost, the ability to linearly control vacuum in phaco mode greatly expands intraoperative options and efficiency; moreover, the range of pedal travel has been increased in both positions 2 and 3, thereby providing enhanced control sensitivity. In the traditional pedal setup, even on the few machines that have linear control of vacuum in the more limited range of position 2's travel, the maximum vacuum preset which was reached at the bottom of position 2's travel was maintained throughout position 3. Therefore, a surgeon had to contend with a single potentially high vacuum level while using various levels of linear ultrasound. In contrast, the Dual Linear pedal allows appropriate titration of the vacuum level for any given amount of linear ultrasound (see Figure 2-12). Although all Dual Linear illustrations in this book depict pitch controlling position 2 (vacuum) and yaw controlling position 3 (ultrasound), these functions can be reversed if desired by the surgeon.

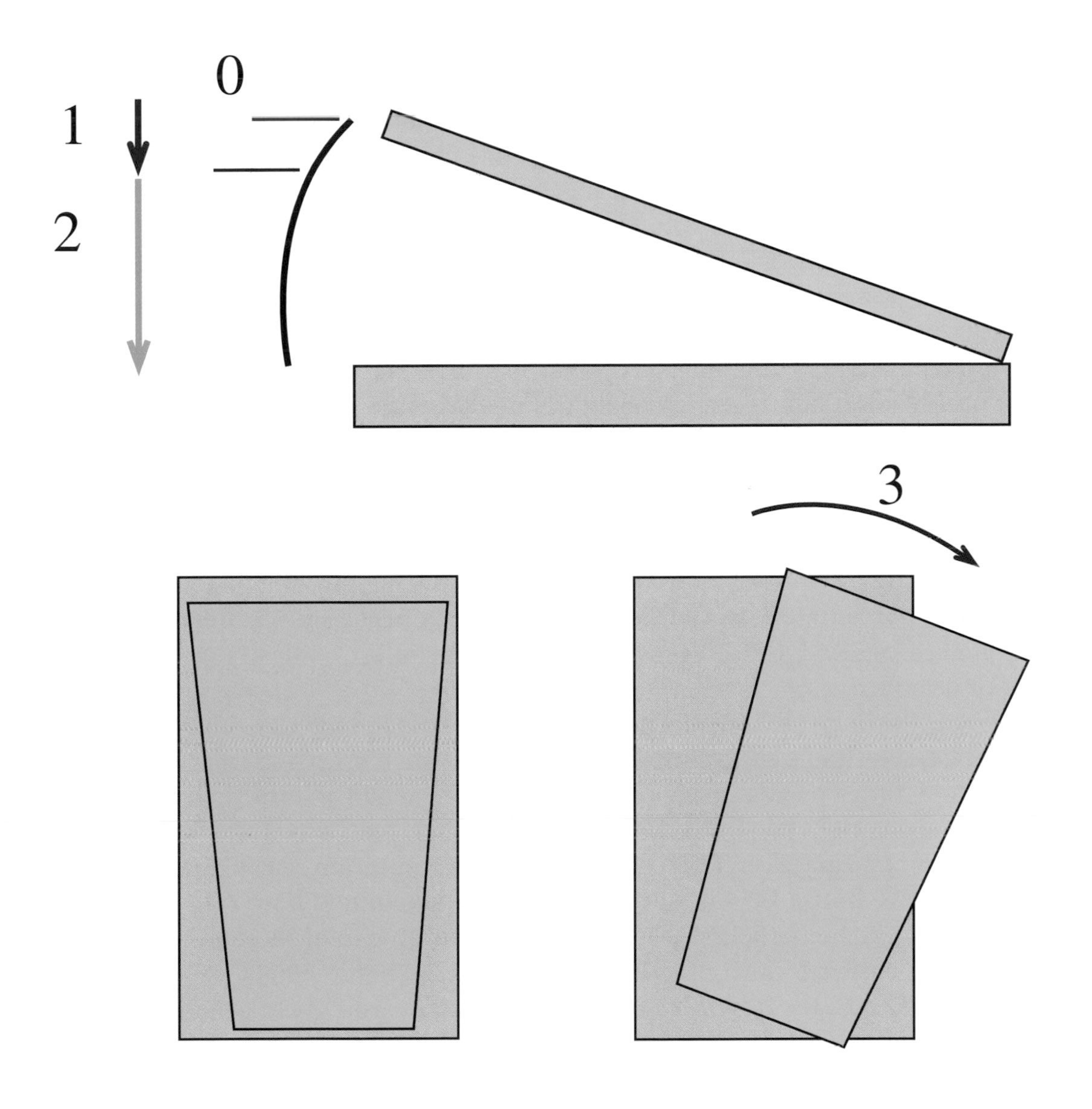

Figure 1-4

Irrigating Bottle

The fluidic circuit is supplied by the elevated irrigating bottle containing an osmotically balanced saline solution; the fluid path then proceeds through the irrigation line, through the irrigation ports on the ultrasonic needle's silicone sleeve, through the anterior chamber, through the aspiration port at the tip of the needle, and then into the aspiration line. The parameter of bottle height has a constant function during all phases of surgery—to keep the chamber safely formed without overpressurization which might stress zonules, misdirect aqueous into the vitreous, or cause excessive incisional leakage. Approximately 11mm Hg pressure (above ambient atmospheric pressure) is produced intraocularly for every 15cm (6 inches) bottle height above the eye (Figure 1-5-1 simplifies the relationship by rounding 11mm Hg to 10mm Hg so that a 45cm bottle height yields an IOP of 30mm Hg); this relationship is accurate for **hydrostatic pressure** in which fluid is present but not moving within the fluidic circuit. However, it is vital that the appropriate bottle height be set **hydrodynamically** with the pump operating (pedal position 2 or 3) and the tip unoccluded so that an adequate pressure head will be established to keep up with the induced aspiration outflow which decreases the IOP from the hydrostatic level present in pedal position 1. If everything else is equal, **the IOP decreases proportionately as the flow rate increases according to Bernoulli's equation** (Figures 1-5-2 and 1-9a); decreasing IOP will manifest clinically as a shallowing anterior chamber.

The flow rate may increase not only as a result of increased pump function but also as a result of decreased fluidic resistance in the circuit (ie, when changing from a small aspiration port to a larger one as in Figure 1-24). If bottle height is insufficient for a given flow rate, the anterior chamber will collapse due to induced vacuum (ie, negative pressure relative to atmospheric). **Therefore, in order to maintain a constant IOP, remember to increase bottle height when increasing a machine's flow rate;** correspondingly, decrease the bottle height when decreasing the flow rate. Moreover, if the surgeon deliberately wishes to lower the IOP by lowering the bottle height (ie, in case of a posterior capsule tear), the flow rate must be decreased accordingly to maintain fluidic balance and avoid an unstable or flat anterior chamber.

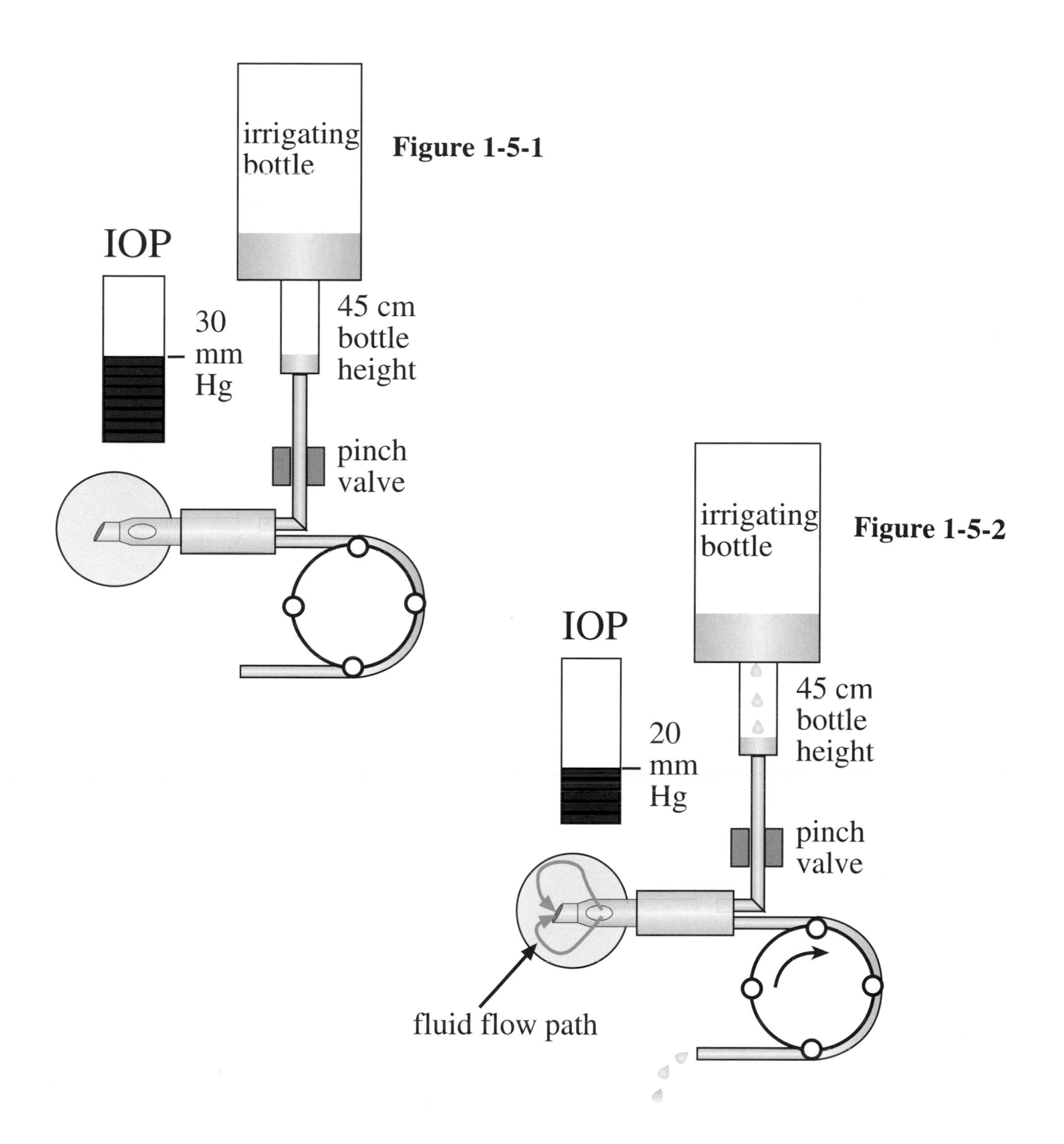
irrigating bottle
Figure 1-5-1
IOP
30 mm Hg
45 cm bottle height
pinch valve
irrigating bottle
Figure 1-5-2
IOP
20 mm Hg
45 cm bottle height
pinch valve
fluid flow path

Figure 1-5

Irrigating Bottle (continued)

When the tip becomes occluded, the IOP will rise to the hydrostatic level established by the bottle height even in position 2 or 3 (Figure 1-6-1) except to the extent that vacuum or ultrasound eventually clears the occlusion in these positions, respectively. Note in Figure 1-6-1 that the pump wheel is rotating but no flow is present; no drops are present at the drain or in the drip chamber. The absence of flow is secondary to the occlusion of the phaco tip's aspiration port by a large piece of nucleus. Occlusion of the aspiration port isolates the anterior chamber from the aspiration line and the pump; this isolation results in identical IOPs of 30mm Hg in both Figures 1-5-1 and 1-6-1 even though the pump is operating in the latter but not in the former. When the pedal is in its baseline non-depressed position 0, the irrigation pinch valve (located on the machine at approximately eye level) is closed, thus isolating the eye from the pressure head established by the column of fluid (bottle height) between the pinch valve and the top of the fluid in the irrigating bottle drip chamber (Figure 1-6-2). The anterior chamber will become shallow in position 0 because of unopposed vitreous pressure; indeed, the IOP approaches 0 to the extent that the incision allows communication with atmospheric pressure. The chamber will collapse without the pressure head provided by the fluid from the elevated irrigating bottle, especially in pedal position 2 or 3; for this reason, the operating room staff must be vigilant in not allowing the bottle to run out during an operation.

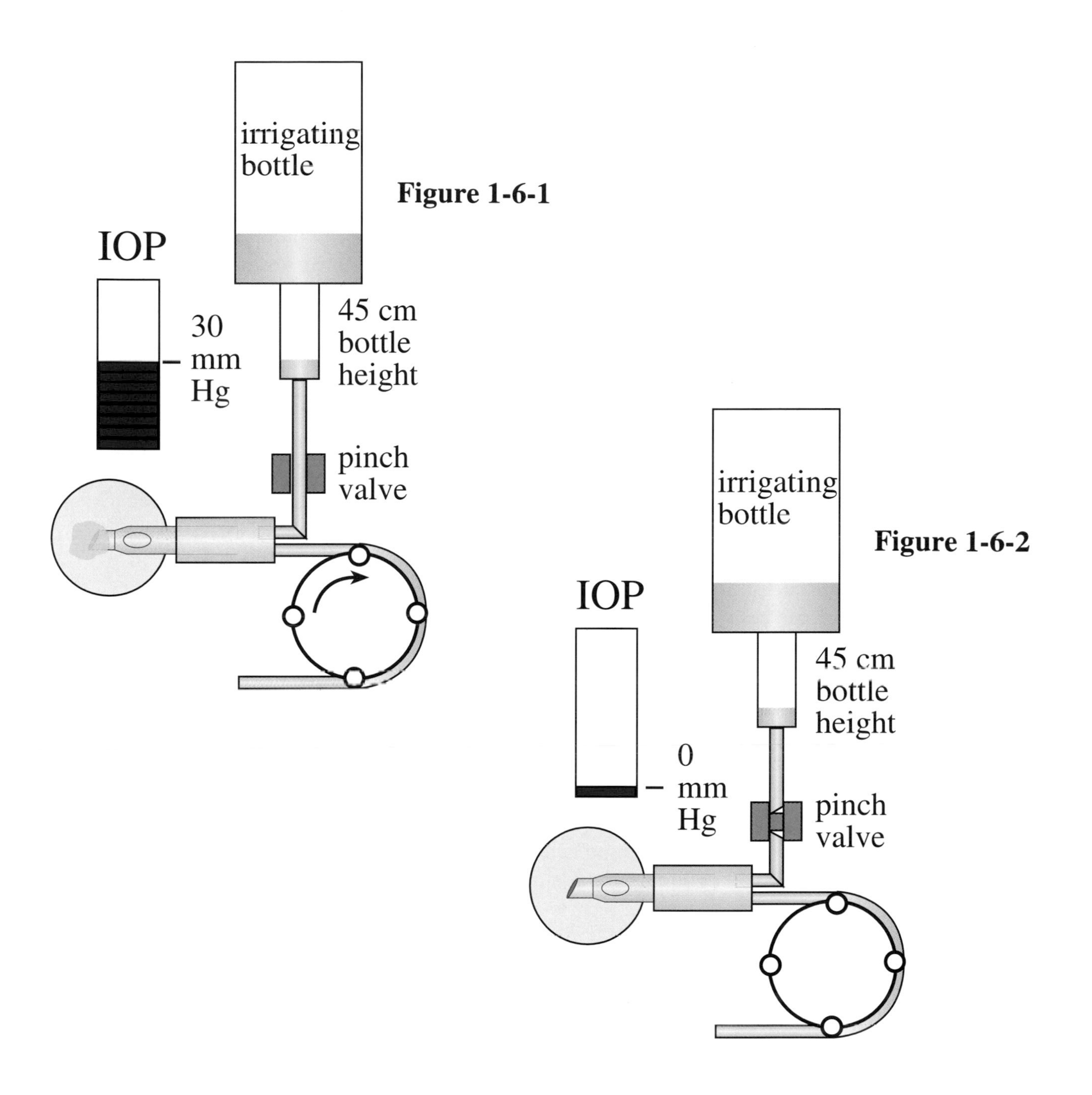
irrigating
bottle
Figure 1-6-1
IOP
30
mm
Hg
45 cm
bottle
height
pinch
valve
irrigating
bottle
Figure 1-6-2
IOP
45 cm
bottle
height
0
mm
Hg
pinch
valve

Figure 1-6

Flow Pumps: Direct Control of Flow; Peristaltic Pump

A discussion of flow and vacuum in phaco surgery must begin with a categorization of the various pumps which are utilized. There are two basic types of pumps in phaco: the flow pump and the vacuum pump. The flow pump, also known as a positive displacement pump, physically regulates the fluid flow in the aspiration line via direct contact between the fluid and a rotating element (pump head) in the pump mechanism; this is in contrast to a vacuum pump, which has an air interface in its drainage cassette which indirectly links the aspiration line fluid to the pump mechanism. With flow pumps, the surgeon commands a given flow rate via the panel preset and/or the pedal position, while aspiration line vacuum levels vary according to different aspiration port sizes and degrees of occlusion, as well as according to the commanded flow rate and vacuum limit preset. **Flow rate**, also known as **aspiration flow rate**, is measured in cc/min and is directly proportional to the rotational speed of the pump head, measured in revolutions per minute (rpm). This relationship is accurate when the aspiration port of a standard phaco needle is unoccluded. Flow ceases when this port is fully occluded, and the rotational speed of the pump head is then inversely proportional to the rise time (see Figure 1-11). Regardless of the state of tip occlusion, adjusting the flow rate control of a flow pump determines the rotational speed of the pump head. **The presence of an independent flow rate control further differentiates a flow pump from all current vacuum pumps used in phaco surgery.**

The two current phaco flow pumps are the peristaltic pump and the scroll pump. Although the scroll pump is the newest example of a flow pump, the **peristaltic pump** is the most commonly employed in current phaco machines and serves as a good schematic example of the flow pump's principles (Figure 1-7). As the pump head rotates, rollers engage the aspiration tubing and collapse it at each point of roller contact. With continued rotation, boluses of fluid are created between rollers and propagated in a peristaltic fashion in the direction of rotation as indicated by the arrows. This fluid flow creates a pressure differential at the beginning of the pump head which draws more fluid from the aspiration tubing.

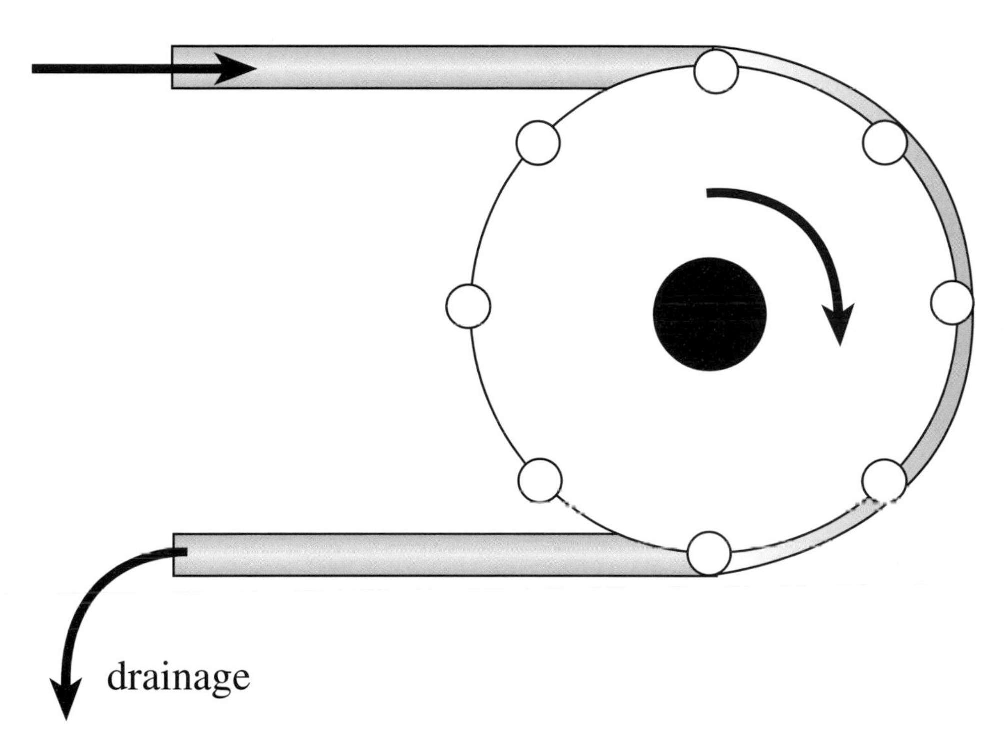

Figure 1-7

Scroll Pump

The peristaltic pump has some liabilities inherent to its basic design. First, fairly compliant aspiration tubing is required so that the pump head rollers can collapse the tubing and milk boluses of fluid through it; however, increased compliance in the fluidic circuit increases the potential for surge problems (see Figure 1-43). Second, the indirect contact between the fluid and rollers via the tubing, as well as imperfect apposition of the collapsed internal tubing walls, allow for pump leakage in which the pump rollers traverse the aspiration line faster than the fluid inside of the line; at a given rotational pump speed, the actual flow rate decreases as resistance to flow (vacuum) increases (see Figure 1-10). The scroll pump design addresses these problems by placing a rigid, orbitally rotating pump element directly within the fluidic circuit (Figure 1-8). The scroll element and pump housing as illustrated are fixed between two rigid flat plates to confine the fluid into the scroll channels. Relative to a peristaltic pump, a scroll pump can utilize less compliant tubing which only needs to be flexible enough to allow ergonomic control of the ultrasonic and IA handpiece; the less compliant tubing has less of a potential for surge problems (see Figures 1-42 and 1-43). Furthermore, by eliminating compliant tubing as an integral pump element, the scroll pump can be manufactured to tighter tolerances which decrease the potential for pump leakage, especially at higher vacuum levels. As a result of its low compliance and minimal leakage, the scroll pump is particularly well suited to having the option of being used in a vacuum emulation mode as discussed with Figure 1-40a.

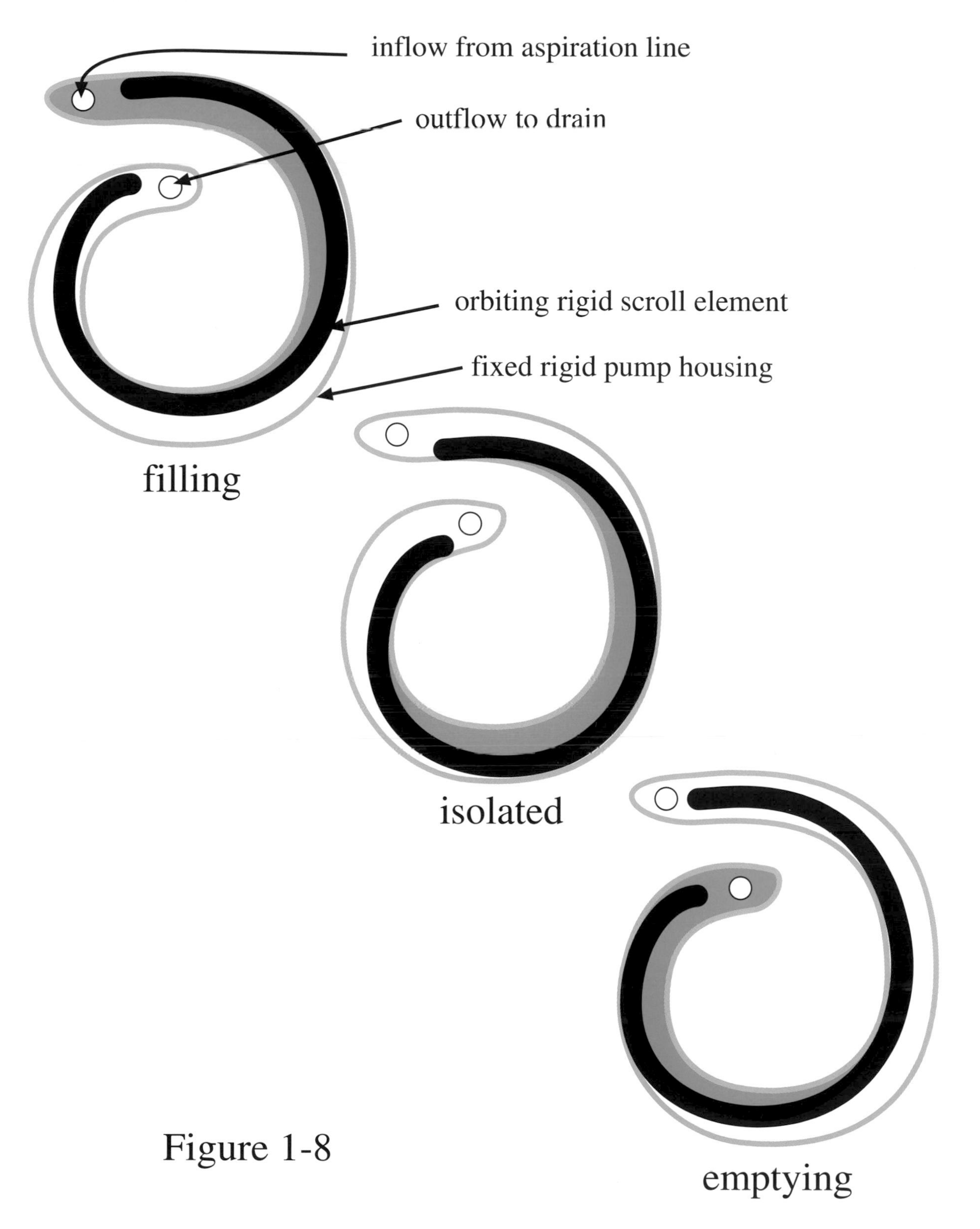
inflow from aspiration line
outflow to drain
orbiting rigid scroll element
fixed rigid pump housing
filling
isolated
emptying

Figure 1-8

Flow Pumps: Indirect Control of Vacuum

The direct control of flow with flow pumps has an indirect but predictable effect on vacuum in the fluidic circuit. When a flow pump is set to a low rotational speed, the subsequent low flow rate does not produce any appreciable vacuum in the aspiration line unless the aspiration port is occluded. Indeed, at lower flow rates with an unoccluded phaco aspiration port, there is a positive pressure in the aspiration line because of the pressure head from the irrigation bottle (Figures 1-9-1 and 1-21); fluid flows as illustrated because of the **pressure differential** between the higher positive pressure of the anterior chamber and the lower (but still positive relative to atmospheric) pressure in the aspiration line. The flow rate is increased in Figure 1-9-2, and **vacuum** (measured in mm Hg below atmospheric pressure, indicated by a negative value on the graph) is produced in the aspiration line because of the resistance induced by the aspiration port (especially with a 0.3mm IA tip or a partially occluded standard 0.9mm phaco tip) and, to a lesser extent, by the aspiration tubing's inherent resistance, which is a function of its length and internal diameter. At slower flow rates, these resistances are negligible. Note that the flow rate can be visually estimated by observing the irrigating bottle's drip chamber. Note also that because the resistances of the aspiration port and tubing are located between the pump and the aspiration port, this is the location of greatest vacuum buildup or **negative pressure** (mm Hg below atmospheric pressure); see also Figure 1-39. The portion of the fluidic circuit between the irrigating bottle and the aspiration port, including the anterior chamber, will have a more positive pressure because of the pressure head from the irrigating bottle. Moreover, this portion of the fluidic circuit will always have a positive value (measured in mm Hg above ambient atmospheric pressure) when the anterior chamber is formed; chamber collapse is indicative of too low a bottle height (not enough positive pressure) or too rapid a flow rate (too much induced vacuum or negative pressure) which results in a net negative pressure.

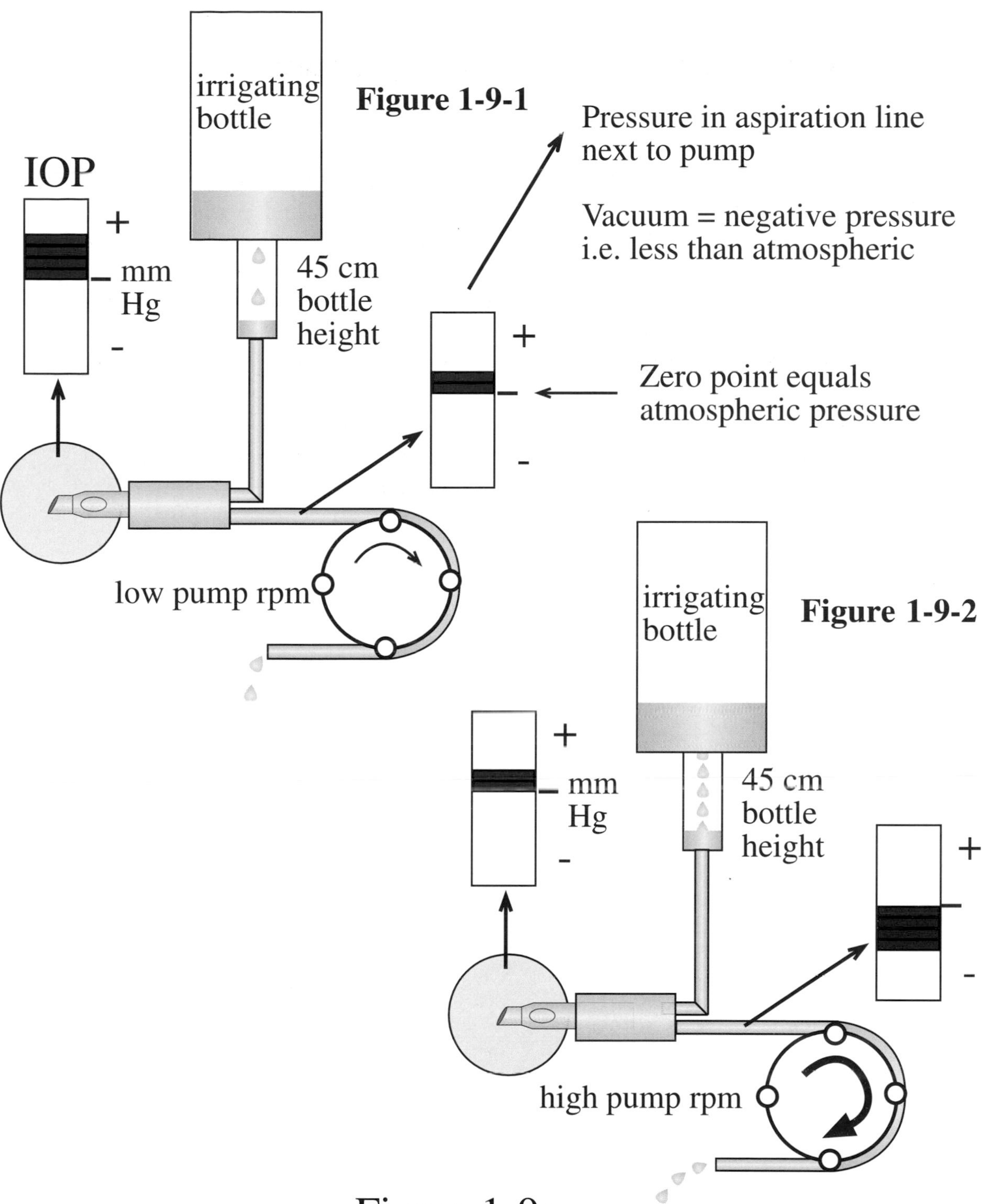

irrigating bottle
Figure 1-9-1
IOP
+
mm Hg
-
45 cm bottle height
Pressure in aspiration line next to pump
Vacuum = negative pressure i.e. less than atmospheric
+
Zero point equals atmospheric pressure
-
low pump rpm
irrigating bottle
Figure 1-9-2
+
mm Hg
-
45 cm bottle height
+
-
high pump rpm

Figure 1-9a

Flow Pumps:
Indirect Control of Vacuum (continued)

If the aspiration line was removed from the pump and simply left open to atmospheric pressure at the same level as the eye, a baseline flow would still be produced because of the pressure head from the elevated irrigating bottle (see Figures 1-37 and 1-38). If the flow pump is then reconnected and driven at a speed which produces a flow greater than the baseline value, the aspiration line pressure (ALP) will be less than the IOP as the pump pulls on the fluid to produce the faster flow (see Figures 1-9-1 and 1-9-2). However, a flow pump can also act as a **flow regulator** in that it can decrease the flow below the baseline level; in this case, the IOP and the ALP are identical (Figure 1-9-3), assuming both the eye and the aspiration line are at the same height below the elevated irrigating bottle, the higher pressure of which is driving the fluidic circuit. Because fluid flow is interrupted where the flow pump head interdigitates with the fluidic circuit (see Figures 1-7 and 1-8), flow cannot occur any faster than the rotational speed of the pump head regardless of how high the bottle is placed.

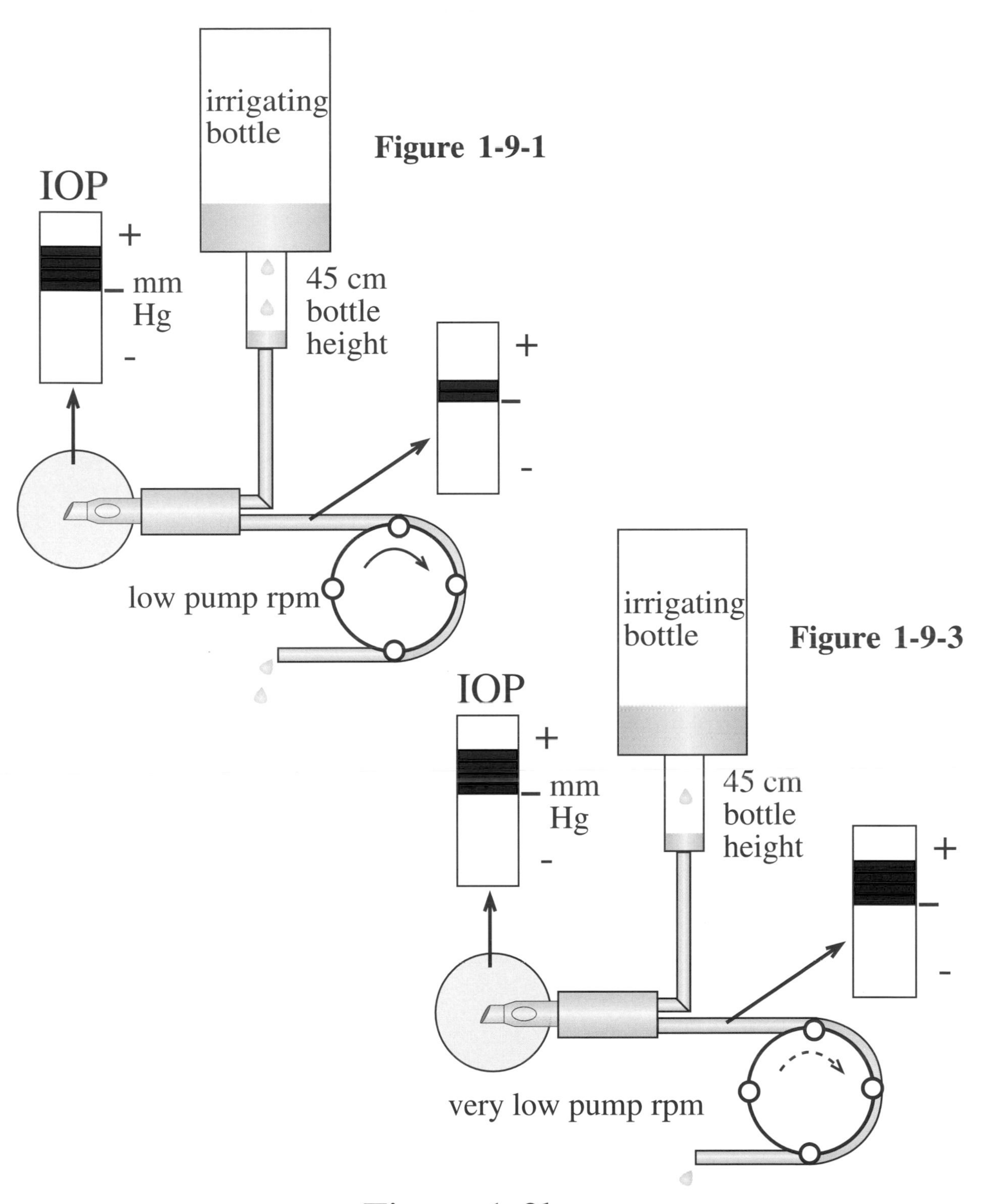
irrigating bottle
Figure 1-9-1
IOP
+
mm
Hg
-
45 cm
bottle
height
+
-
low pump rpm
irrigating bottle
Figure 1-9-3
IOP
+
mm
Hg
-
45 cm
bottle
height
+
-
very low pump rpm

Figure 1-9b

Flow Pumps: Tip Occlusion

Actual fluid flow is dependent on the degree of aspiration port occlusion; this is especially true for peristaltic pumps, which often have more pump leakage than scroll pumps. Flow rate decreases with increasing tip occlusion (ie, decreased effective aspiration port surface area) until flow ceases completely with complete tip occlusion even though the pump head may continue to rotate (Figure 1-10). This scenario assumes sufficient density of the tip-occluding fragment such that it is not deformed and aspirated into the tip by the given vacuum preset. The activity in the drip chamber is a gauge of fluidic circuit flow, and therefore mirrors the strength and rapidity of currents in the anterior chamber. Note in the middle diagram that a given aspiration port surface area which causes a given resistance to flow could be produced either by a partially occluded phaco tip or an unoccluded IA tip. Note also that aspiration line vacuum (mm Hg below atmospheric, shown here as a positive meter reading) increases as the pump attempts to draw fluid through an increasing resistance as the effective aspiration port surface area decreases; correspondingly, the IOP increases as actual flow rate decreases (see also Figure 1-35b). The middle diagram also illustrates how actual vacuum is unable to reach the vacuum limit preset in the absence of complete aspiration port occlusion (see also Figures 2-5 and 2-6). Finally, note in the bottom right schematic in Figure 1-10 that the vacuum does not build past the preset limit (green bar) even though the pump head is still turning; this vacuum regulation is made possible by a **venting mechanism** (see Figures 1-13 and 1-41). In actual practice, most current machines augment the venting mechanism by slowing and/or stopping the pump head when the preset vacuum limit is reached.

Aspiration flow control on the phaco machine is still important with complete tip occlusion in that it controls the rotational speed of the pump head, and even though no actual flow exists with complete occlusion, the surgeon can control the speed of vacuum buildup via pump speed control. The amount of time required to reach a given vacuum preset, assuming complete tip occlusion, is defined as **rise time**.

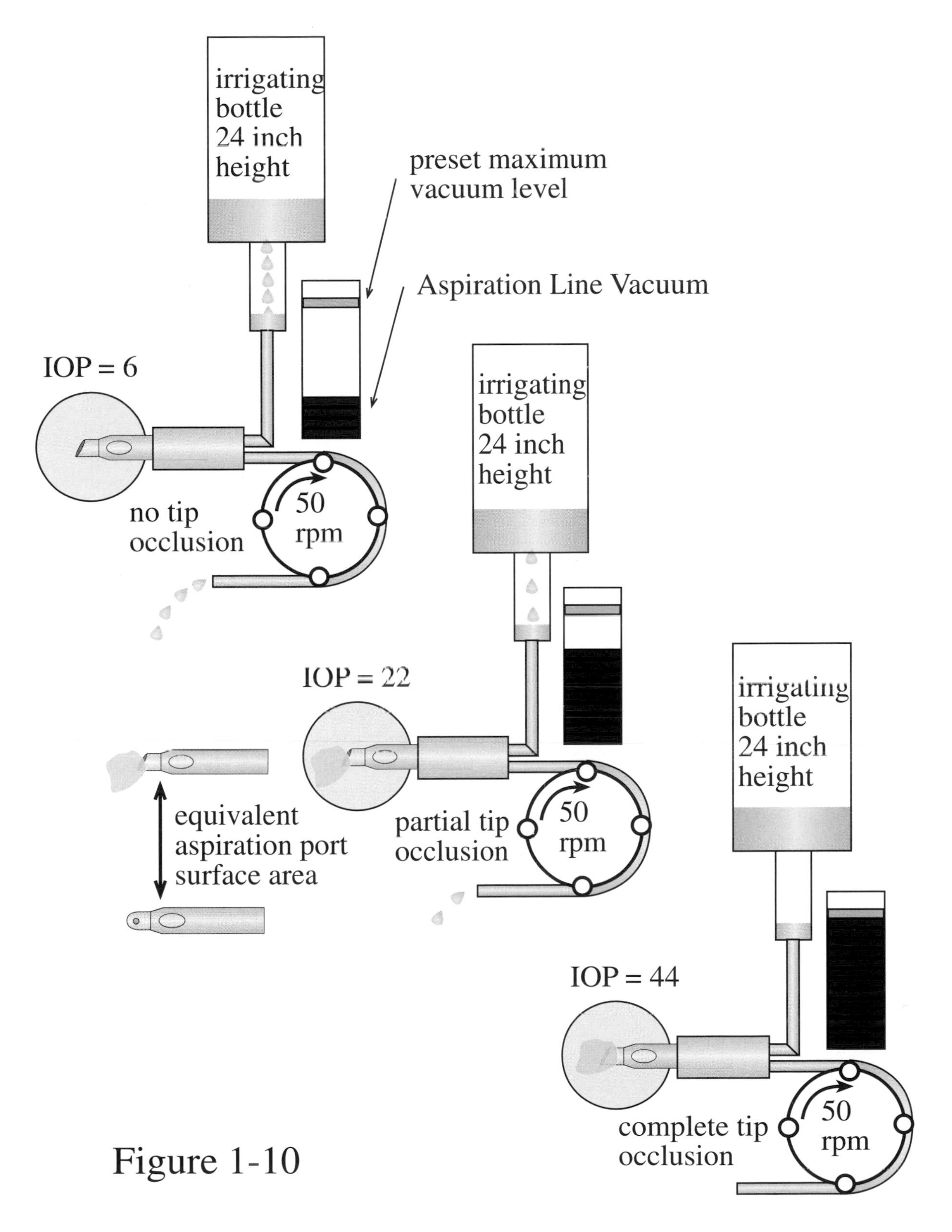
irrigating bottle 24 inch height
preset maximum vacuum level
Aspiration Line Vacuum
IOP = 6
no tip occlusion
50 rpm
irrigating bottle 24 inch height
IOP = 22
partial tip occlusion
50 rpm
equivalent aspiration port surface area
irrigating bottle 24 inch height
IOP = 44
complete tip occlusion
50 rpm

Figure 1-10

Rise Time: Flow Pumps

Rise time is inversely proportional to the rotational speed of the pump head (Figure 1-11). All graphs represent the same hypothetical phaco machine (with occluded aspiration port), but note that when the flow rate is cut in half (from 40 to 20cc/min), the rise time is doubled (from 1 to 2 sec). Rise time is doubled again to 4 sec when flow rate is halved again to 10cc/min. A longer rise time gives the surgeon more time to react in cases of inadvertent incarceration of iris, capsule, or other unwanted material; in such cases, the pedal can be raised to position 1 (for venting; see Figure 1-13) or even refluxed if necessary before dangerously high levels of vacuum are reached, which could, for example, rupture the capsule. Although a useful setting for training residents, even experienced surgeons appreciate the enhanced safety margin afforded by a longer rise time. Safety and time efficiency are conflicting objectives with respect to rise time, with longer rise times delaying parts of the procedure which require vacuum buildup, such as thick cortical removal or gripping the nucleus while chopping off a fragment with a second instrument; moderate flow rates of around 28cc/min represent a good compromise. Some machines offer a programmable rise time in that the pump speed can be set to increase or decrease upon aspiration port occlusion, as sensed by passing a programmed threshold vacuum level; examples of this include the AMO Diplomax's Occlusion Mode Phaco as well as Surgical Design's Adjustable Rise Time.

Some points should be made about the preceding discussion on rise time. First, rise time was adjusted via manipulation of the machine's flow rate control. However, as discussed previously, no actual flow exists with complete occlusion, which is necessary to efficiently build vacuum at the phaco tip. Adjusting the machine's flow parameter, measured in cc/min, actually determines the rotational speed of the pump head. Vacuum builds more quickly as the pump head more rapidly pushes against the fluid in the aspiration line tubing (peristaltic) and cassette (scroll), even though no additional fluid is removed from the anterior chamber through the occluded phaco tip.

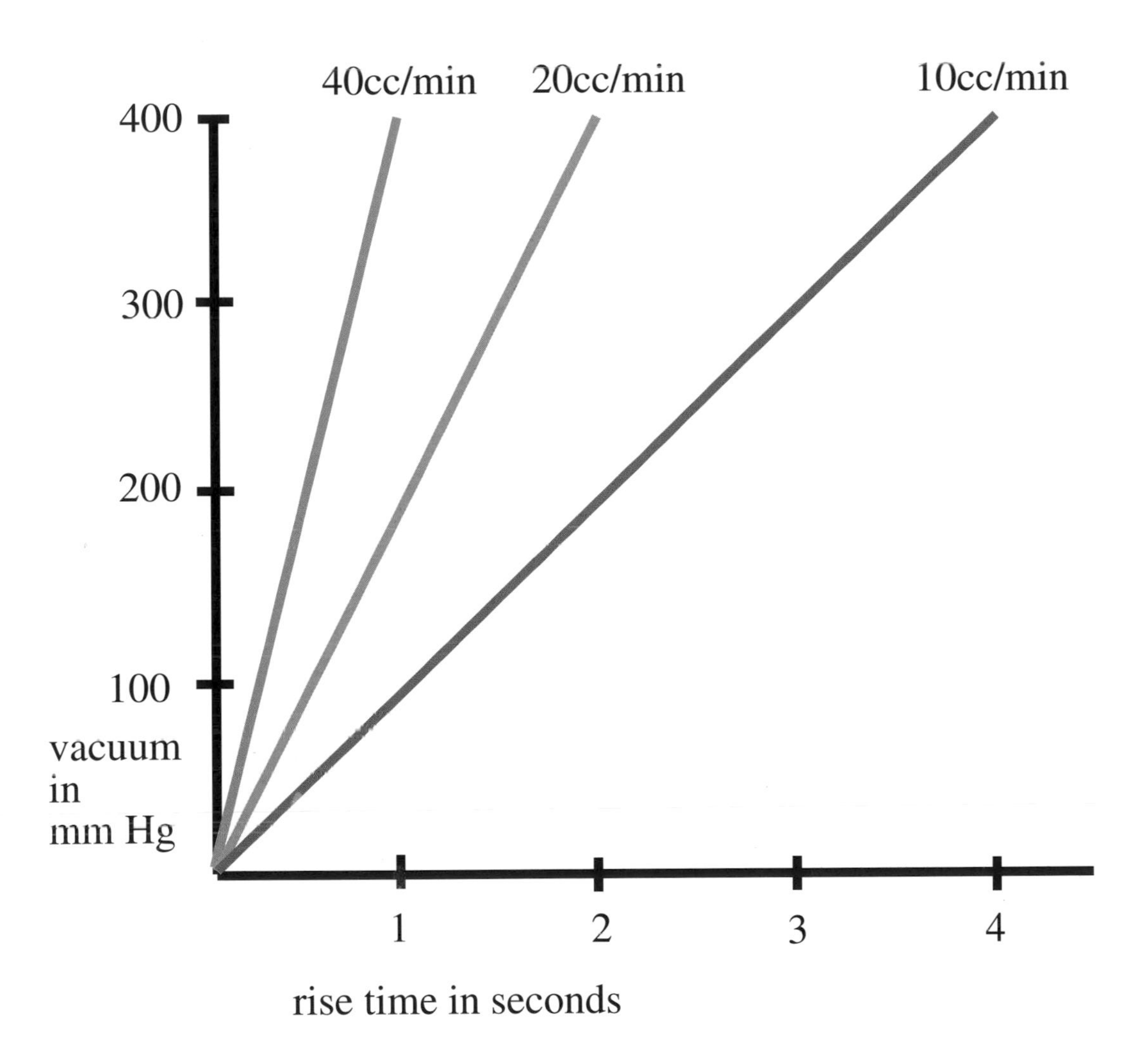
40cc/min
20cc/min
10cc/min
400
300
200
100
vacuum
in
mm Hg
1
2
3
4
rise time in seconds

Figure 1-11

Rise Time: Flow Pump Compliance

Another point regarding the rise time discussion concerns the fact that although no fluid flows from the eye with tip occlusion, a minute amount of fluid is pumped from the aspiration line tubing as vacuum is built up, thus accounting for the relation of pump speed to rise time. Because fluid is noncompressible and nonexpansile, theoretically no change in aspiration line fluid volume would occur as the pump head exerted pressure on the fluid. However, two factors account for this not being true with peristaltic pumps. First, the use of the aspiration line tubing as a conduit for transmitting the pump rollers' force results in some inefficiency in the form of leakage both between the pump rollers and the tubing, as well as in between the opposed internal surfaces of the aspiration line tubing. Second, the mechanism of action of a peristaltic pump requires enough aspiration line tubing compliance to allow for collapse by the pump rollers. **Compliance**, defined as a change in volume in response to a change in pressure, results in some tubing constriction as some fluid is removed from the line (not the eye) by the pump even with complete tip occlusion (Figure 1-12). Higher compliance in a fluidic circuit generally results in longer rise times as the pump has to work first to overcome the compliance before working to build vacuum against an occluding fragment at the aspiration port. The most modern peristaltic pumps minimize the system's compliance to the minimum level compatible with the functioning of the pump, thereby attaining fairly rapid potential rise times. By placing the pump element directly in the aspiration fluid path, a scroll pump further reduces the need for aspiration line compliance to the minimum amount required for ergonomic handpiece control; this type of pump can therefore achieve the tightest potential control of rise time with the most rapid vacuum buildup attainable.

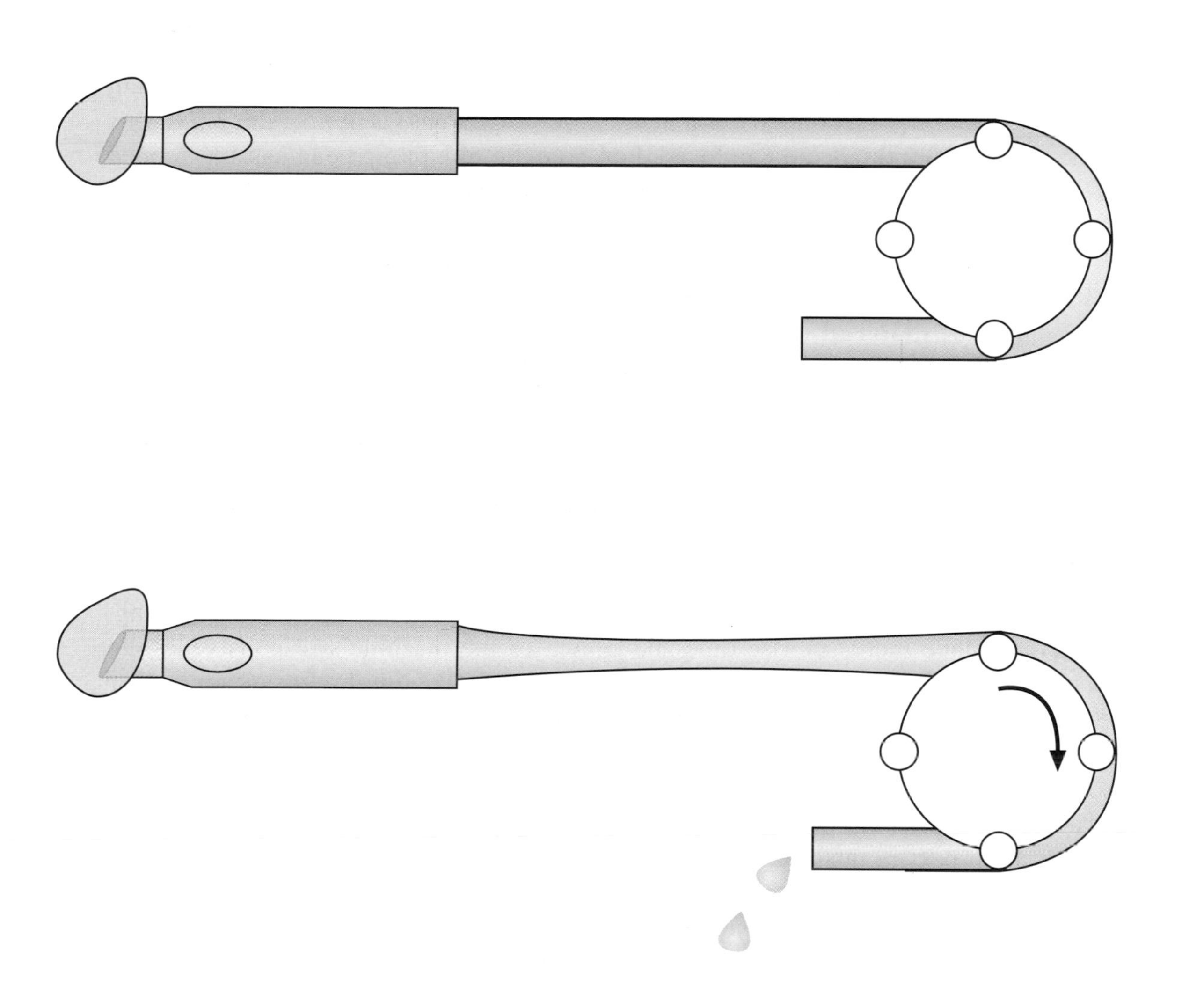

Figure 1-12

Rise Time: Flow Pump Venting and Vacuum Limit Preset

The final point concerning rise time and flow pumps is the fact that a maximum vacuum limit can be preset on the machine. In order to prevent vacuum buildup past this level, a variety of methods are employed. For example, the pump head can be stopped when the preset value is reached; some newer machines progressively decrease the pump speed as the vacuum limit is approached. Alternatively, or additionally, **vacuum can be regulated with a moving pump head by venting air or fluid into the aspiration line if the preset value is exceeded. Venting is also employed if the surgeon wishes to release material (eg, inadvertently incarcerated material such as iris or capsule) which is held to the phaco tip with vacuum; in this case, venting is engaged automatically on most modern phaco machines (both flow and vacuum pumps) by simply raising the foot pedal out of position 2 and into position 1 or 0.** Figure 1-13-1 illustrates a nuclear fragment firmly gripped by the phaco tip with high vacuum, whereas Figure 1-13-2 shows the fragment still in position but not held with any force after the air from the vent valve purged the trapped vacuum; the fragment could be easily removed at this point with either a second instrument or with reflux. Air venting has the disadvantage of increasing the fluidic circuit's compliance relative to fluid venting. Higher compliance increases rise time and decreases the machine's responsiveness to foot pedal vacuum control (see Figures 1-41 and 1-42). **By employing either air or fluid venting to regulate vacuum buildup, a flow pump therefore directly controls flow but also allows indirect control of vacuum.**

One way to evaluate a machine's venting performance is to utilize a porcine wet lab. The contra-incisional posterior iris surface is engaged by the (bevel-up) phaco needle's aspiration port in position 2 while the anterior iris surface is observed to dimple into the port. After waiting for rise time to build to the vacuum preset limit (eg, 100 to 200mm Hg), the pedal is then raised into position 1 (or into position 0 if a continuous irrigation mode has been engaged—see discussion with Figure 1-2). Ideally, the surgeon should observe an immediate gentle release of the incarcerated iris as the anterior surface resumes its normal flat architecture. Examples of poor venting performance would be a failure to release the iris (eg, anterior dimple does not flatten out), an overly forceful release of the iris (eg, the anterior iris surface momentarily bulges anteriorly upon release), or an immediate regrabbing of the iris after a momentary release (ie, reformation of the anterior iris dimple after a momentary flattening).

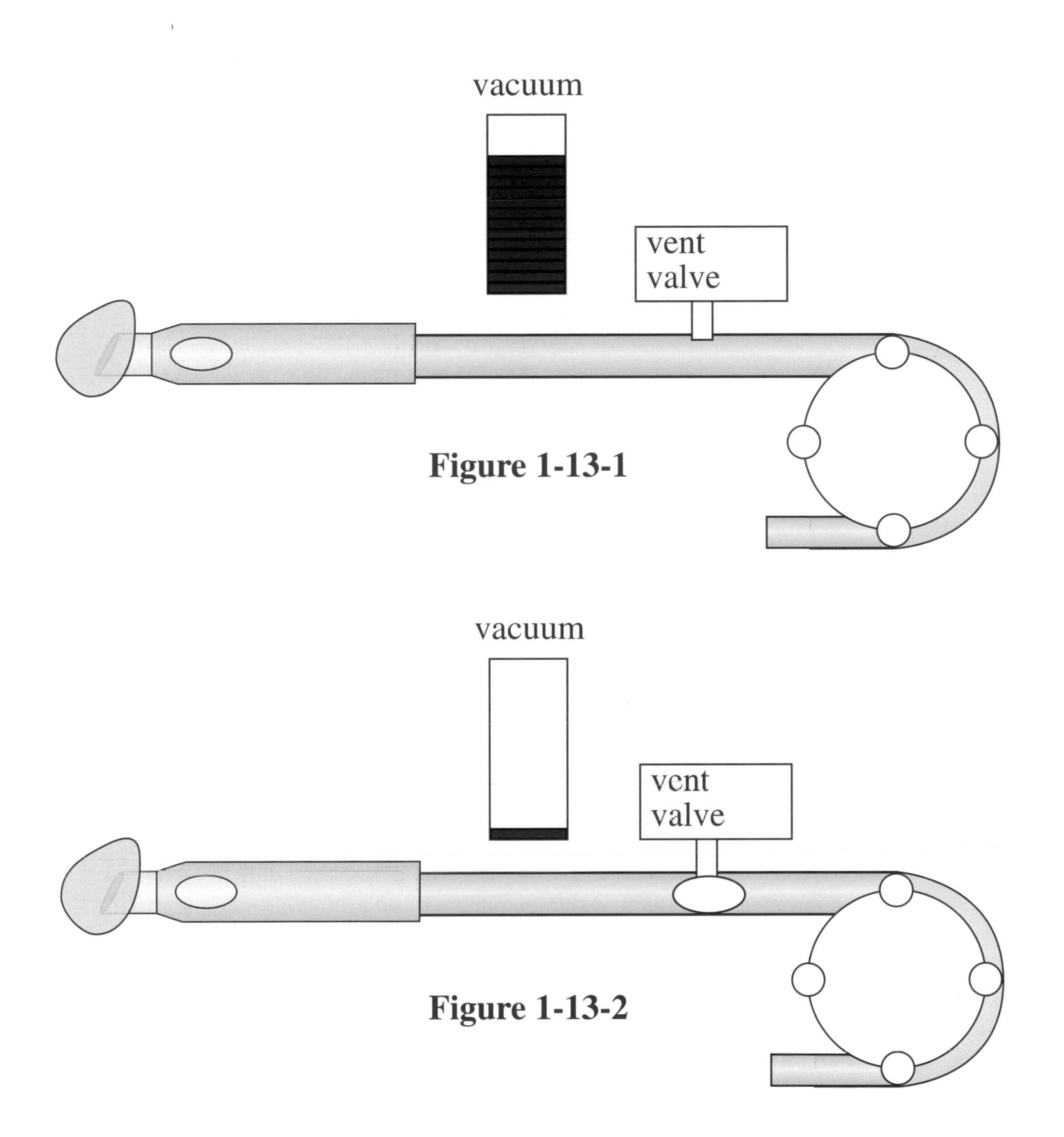

Figure 1-13-1

Figure 1-13-2

Figure 1-13

Schematic Machine: Flow Pump

The original schematic from Figure 1-1 will now be enhanced in order to expand on the previously discussed concepts regarding rise time. A Dual Linear pedal is seen in side view (see Figure 1-4). Note the new displays on this schematic (Figure 1-14).

Pump flow is also know as **aspiration flow rate** or just simply flow rate. The machine display will typically be in cc/min, but recall that this will be valid only for an unobstructed fluidic circuit (see Figure 1-10). When adjusting this parameter, the surgeon is actually adjusting the rotational speed of the pump head, and if the aspiration port is occluded, then increasing the pump speed will decrease rise time (see Figure 1-11). Increasing the flow rate with an unobstructed tip will produce stronger and more rapid anterior chamber currents which will more readily attract material to the aspiration port, such as nuclear fragments and cortex, as well as iris and capsule.

Maximum vacuum, measured in mm Hg, is preset by the surgeon. It represents the highest vacuum obtainable given complete occlusion of the aspiration port. Without this limiting set point, a rotating flow pump would continue to build vacuum to dangerous levels. Once again, the speed with which this level is reached is proportionately determined by the flow rate setting.

Actual vacuum indicates the real-time vacuum pressure at the machine's **pressure transducer**, which is usually located at or within the pump housing. With an unoccluded tip and an operating pump (pedal position 2 or 3), vacuum decays (ie, pressure becomes more positive) in the fluidic circuit from the pump toward the anterior chamber (see Figure 1-9a); however, with an occluded tip, the actual vacuum at the pump is the same as the vacuum holding the occluding material to the aspiration port (see Figure 1-25—these concepts are valid for both flow and vacuum pumps). The actual vacuum is a percentage of the maximum vacuum; variables that influence it include the maximum vacuum preset, the pump flow, the size of the aspiration port, the length and internal diameter of the aspiration line tubing, the degree of tip occlusion, and the position of the foot pedal when linear control is used. **Note that the machine is placed at the patient's eye level to standardize not only the vacuum transducer readings, but also the amount of irrigating bottle elevation.**

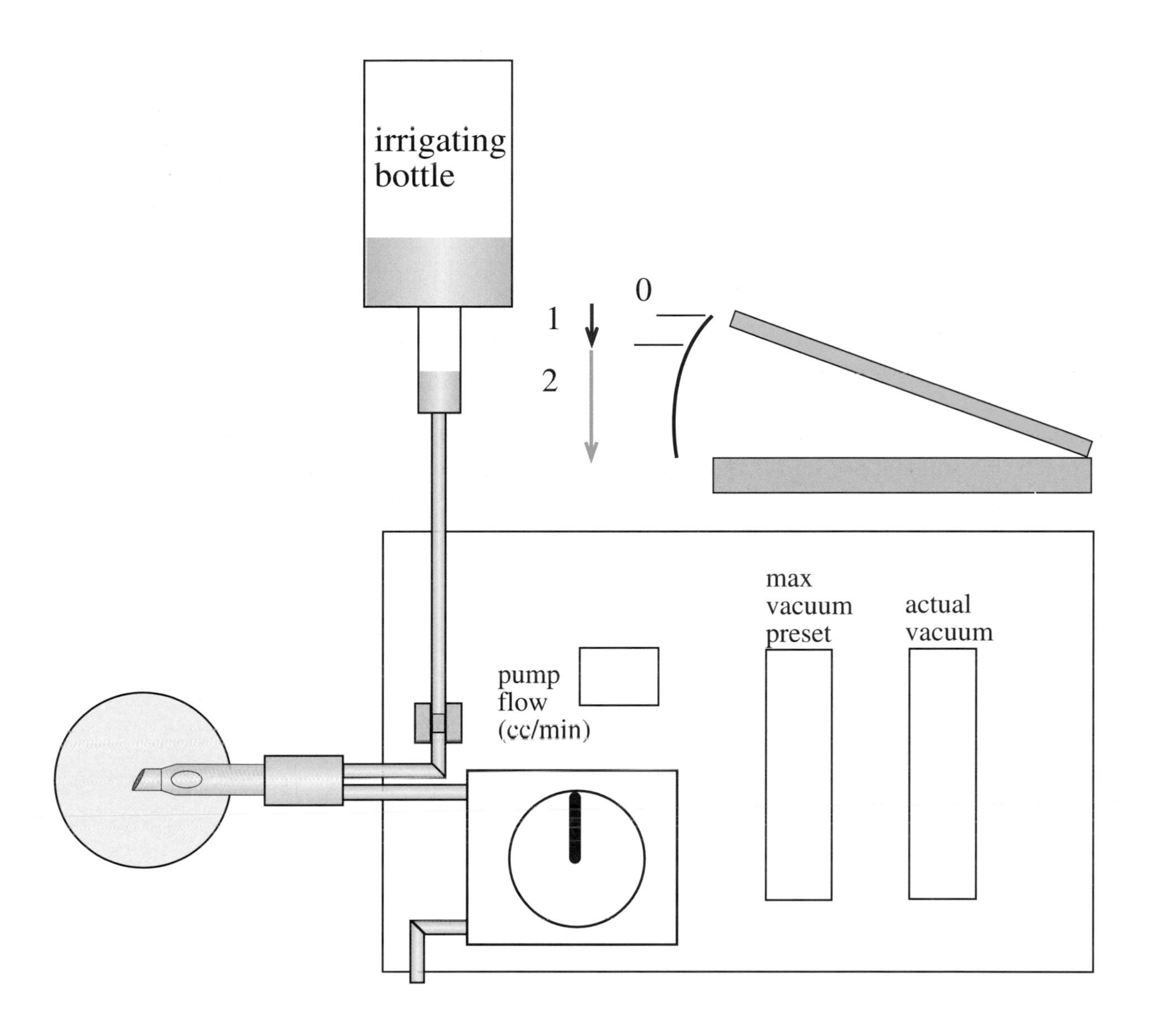
irrigating
bottle
0
1
2
max
vacuum
preset
actual
vacuum
pump
flow
(cc/min)

Figure 1-14

Relationship Among Flow Rate, Rise Time, and Vacuum

The following schematics illustrate how increasing the flow rate decreases rise time (see Figure 1-11). The time displays utilize zero as the time when the tip is occluded and pump action is initiated by abruptly pushing the foot pedal from position 0 to the bottom of position 2. Because the pump starts right at time zero with complete occlusion of the aspiration port, the following schematics do not demonstrate any vacuum preload due to resistance to flow at higher flow rates (see Figure 1-9a). Therefore, the mechanism of shorter rise times with faster flow rate settings is due to the more rapid rotational speed of the pump head more rapidly driving the aspiration line fluid and thus building vacuum more quickly.

Figure 1-15: *20cc/min pump flow. Time: 0.1 sec.* At this instant just after complete occlusion, actual vacuum has not had a chance to build yet. However, because the tip is completely occluded, no fluid is aspirated from the eye (note the lack of drainage from the machine). Consequently, because of the sealed anterior chamber, irrigation also ceases (note the lack of activity in the drip chamber).

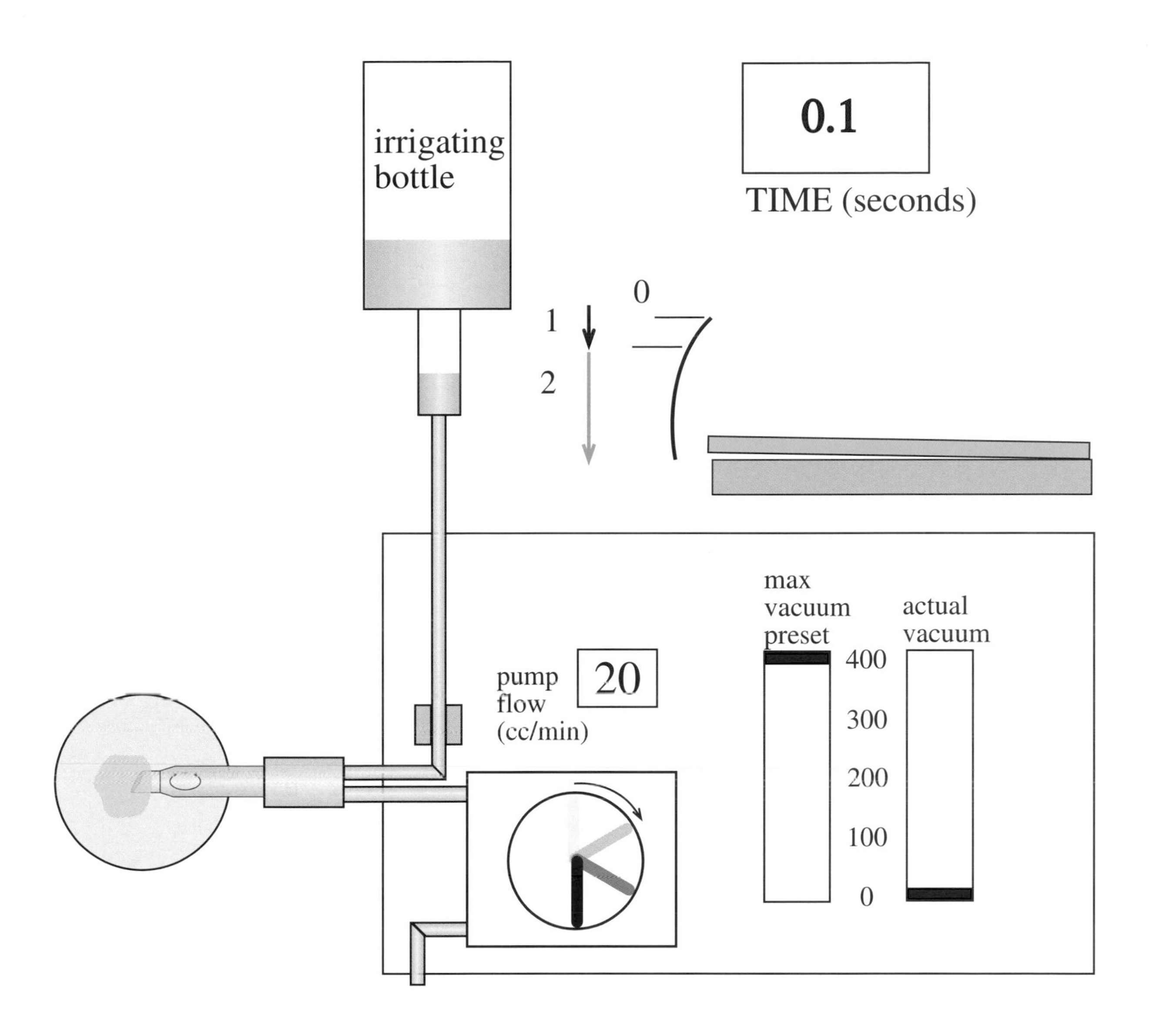
irrigating
bottle
0.1
TIME (seconds)
0
1
2
max
vacuum
preset
actual
vacuum
400
300
200
100
0
pump
flow
(cc/min)
20

Figure 1-15

Relationship Among Flow Rate, Rise Time, and Vacuum (continued)

Figure 1-16: *20cc/min pump flow. Time: 2 sec.* As the pump head continues to drive infinitesimally small amounts of fluid through the aspiration tubing, actual vacuum begins to rise. After 2 sec, it has reached a level of 200mm Hg on this particular machine. As the pump is building vacuum, it is overcoming any fluidic circuit compliance (see Figures 1-12, 1-41, and 1-42).

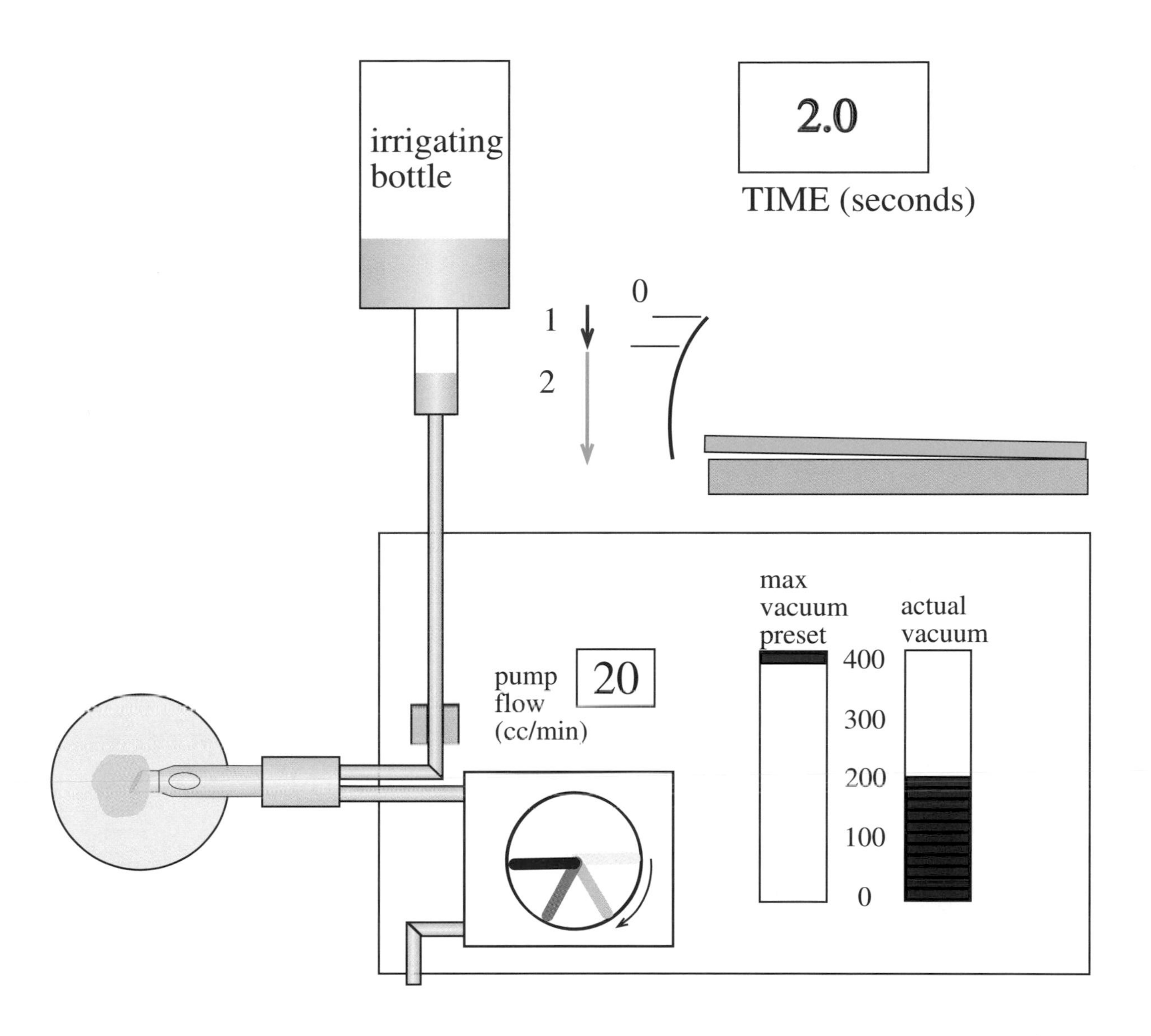
irrigating bottle
2.0
TIME (seconds)
0
1
2
max vacuum preset
actual vacuum
400
300
200
100
0
pump flow (cc/min)
20

Figure 1-16

Relationship Among Flow Rate, Rise Time, and Vacuum (continued)

Figure 1-17: *20cc/min pump flow. Time: 4 sec.* The actual vacuum has now reached the maximum preset value of 400mm Hg.

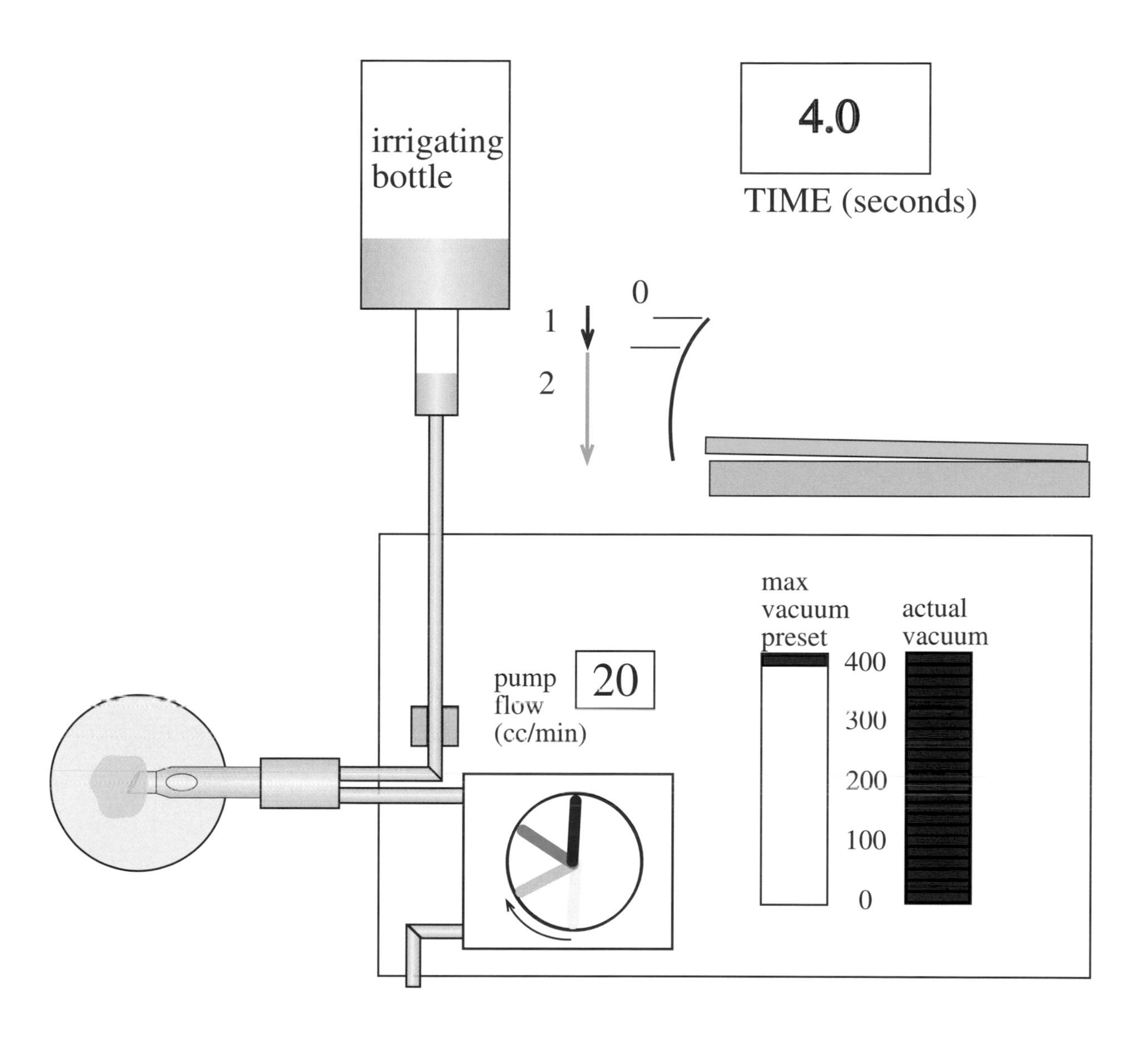

irrigating bottle
4.0
TIME (seconds)
0
1
2
max vacuum preset
actual vacuum
400
300
200
100
0
pump flow (cc/min)
20

Figure 1-17

Relationship Among Flow Rate, Rise Time, and Vacuum (continued)

Figure 1-18: *40cc/min pump flow. Time: 2 sec.* For this illustration, the machine had been reset to 40cc/min flow; at time zero, the tip was completely occluded, the actual vacuum was zero, and the foot pedal was abruptly depressed from position 0 to the bottom of position 2. By doubling the pump flow (therefore doubling the rotational speed of the pump head), the time required to reach the maximum vacuum (ie, rise time) has been cut in half (compare to Figure 1-17). At 40cc/min flow rate on this machine, vacuum rises at a rate of 100mm Hg every 0.5 sec.

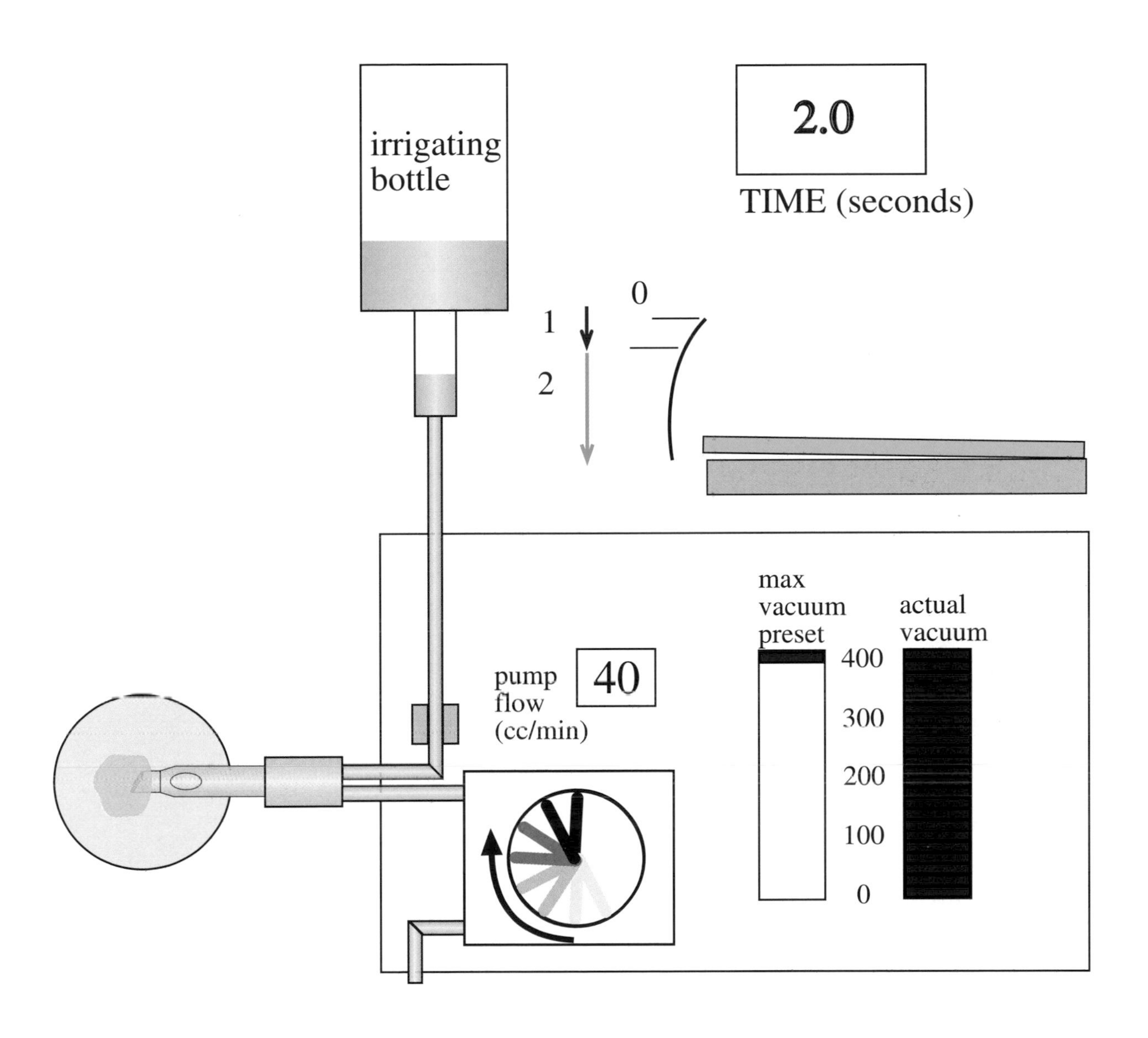
irrigating
bottle
2.0
TIME (seconds)
0
1
2
max
vacuum
preset
actual
vacuum
pump
flow
(cc/min)
40
400
300
200
100
0

Figure 1-18

Relationship Among Flow Rate, Rise Time, and Vacuum (continued)

Figure 1-19: *40cc/min pump flow. Time: 2 sec.* The machine has again been reset for this illustration. Time zero begins with complete tip occlusion, zero vacuum, and the foot pedal being abruptly depressed from position 0 to a point halfway into position 2, which on this particular **linear control** machine yields a maximum potential vacuum of half of the maximum preset vacuum (ie, 200mm Hg). Although the time reading is 2 sec, the actual vacuum of 200mm Hg was reached after 1 sec. Recall that a 40cc/min pump flow setting on this particular machine increases vacuum by 100mm Hg every 0.5 sec with occlusion of the aspiration port (see Figure 1-18). Between the time readings of 1 and 2 sec, this machine was **venting** (see Figure 1-13), a combination of intermittent pump cessation coupled with air (or fluid) introduction into the aspiration line which serves to prevent the actual vacuum from increasing past 200mm Hg as determined by pedal position and the maximum vacuum preset.

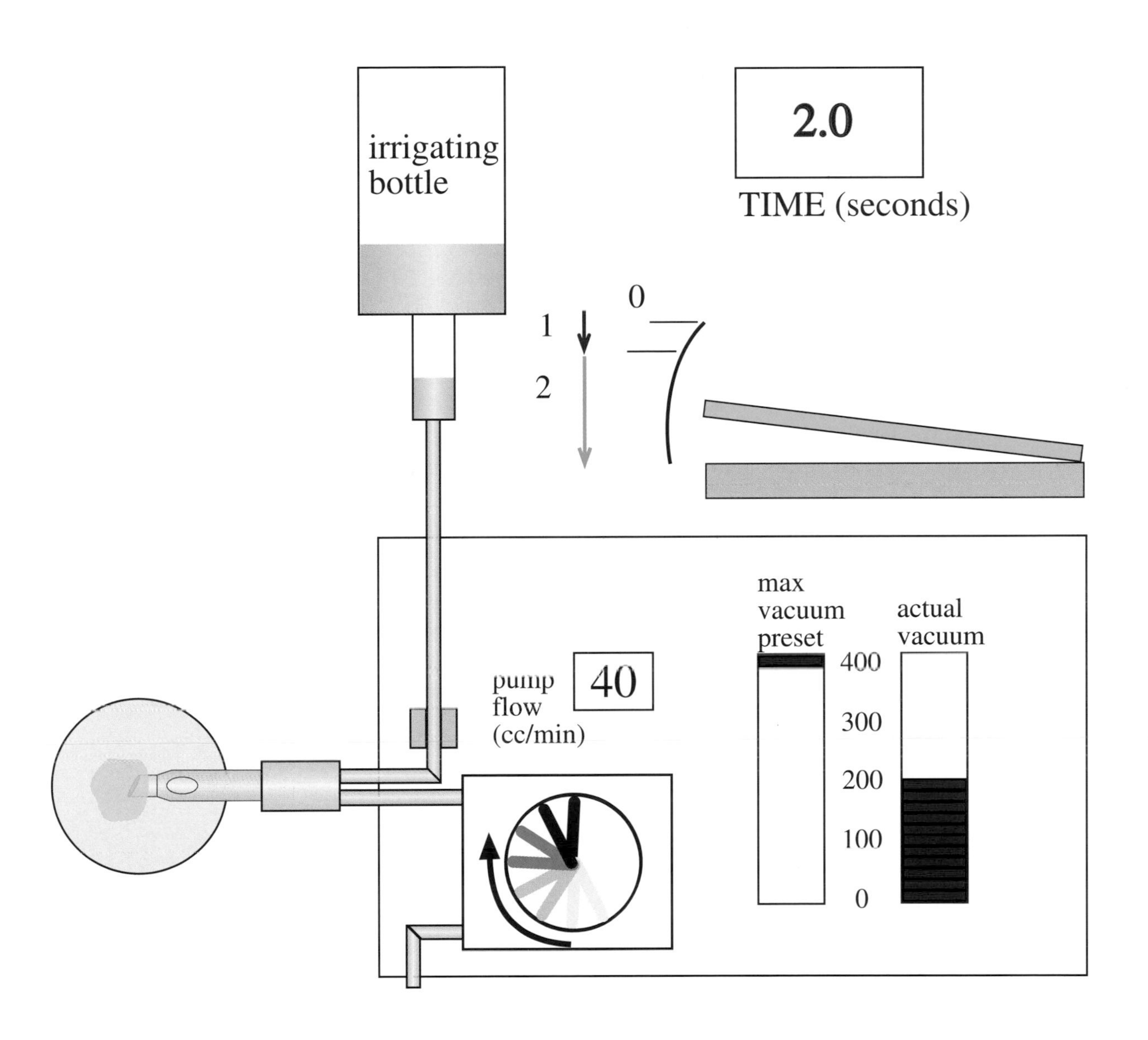
irrigating bottle
2.0
TIME (seconds)
0
1
2
max vacuum preset
actual vacuum
pump flow (cc/min)
40
400
300
200
100
0

Figure 1-19

Relationship Among Flow Rate, Rise Time, and Vacuum (continued)

Figure 1-20: *40cc/min pump flow. Time: 0.5 sec.* Again, the machine has been reset so that time zero begins with complete occlusion, zero vacuum, and the pedal being abruptly depressed from position 0 to a point halfway into position 2's travel. With a maximum vacuum preset of 400mm Hg and the linear control pedal halfway into position 2, the maximum potential vacuum (MPV) is 200mm Hg. However, after just 0.5 sec, the actual vacuum is only 100mm Hg (recall that a 40cc/min flow setting yields a rise time rate of 100mm Hg/0.5 sec on this machine—see Figure 1-18). Remember this **rise time lag** when clinically evaluating vacuum level, especially when using lower flow rates which produce correspondingly longer rise times. For example, if your goal is to aspirate the material occluding the tip or to firmly grip the nucleus prior to chopping, allow sufficient rise time for vacuum to build to the MPV before depressing the pedal still further, assuming the material does not aspirate at the MPV level.

Note that the rate of vacuum increase (rise time) is dependent only on the flow setting, which determines pump head rotational speed. The machine and time readings shown in Figure 1-20 would be identical whether the pedal was halfway or fully into position 2 because the pedal on this hypothetical machine allows linear control of vacuum, not flow. Some machines do offer linear flow control, which decreases rise time by increasing flow rate (pump speed) with increased pedal depression. Also, some machines (such as the Surgical Design machine and the AMO Diplomax) can be programmed to change pump speed (and therefore rise time) upon occlusion, which is sensed as the passing of a programmed threshold vacuum level.

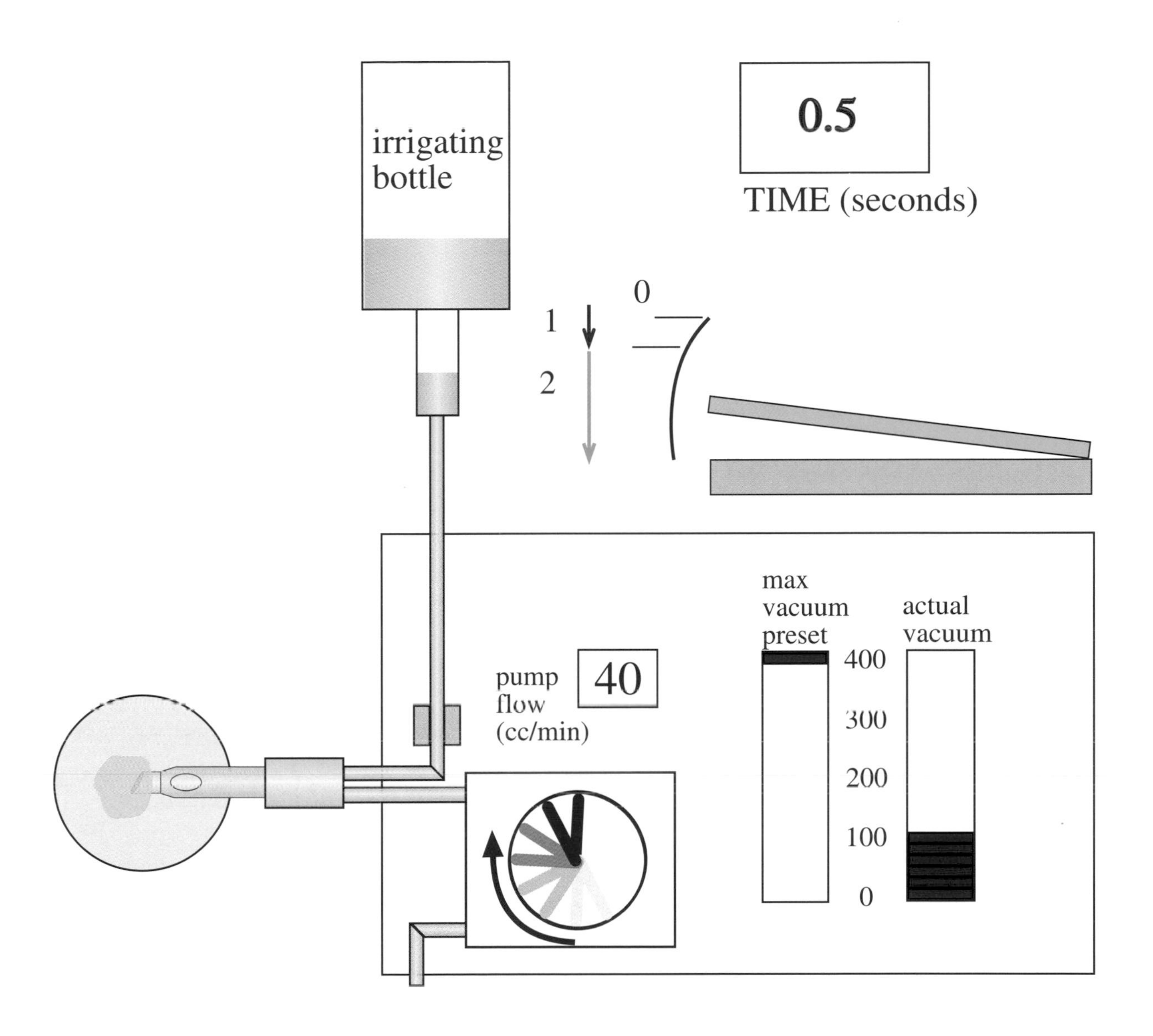
irrigating
bottle
0.5
TIME (seconds)
0
1
2
max
vacuum
preset
actual
vacuum
400
300
200
100
0
pump
flow
(cc/min)
40

Figure 1-20

Relationship Between Flow and Vacuum 1

Figure 1-21 is measuring **IOP** and **ALP** (aspiration line pressure) in a machine with a phaco handpiece (standard tip, **no occlusion**) and a bottle height of 24 inches above the handpiece test chamber; this bottle height produces an IOP of 44mm Hg hydrostatic pressure (see Appendix C). The vacuum limit is preset to 120mm Hg. Zero mm Hg is calibrated to ambient room air atmospheric pressure; by convention, pressures below atmospheric are negative numbers (ie, -200mm Hg **pressure** = +200mm Hg **vacuum**, see Appendix C).

Position 1: There is open communication in the fluid circuit from the irrigation bottle to the test chamber (IOP) to the aspiration line to the pump (see Figures 1-1 and 1-2). The IOP and ALP are the same (44mm Hg) since the test chamber and the aspiration line are on the same tray; both of them are identically pressurized by the 24-inch column of water from the irrigation bottle.

Position 2 (10cc/min): The pump is now removing fluid from the aspiration line quickly enough to reduce the ALP to 15mm Hg. The IOP is reduced only to 30mm Hg because the phaco handpiece/needle combination is acting as a **flow restriction (or fluidic resistor)** between the test chamber and the aspiration line (see also Figure 1-35b). Indeed, it is this resistance which enables the pump to build vacuum. "Vacuum" is of course a relative term and not always negative; even though both IOP and ALP are positive values in this case, flow exists because of the difference in pressure between them (see discussion of **pressure differential** with Figure 1-9a).

Position 2 (20cc/min): ALP has now dropped to -20mm Hg, while IOP has decreased to +20mm Hg.

Position 2 (30cc/min): ALP is down to -50mmHg, while IOP has dropped to +10mm Hg.

Position 2 (40cc/min): ALP has decreased to -90mm Hg, while IOP hovers around 0mm Hg. At this IOP level, the anterior chamber would be shallow and unstable; it is likely to collapse under the equivalent atmospheric pressure and especially the greater vitreous pressure. Bottle height should be increased at this flow rate in order to raise the IOP, thereby deepening and stabilizing the anterior chamber.

Note that, contrary to some previous teachings, a peristaltic (flow) pump does build vacuum without occlusion (see the negative ALPs at flow rates of 20cc/min and greater). Even at lower flow rates, a **relative vacuum** (pressure lower than IOP) is developed in the aspiration line due to the resistance to flow from the phaco tip, as well as the aspiration line itself.

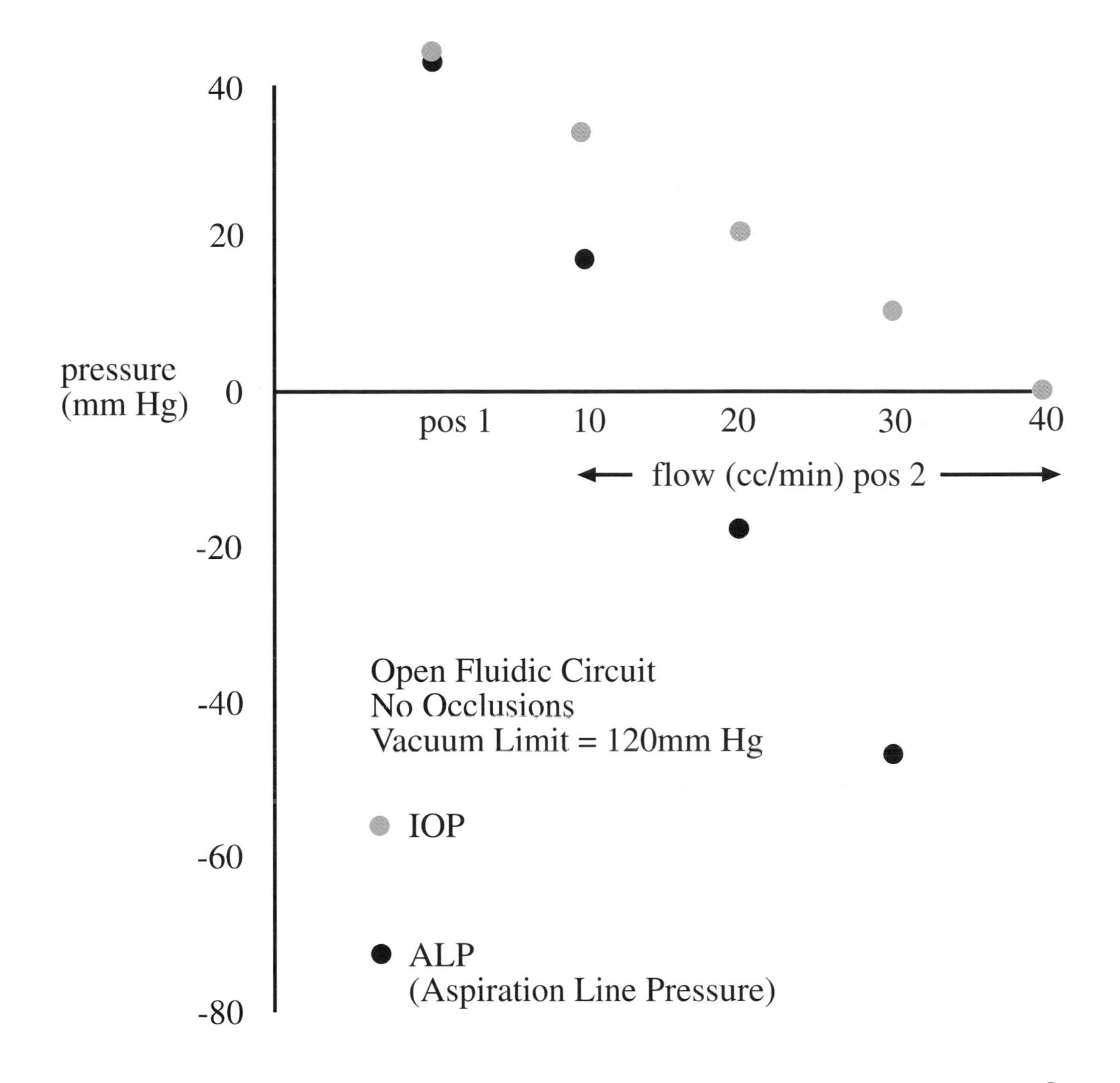
40
20
0
-20
-40
-60
-80
pressure
(mm Hg)
pos 1
10
20
30
40
flow (cc/min) pos 2
Open Fluidic Circuit
No Occlusions
Vacuum Limit = 120mm Hg
IOP
ALP
(Aspiration Line Pressure)

Figure 1-21

Relationship Between Flow and Vacuum 2

Recall that in position 0, a pinch valve on the machine occludes the irrigation line, thereby separating the test chamber (anterior chamber) from the full pressure of the bottle height. If the handpiece in this setup is on a tray 6 inches below the machine's pinch valve, then the IOP/ALP (aspiration line pressure) is the result of the corresponding 6-inch column of water above the test chamber (approximately 11mm Hg). Compare this to position 1 (Figure 1-22) in which the pinch valve is open, thus allowing communication between the test chamber/aspiration line and the full 24-inch column of water between the test chamber and the irrigation bottle; this four-fold increase in water column height (24 vs 6 inches) produces a corresponding four-fold increase in IOP/ALP (44mm Hg vs 11mm Hg). This pressure differential between position 1 and 0 is readily apparent clinically whereby the anterior chamber is noted to become shallow when changing from position 1 to position 0 as a result of vitreous pressure having less opposition in position 0.

Note the effect of a total aspiration port occlusion while in pedal position 2 (see Figure 1-22). Because the test chamber/anterior chamber is now isolated from the active pump by the occlusion, the IOP is simply a function of the bottle height, just as in position 1. However, with total resistance to flow, the ALP drops to the vacuum preset level (-50mm Hg in this case). **Whether you are using a flow pump or a vacuum pump, total tip occlusion is necessary to build up holding power to the maximum preset vacuum**; an important example would be stabilizing the nucleus with the phaco tip while performing a phaco chop maneuver.

The effect of the tip/resistor is greater with increasing flow rates, shown schematically as increasing distance between IOP and ALP (see also Figure 1-35b). A higher resistance IA tip produces even greater pressure differentials with ALPs being lowered more and IOPs not being lowered as much relative to the phaco tip resistor. **In unoccluded hydrostatic states without flow (positions 0 and 1), IOP is equal to ALP regardless of the tip/resistance in the fluid circuit.**

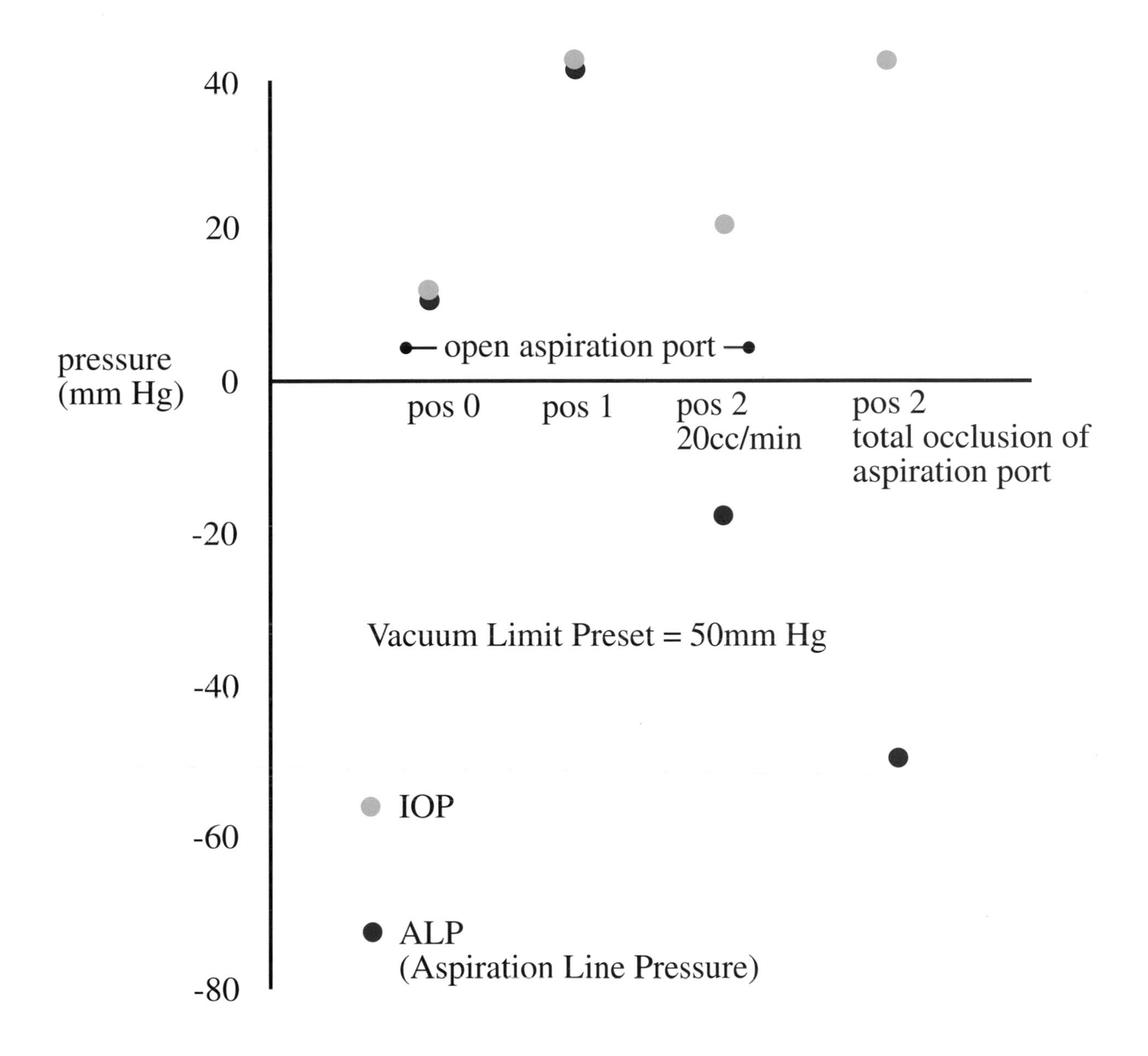

40
20
0
-20
-40
-60
-80
pressure
(mm Hg)
open aspiration port
pos 0
pos 1
pos 2
20cc/min
pos 2
total occlusion of
aspiration port
Vacuum Limit Preset = 50mm Hg
IOP
ALP
(Aspiration Line Pressure)

Figure 1-22

Vacuum Pumps: Indirect Control of Flow

As opposed to a flow pump, a vacuum pump directly controls vacuum in the fluidic circuit while it indirectly controls flow. In other words, the surgeon commands a given aspiration line vacuum level with the panel preset and/or the pedal position, while the flow varies according to aspiration port size and degree of occlusion, as well as according to the level of commanded vacuum. Vacuum pumps represent the second main category of phaco pumps, with examples being the rotary vane pump, the diaphragm pump, and the venturi pump. These three pumps have in common a rigid drainage cassette which connects the pump to the aspiration line tubing; contrast this arrangement to that of a flow pump, in which the pump connects the aspiration line to the drainage pouch. As opposed to the typical flexible drainage pouch used in flow pumps, the cassette's rigid walls allow it to maintain a commanded vacuum without collapsing; this vacuum proportionately induces flow when the aspiration port is unoccluded, thereby indirectly controlling flow by directly controlling vacuum. This indirect control of flow is particularly significant because no current vacuum pump phaco machine has an actual flow rate adjustment control; contrast this to flow pumps, which do have an independent flow rate control. Both types of pumps have a maximum vacuum limit control.

As vacuum substantially increases in the drainage cassette in Figure 1-23, the flow rate correspondingly increases; note the increased number of drips in the drip chamber and drainage cassette in Figure 1-23-2 relative to 1-23-1. Although the vacuum level just inside the phaco tip also increases, it does so to a lesser extent because the relatively large 0.9mm standard needle aspiration port offers little resistance to low flow of the low viscosity irrigating fluid (see Figure 1-35b). Therefore, the force of the vacuum in the drainage cassette is mostly expended in producing the faster flow rather than a higher vacuum at the tip; this phenomenon can be measured as a vacuum degradation along the aspiration line with increasing distance from the pump (see Figure 1-39).

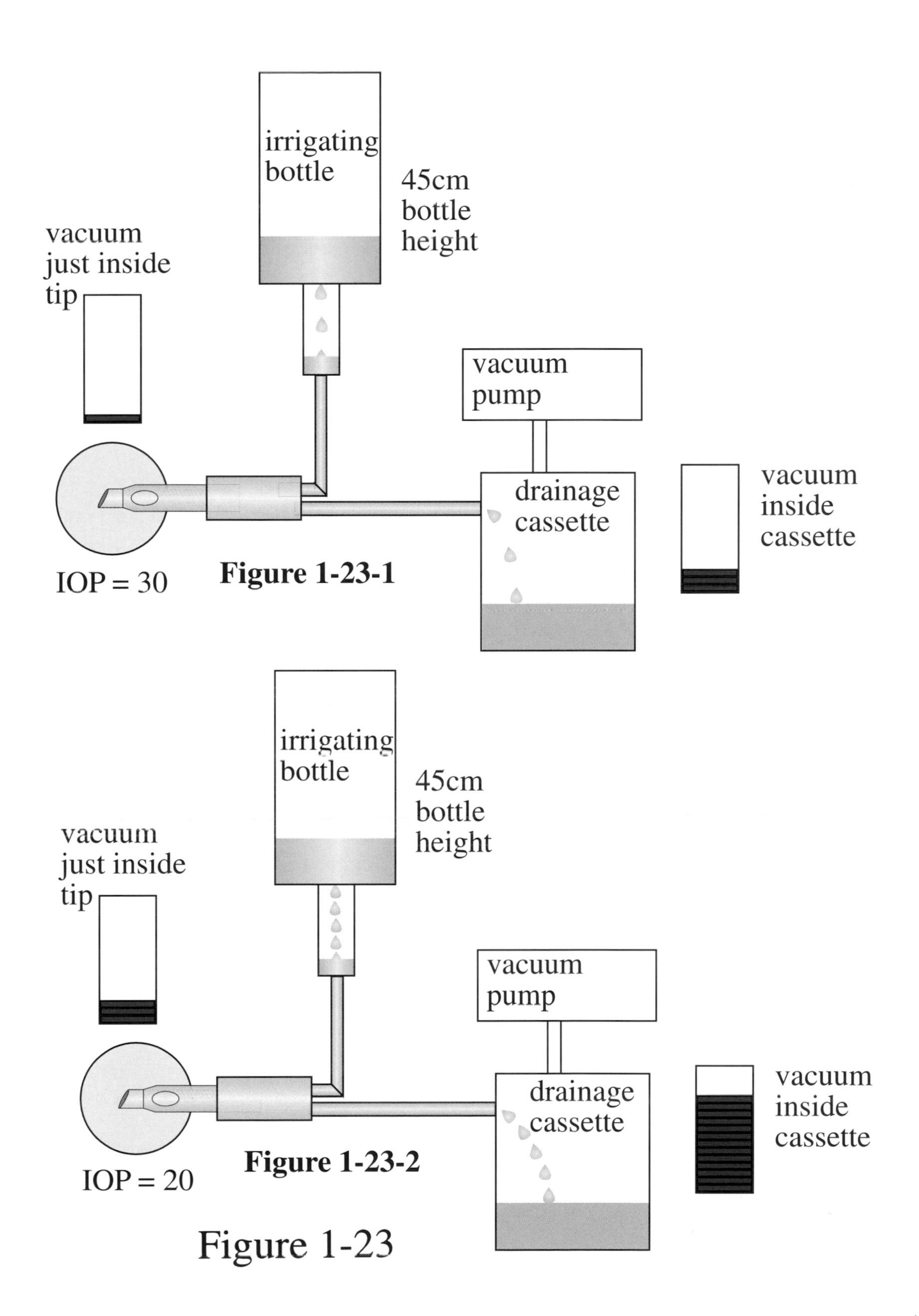
irrigating bottle
45cm bottle height
vacuum just inside tip
vacuum pump
drainage cassette
vacuum inside cassette
IOP = 30
Figure 1-23-1
irrigating bottle
45cm bottle height
vacuum just inside tip
vacuum pump
drainage cassette
vacuum inside cassette
IOP = 20
Figure 1-23-2

Figure 1-23

Vacuum and Flow Pumps: Flow Resistance

If a higher resistance 0.3mm diameter aspiration port (ie, an IA tip) was substituted for the phaco tip in Figure 1-23-2, the vacuum inside the tip would be higher (but still not as high as in the cassette) and the flow would be lower (Figures 1-24 and 1-35a). This principle of decreased flow caused by decreased effective aspiration port surface area holds true for flow pumps as well as vacuum pumps (albeit not to the same degree; see the bottom of Figure 1-35a); note in Figure 1-10 how the surface area of the aspiration port is effectively decreased by partial and then complete occlusion of a nuclear fragment, a scenario which would similarly affect a vacuum pump. Also, a flow pump attempting to pull fluid through a higher resistance, smaller aspiration port will result in higher vacuum at the tip and in the aspiration line relative to a larger aspiration port with lower resistance (see Figures 1-10 and 1-35b).

Note how the IOP increases as a result of the decreased flow rate produced by the smaller, higher resistance aspiration port on the IA tip (Figure 1-24-1); note also how this identical fluidic result would be produced by a phaco needle with its aspiration port size effectively reduced to IA port size by a partially occluding nuclear fragment (see Figure 1-24-1). Compare Figures 1-24-1 and 1-23-1; note how a constant flow rate (illustrated by the drip chamber and drainage cassette activity) and bottle height result in the same IOP regardless of the particular aspiration port (resistance) and pump setting combination which produced the flow rate. Note that this IOP is 30mm Hg rather than a predicted hydrostatic pressure of 33mm Hg (3 x 11mm Hg per 15cm bottle height), with the difference being due to the hydrodynamic state with a modest flow rate as opposed to a hydrostatic state without any flow. Recall also Figure 1-9a, which illustrates how IOP decreases as increased pump function causes an increased flow rate. Both Figures 1-9a and 1-24 assume a constant bottle height; **in order to maintain a given IOP as the flow rate is varied, the bottle height must be adjusted accordingly (eg, lowering the bottle height when decreasing the flow rate).**

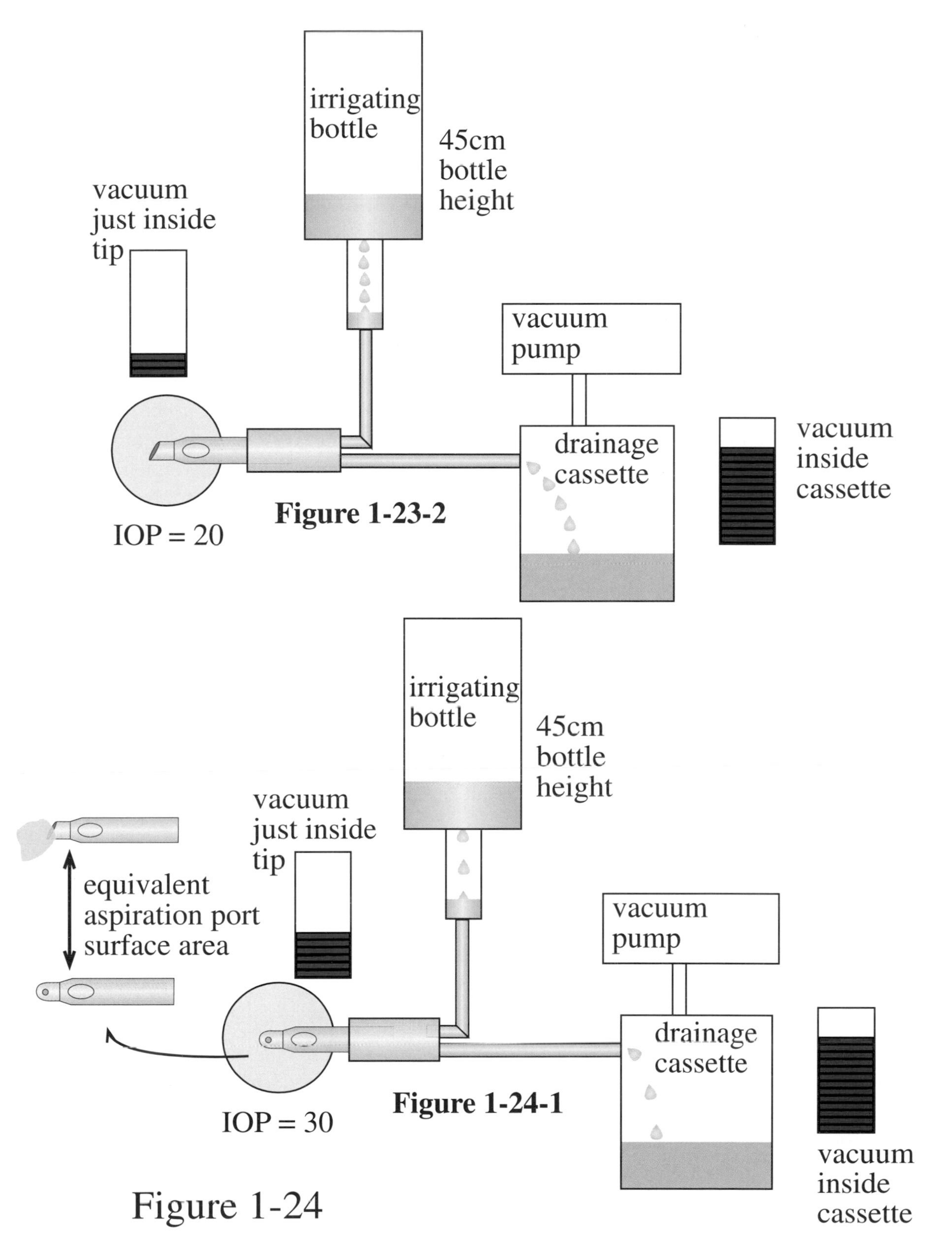

Figure 1-23-2

Figure 1-24-1

Figure 1-24

Vacuum Pumps: Vacuum Transfer Upon Tip Occlusion

By allowing indirect control of flow when the phaco tip is unoccluded (see Figure 1-23), the vacuum pump allows the surgeon to titrate intraocular currents in order to attract material (ie, a chopped nuclear fragment) to the tip's aspiration port. Once the port is occluded by such a fragment, flow is interrupted; vacuum then rapidly transfers from the drainage cassette along the aspiration line to the occluded aspiration port, where it grips the occluding fragment in direct proportion to the level of vacuum (Figure 1-25). **Both flow and vacuum pumps require complete occlusion of the aspiration port in order to build vacuum at the port to the maximum preset level.** The one exception to this rule is when a flow pump is driven at a sufficient pump speed through a high resistance (eg, IA) unoccluded aspiration port such that vacuum builds in the aspiration line (see Figure 1-35b) to a level which might reach a given vacuum limit preset. However, this vacuum is just inside of the aspiration port, and a fragment must still completely cover and occlude the port in order for the vacuum to grip it and hold it firmly to the tip with a force that is proportionate to the amount of vacuum; this is also true for both flow and vacuum pumps.

An easy experiment that illustrates the above principles utilizes a common household canister-type vacuum cleaner, which typically houses a vacuum-type pump. If the round plastic nozzle at the end of the hose (without any brush or other attachments) is placed against the corner of a small (eg, 2 x 4 x 4 inch) wooden block, the nozzle will be unable to pull the block. However, if the nozzle is simply placed perpendicular against one of the block's flat surfaces so that the nozzle is completely occluded, sufficient grip will ensue which will allow the block to be pulled along the surface on which it rests.

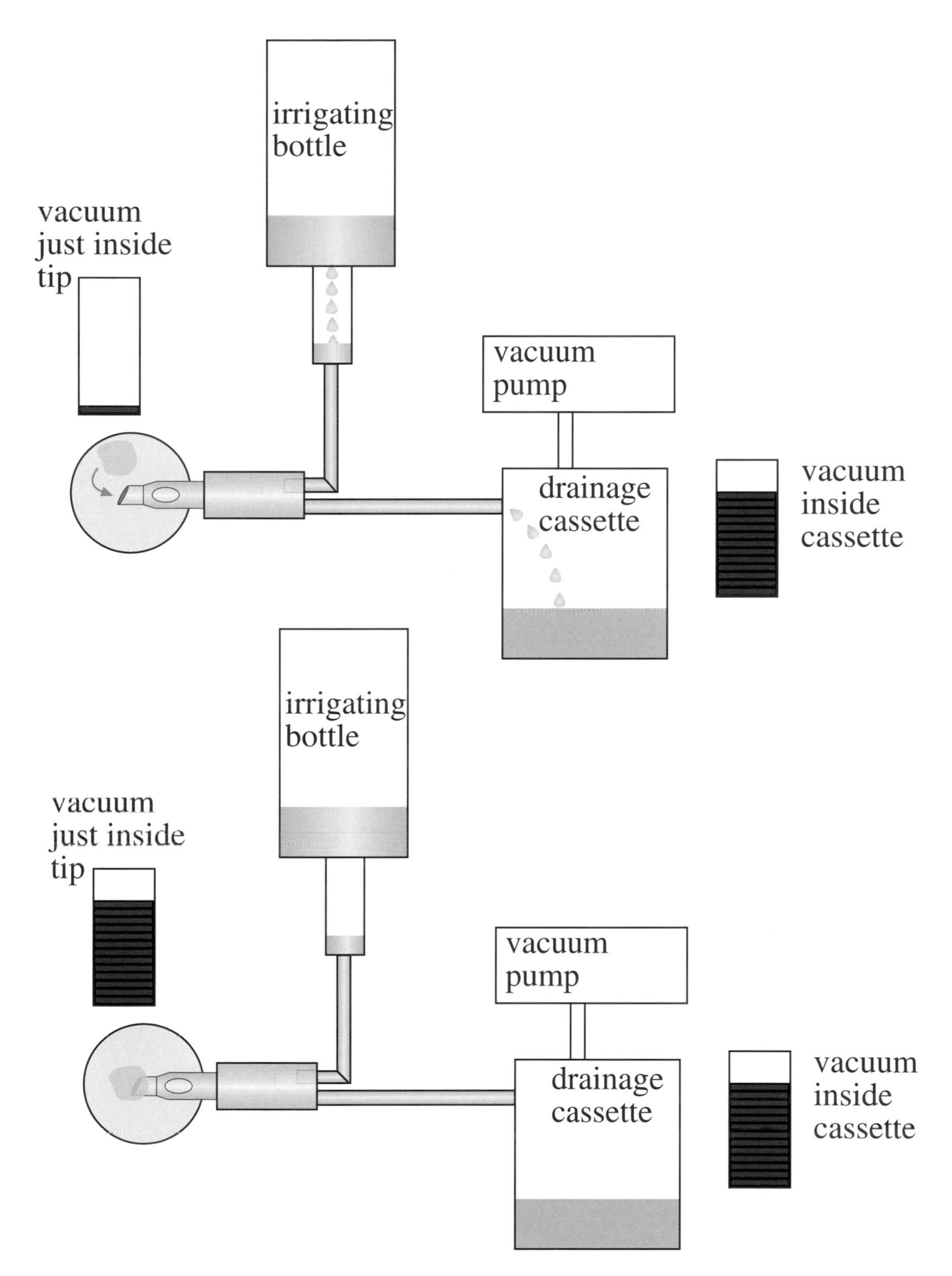
irrigating bottle
vacuum just inside tip
vacuum pump
drainage cassette
vacuum inside cassette
irrigating bottle
vacuum just inside tip
vacuum pump
drainage cassette
vacuum inside cassette

Figure 1-25

Vacuum Pumps: Direct Control of Vacuum

With tip occlusion and vacuum transfer from the cassette to the tip (see Figure 1-25), the level of vacuum is the same along this portion of the machine's fluidic circuit between these two points. Note the identical vacuum meter readings both at the cassette and just inside the tip. At this point, the surgeon can titrate the amount of grip appropriately by titrating the pump vacuum with linear pedal control (Figure 1-26); the vacuum at the tip will promptly respond proportionately according to **Pascal's Principle**, which states that any change in pressure applied to an enclosed fluid will be transmitted undiminished to all parts of that fluid as well as its enclosing surface, including in this case the nuclear fragment. Linear pedal control of vacuum in phaco mode is unfortunately quite uncommon in current vacuum pump machines, with the Chiron Catalyst (rotary vane) and the Dual Linear Storz Millennium (with venturi pump module) being notable exceptions. This feature can be emulated on a flow pump by directly controlling flow at the pump head in order to indirectly control vacuum with an occluded aspiration port; a feedback algorithm from the aspiration line pressure transducer accordingly drives the pump head to achieve the commanded vacuum (see Figure 1-40a). Unfortunately, this feature is also rare on flow pumps, with the Storz Millennium (with scroll pump module) and the Gevoer machine being notable exceptions. The AMO Prestige (peristaltic pump) is another exception, albeit with the limitations of a standard pedal setup as opposed to Millennium's Dual Linear control (see Figures 1-2 through 1-4). Furthermore, the Prestige only allows linear control of the vacuum limit preset as opposed to the Millennium scroll pump's true commanded vacuum mode emulation (see Figure 1-40a).

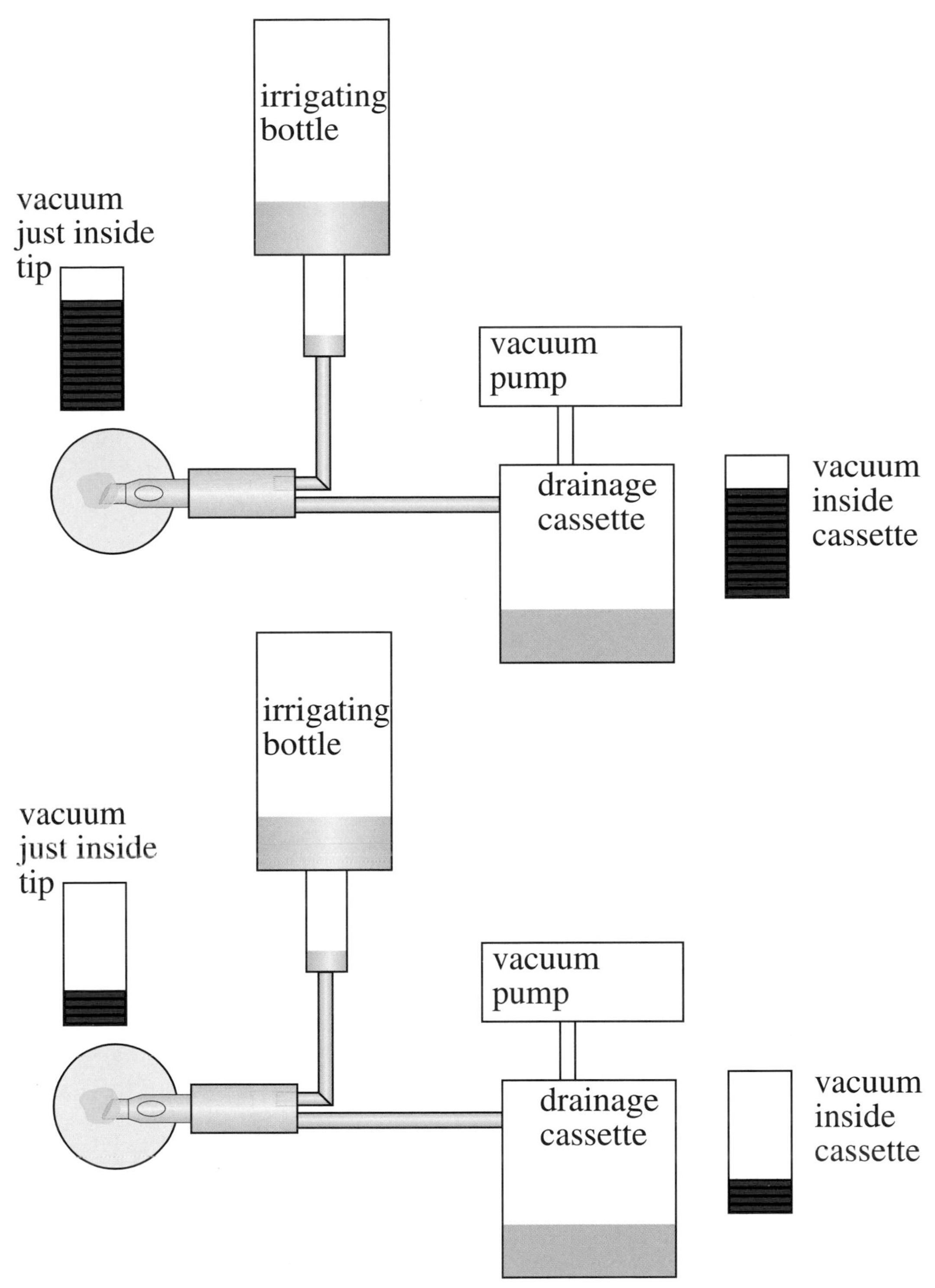
irrigating bottle
vacuum just inside tip
vacuum pump
drainage cassette
vacuum inside cassette
irrigating bottle
vacuum just inside tip
vacuum pump
drainage cassette
vacuum inside cassette

Figure 1-26

Venturi Pump

As mentioned previously, there are currently three types of vacuum pumps utilized in phaco machines, with the venturi being perhaps the most prevalent (Figure 1-27). This pump is driven by compressed gas (nitrogen or air), which is directed through the main pump housing B. By varying the size of opening A, the volume of gas through chamber B is proportionately controlled. The gas flow over the opening of tube C into chamber B creates a pressure differential via a venturi effect with air flow as indicated by the green arrows. This air flow and pressure differential in tube C create a vacuum in the rigid drainage cassette D which pulls fluid in from the aspiration tubing in proportion to this vacuum level when the aspiration port is unoccluded. As discussed previously (see Figure 1-26), the vacuum level in D controls the amount of grip of a fragment that occludes the aspiration port.

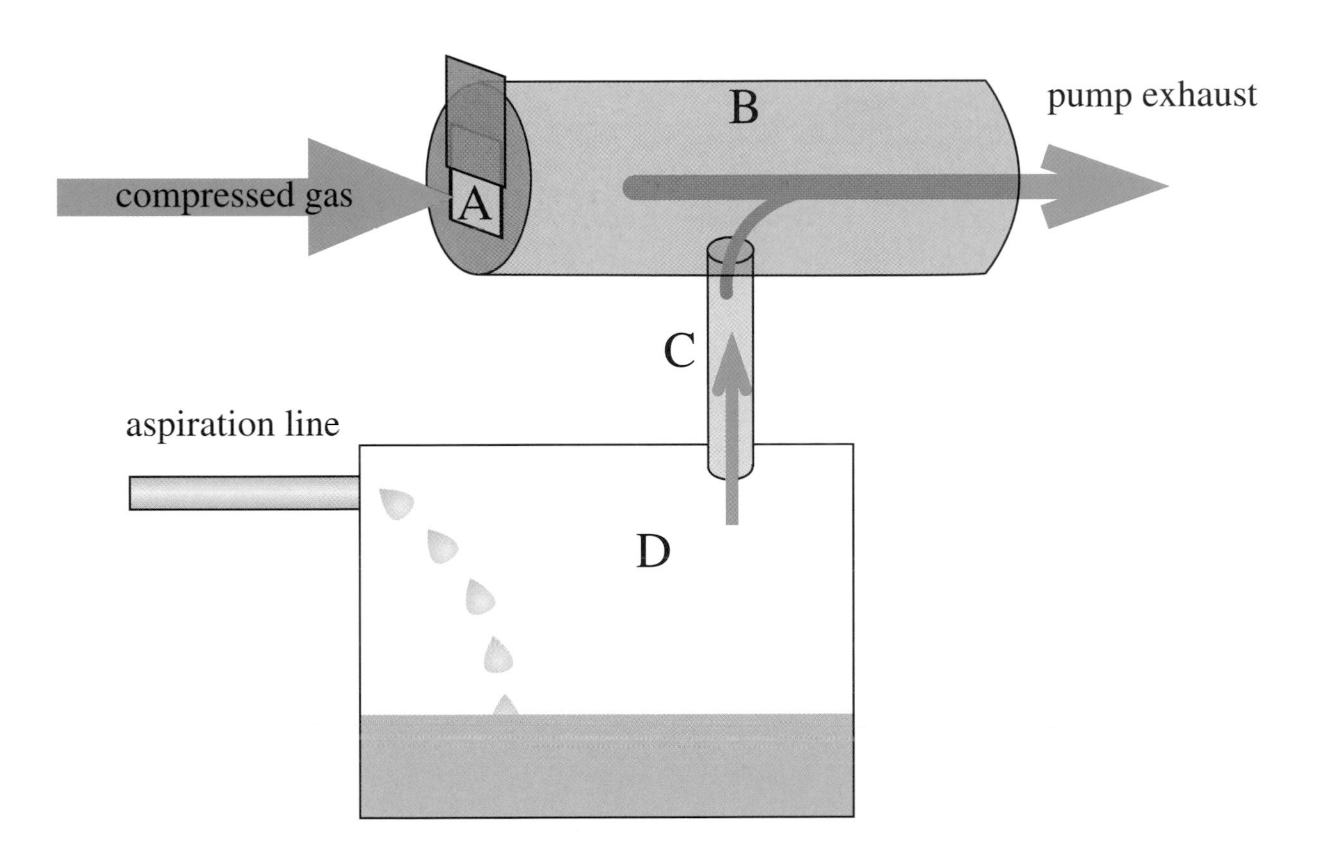

Figure 1-27

Diaphragm Pump

This is the type of pump commonly found in vacuum cleaners. Figure 1-28 illustrates a flexible diaphragm A which is alternately pushed in and pulled out by a rod connected to an electric motor rotating as indicated. When the diaphragm is pulled out, pressure is decreased in chamber B relative to chambers E and F. This pressure differential causes valve C to open with corresponding movement of air and fluid as illustrated. Valve D cannot open into chamber B, so chamber F is unaffected during this phase. When the diaphragm is pushed in, pressure is increased in chamber B. This pressure differential opens valve D and exhausts the air pulled in from chamber E during the previous phase. This exhaust is vented into chamber F and then out of the pump. Chamber E is unaffected during this phase because valve C, like valve D, is one-way only. The amount of vacuum created is directly proportional to the pump's motor speed. For the sake of simplicity, the rigid drainage cassette, which is common to all vacuum pumps, has been incorporated into this pump schematic in the form of chamber E; in actual practice, the cassette would be linked to the pump via a tube where the aspiration line is shown, and chamber E would not have any fluid.

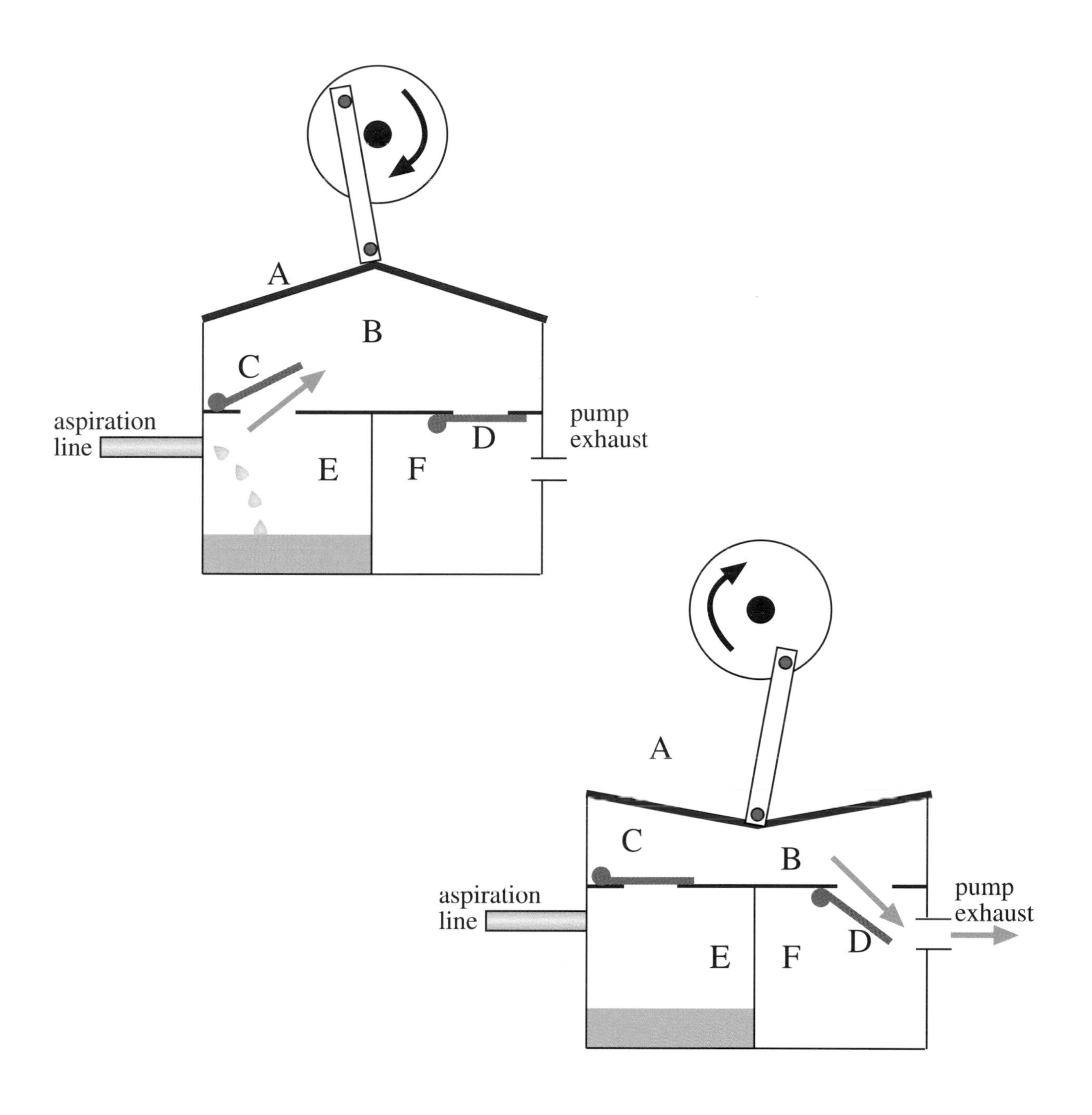
A
B
C
aspiration line
D
pump exhaust
E
F
A
C
B
aspiration line
pump exhaust
D
E
F

Figure 1-28

Rotary Vane Pump

The rotor, which contains freely sliding flat vanes, is mounted eccentrically in the pump housing and is driven by an electric motor. As a vane passes through the expanding volume of inlet area A, vacuum is created which translates to the rigid drainage cassette through the connecting tube as shown. The trapped air is swept through area B, and then is compressed through the decreasing volume of area C so that it is vented out through the pump exhaust. As with the diaphragm pump, the amount of vacuum created is directly proportional to the pump motor speed.

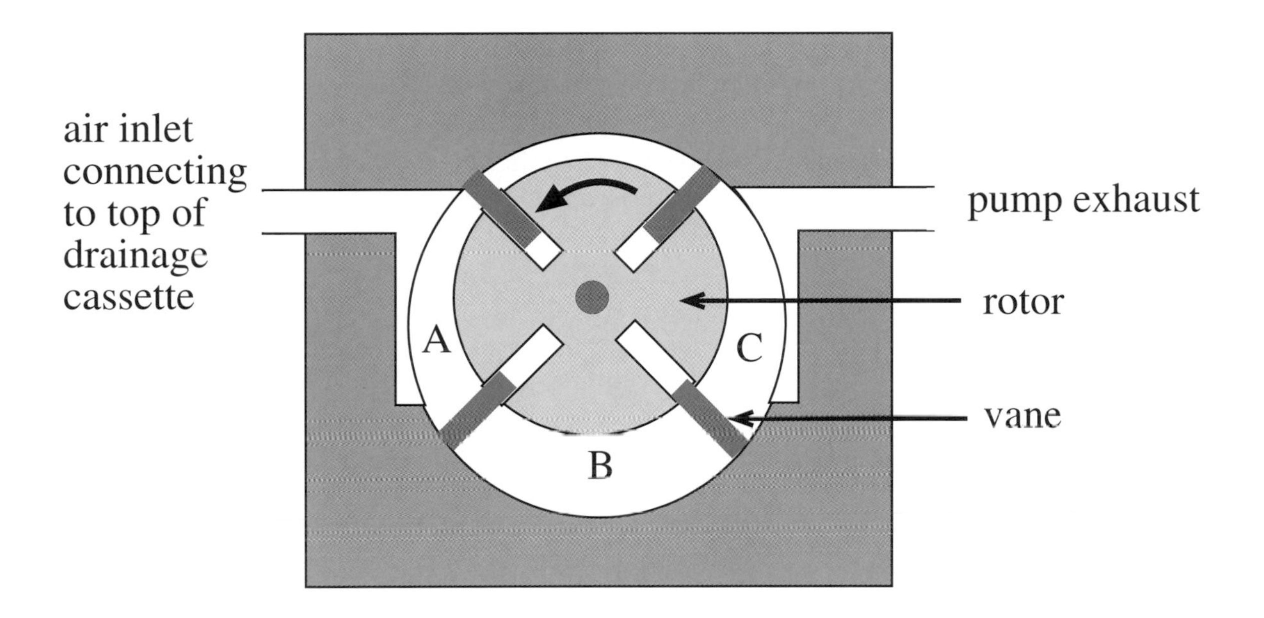
air inlet connecting to top of drainage cassette
pump exhaust
rotor
vane
A
B
C

Figure 1-29

Rise Time: Vacuum Pumps

Because no rollers are required to collapse the tubing as with peristaltic pumps, vacuum pumps can employ more rigid tubing with less compliance. This lower compliance coupled with these pumps' inherently rapid vacuum production, as well as the short times needed for vacuum transfer from the cassette to the phaco (or IA) tip, result in low rise times with most vacuum pumps.

Low rise times can be a potential liability when using high vacuum techniques. If unwanted material is inadvertently incarcerated in the aspiration port, the surgeon has little time to react before potentially permanent damage occurs. Recall that when using a flow pump with a high vacuum preset, a low flow rate can be set to produce longer rise times which give the surgeon more time to react to unwanted occlusions (see Figure 1-11). Most vacuum pumps do not allow attenuation of rapid rise times, although the Storz venturi machines are exceptions. These pumps allow the surgeon to set a time delay for full commanded vacuum buildup which starts when the surgeon enters pedal position 2. However, once this delay has elapsed, any subsequent engagement of material will be exposed to a typically rapid vacuum pump rise time. An even better solution to this issue is the previously discussed Dual Linear foot control on the Storz Millennium (see Figure 1-4). With linear control of vacuum in phaco mode, the surgeon can approach material with safer lower vacuum levels and increase it only after desired material is positively engaged. Furthermore, the rise time in this case will be determined by the physical speed of pedal movement through its linear vacuum travel; attenuation of rapid vacuum pump rise times is accomplished simply by slowly advancing the pedal (Figures 1-30 and 1-34).

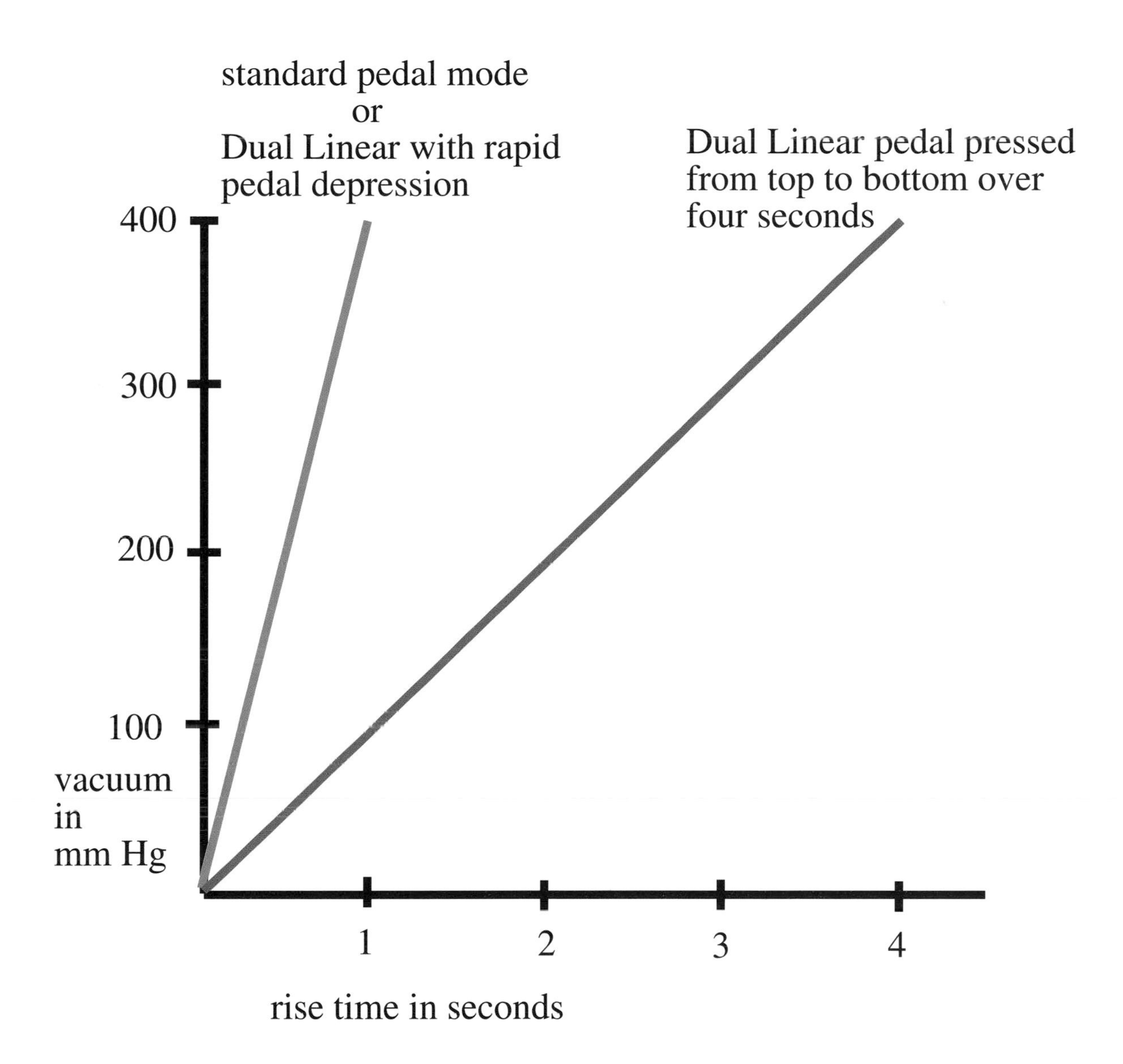
standard pedal mode
or
Dual Linear with rapid
pedal depression
Dual Linear pedal pressed
from top to bottom over
four seconds
400
300
200
100
vacuum
in
mm Hg
1
2
3
4
rise time in seconds

Figure 1-30

Vacuum Pumps: Relationship Between Rise Time and Vacuum

Note how Figure 1-31 differs from the flow pump schematics (eg, Figure 1-14) with regard to the lack of a flow rate parameter adjustment; this is arguably a clinically arbitrary omission in that flow can be indirectly controlled by applied vacuum if the aspiration port is not completely occluded (see Figure 1-23). Furthermore, just as rise time (with an occluded tip) can be varied with a flow pump by changing the flow rate parameter adjustment (pump speed), rise time can be controlled without flow rate adjustment on a vacuum pump if the surgeon utilizes Dual Linear pedal control (see Figures 1-30 and 1-34). Recall that the actual vacuum on these schematics is measured by the machine's pressure transducer which is typically connected to the drainage cassette; it is therefore not an accurate reflection of vacuum just inside the aspiration port unless the port is completely occluded (see Figures 1-25 and 1-39).

At time zero, the tip is occluded and the linear control pedal is abruptly pushed from position 0 to a halfway point in position 2; this pedal position coupled with a maximum vacuum preset of 400mm Hg will yield a maximum potential vacuum of 200mm Hg, but at time 0.25 sec, vacuum has only risen to 100mm Hg (assuming a rise time of 200mm Hg/0.5 sec as shown in Figure 1-30). Just as with the foregoing flow pump rise time examples, flow has stopped since the aspiration port is completely occluded. There is no dripping in either the drip chamber or the drainage cassette; the arrow in the drainage cassette represents the pulling force exerted on the aspiration line fluid by the vacuum pump.

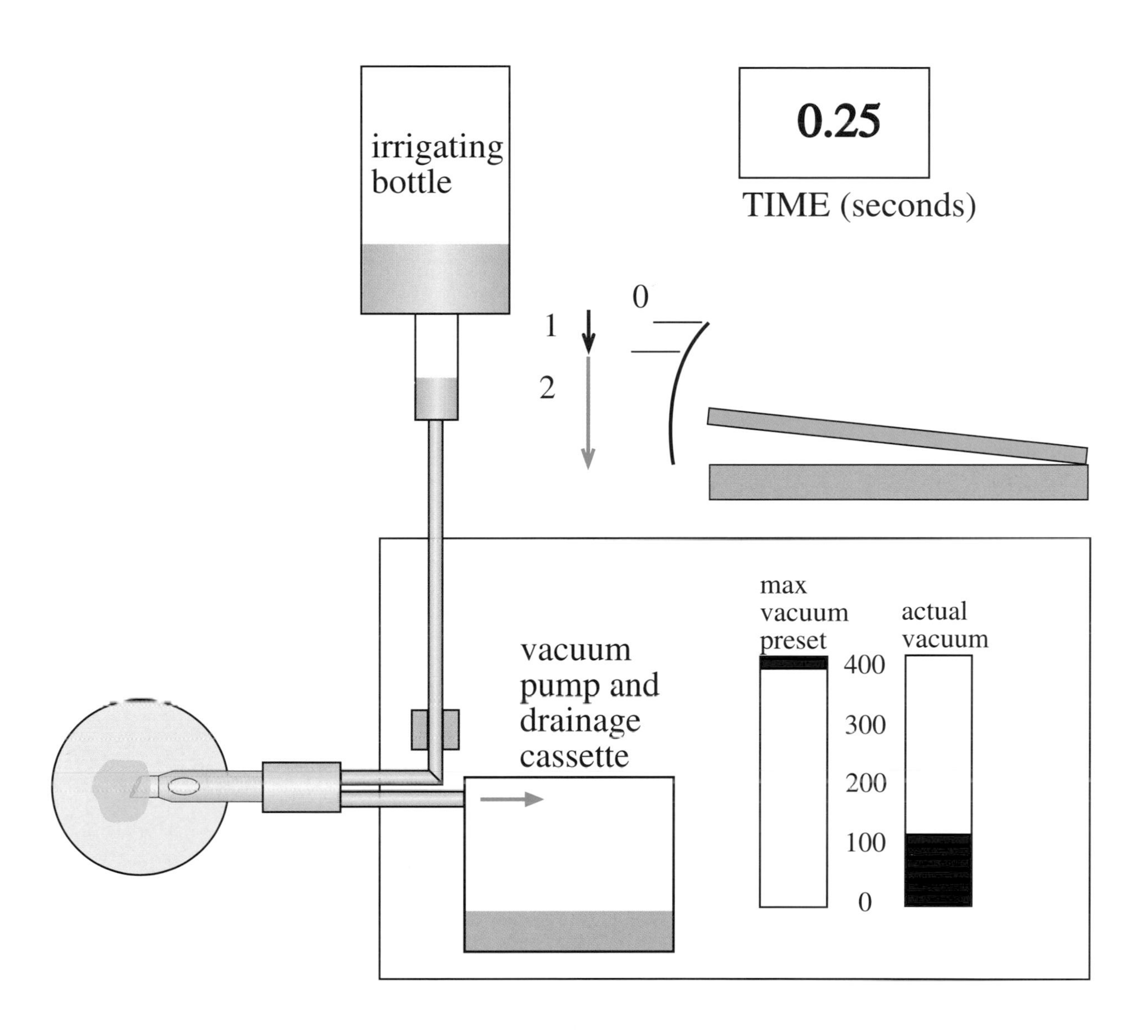
irrigating bottle
0.25
TIME (seconds)
0
1
2
max vacuum preset
actual vacuum
vacuum pump and drainage cassette
400
300
200
100
0

Figure 1-31

Vacuum Pumps: Relationship Between Rise Time and Vacuum (continued)

Figure 1-32: At time 0.5 sec after tip occlusion and pedal actuation, actual vacuum has now reached 200mm Hg, which is the maximum potential vacuum for this combination of pedal position and maximum vacuum preset.

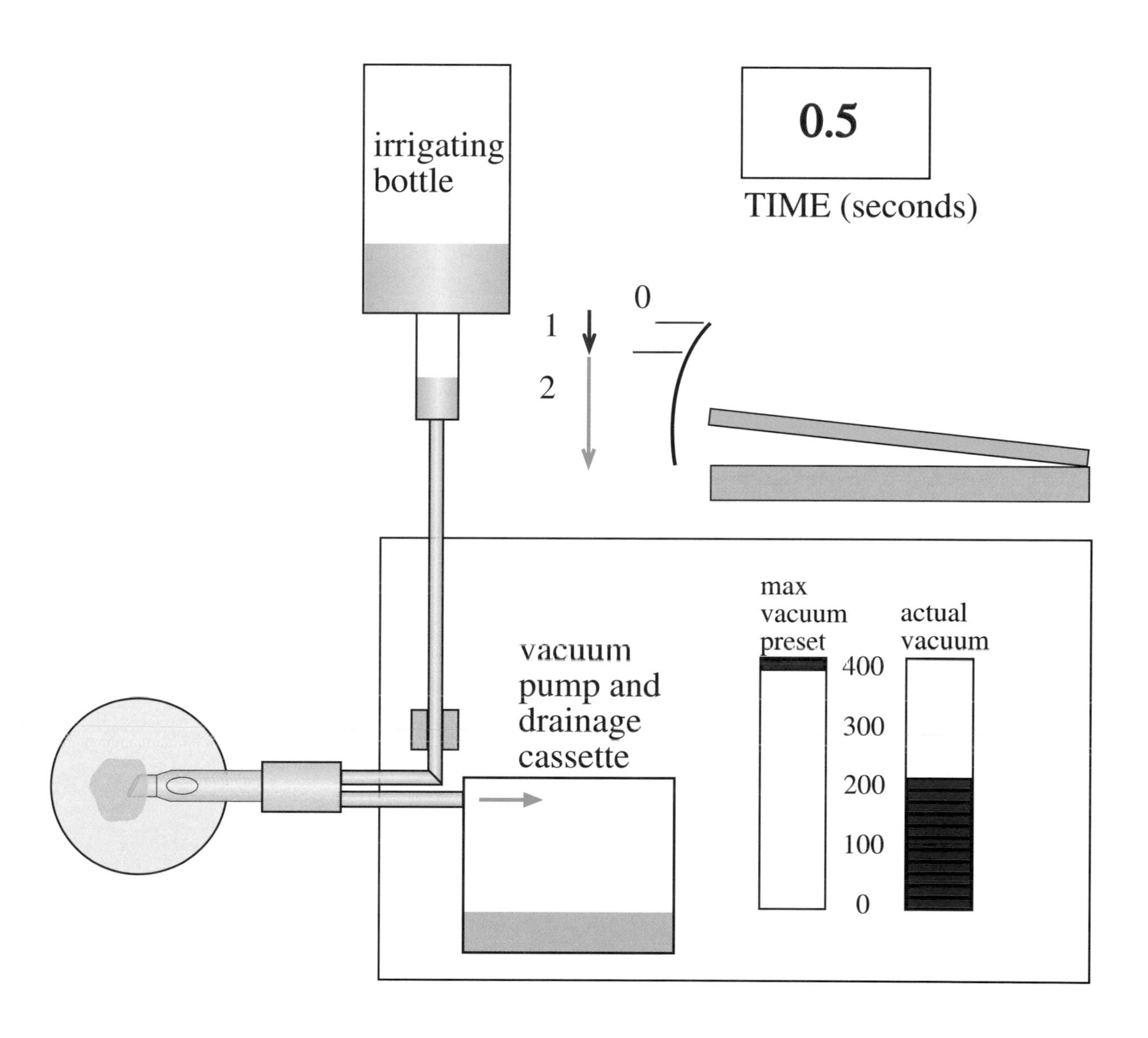
irrigating bottle
0.5
TIME (seconds)
0
1
2
max vacuum preset
actual vacuum
vacuum pump and drainage cassette
400
300
200
100
0

Figure 1-32

Vacuum Pumps: Relationship Between Rise Time and Vacuum (continued)

Figure 1-33: At time 0.5 sec in Figure 1-32, suppose the pedal was abruptly fully depressed from its original position which was only halfway into position 2. Given the rise time rate of 200mm Hg/0.5 sec and the starting point of 200mm Hg, it will take an additional 0.5 sec to reach 400mm Hg; therefore, the total elapsed time will be 1 sec as illustrated here. Remember to allow for this delay of rise time (see also Figure 1-20) when changing the pedal position to increase linear vacuum.

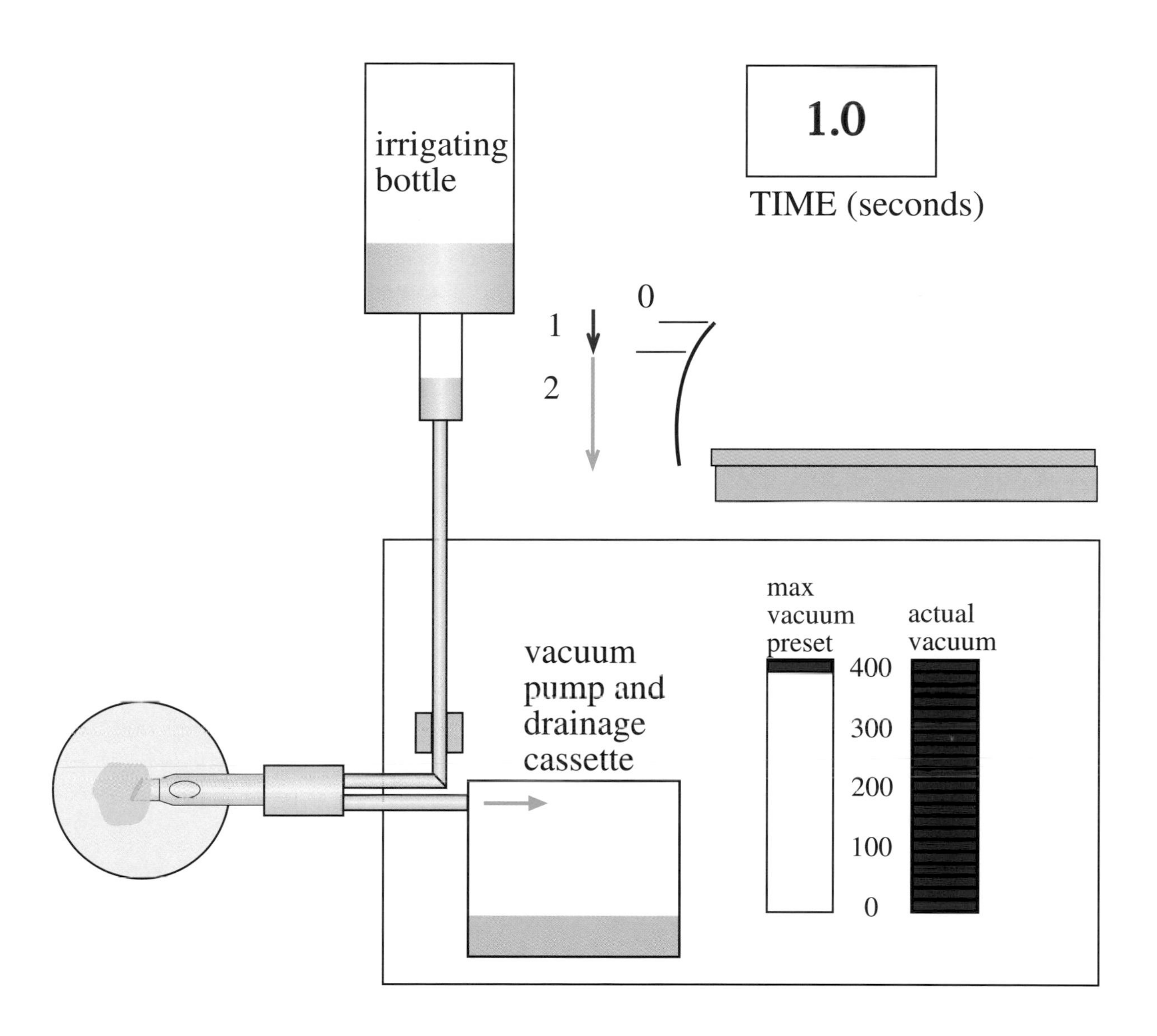
irrigating
bottle
1.0
TIME (seconds)
0
1
2
max
vacuum
preset
actual
vacuum
vacuum
pump and
drainage
cassette
400
300
200
100
0

Figure 1-33

Vacuum Pumps: Relationship Between Rise Time and Vacuum (continued)

Figure 1-34: The rise time lag alluded to in Figure 1-33 is usually clinically insignificant with vacuum pumps or with flow pumps operating at a fast flow rate (rotational pump head speed). Indeed, the fast rise times in these cases can be a liability in that the surgeon has little time to react in case of inadvertent incarceration of unwanted material in the aspiration port before dangerously high levels of vacuum build up. By accepting the compromise of a longer rise time with correspondingly slower pedal responsiveness, a surgeon can set a slower flow rate when using a flow pump, thus intentionally inducing a rise time lag. When using a machine with linear control of vacuum in phaco mode (ie, Chiron Catalyst, Storz Millennium, or AMO Prestige), the rise time can be lengthened by moving the pedal more slowly through its linear range of travel. This mechanical control of rise time can be used on both flow pumps as well as vacuum pumps, and is particularly effective when using Dual Linear control with its larger range of travel in position 2 (see Figure 1-34). Compare the rise time of 4 sec in this figure to the rise time of 1 sec in Figure 1-33 which would have been produced with abrupt, full depression of the foot pedal (see also Figure 1-30).

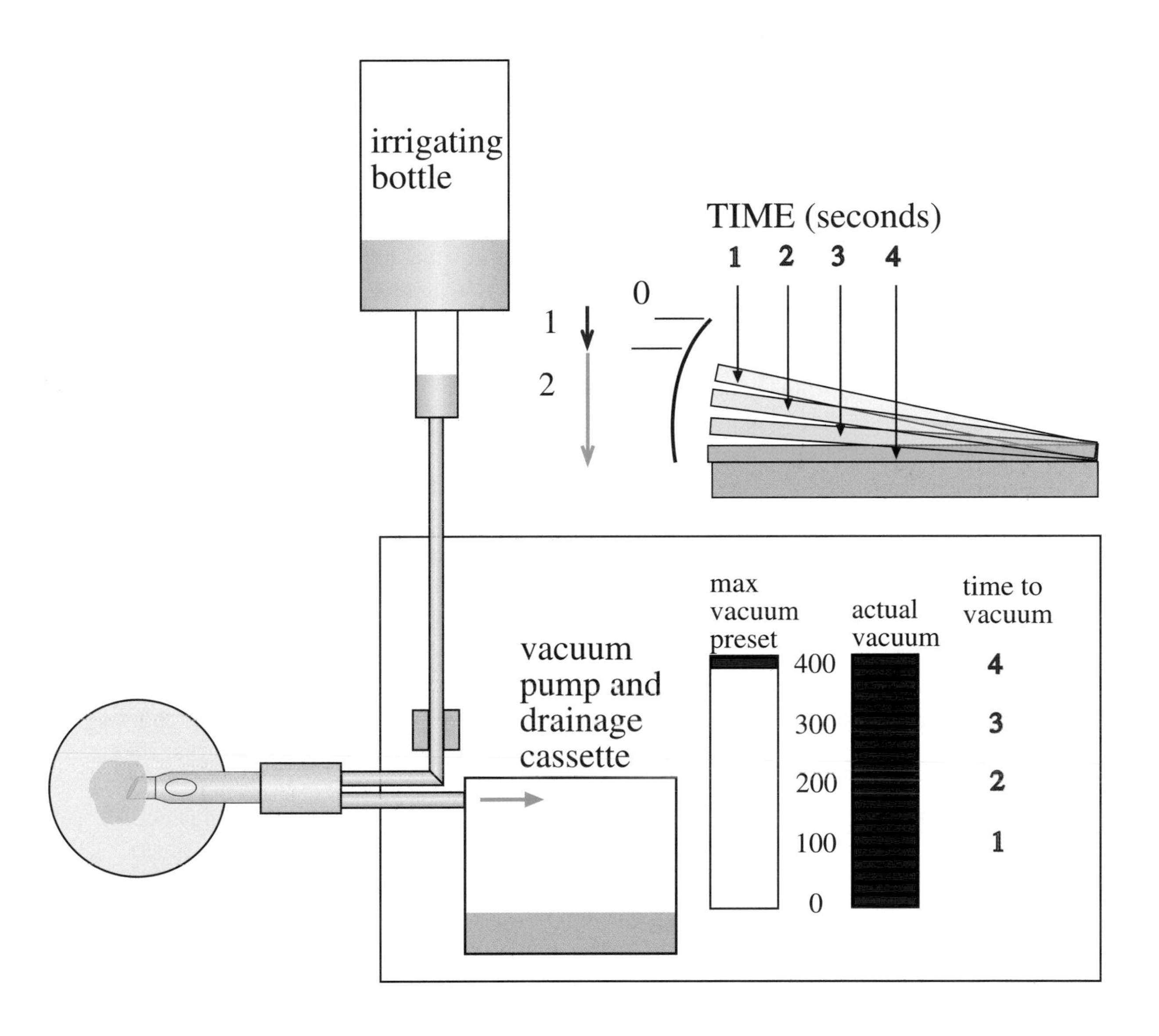
irrigating bottle
TIME (seconds)
1 2 3 4
0
1
2
max vacuum preset
actual vacuum
time to vacuum
vacuum pump and drainage cassette
400
300
200
100
0
4
3
2
1

Figure 1-34

Fluidic Resistors Affecting Flow

As was illustrated in Figure 1-23, the direct linear control of vacuum in the drainage cassette of vacuum pumps allows indirect linear control of flow. However, this indirect flow control means that these pumps are more sensitive to restrictive variances in the fluidic circuit. One component of this "restrictance" (resistance) is the length and internal diameter of the tubing. Another especially important point of resistance is the diameter of the aspiration port, which is usually the smallest diameter of the fluidic circuit. The top diagram in Figure 1-35a illustrates a venturi machine with a 24-inch bottle height; when aspiration ports are present, they are unoccluded. Note how higher vacuums produce higher flow rates, as illustrated in Figure 1-23. Also note how the flow rate at a given vacuum decreases from the setup with no handpiece (lowest resistance) to the setup with the 0.9mm standard phaco tip port (medium resistance) to the setup with the 0.5mm inner diameter MicroFlow phaco tip (higher resistance) to the setup with the 0.3mm IA port (highest resistance). It should be noted that a partially occluded standard phaco tip (ie, during sculpting) might have a flow profile similar to the MicroFlow or IA tip because of the smaller effective aspiration port surface area resulting from partial occlusion (see the middle diagram in Figure 1-10).

Another way to think about this phenomenon is in terms of percentages. For example, if the vacuum and bottle height on a particular venturi machine (without a handpiece) are adjusted to produce 40cc/min measured outflow in the drainage cassette, then adding a phaco handpiece to the fluid circuit will decrease the flow rate to 30cc/min, a 25% drop. Similarly, using an IA tip will decrease flow by 70% because of the greater resistance across the 0.3mm IA port. Note in the bottom section of Figure 1-35a that the same phaco and IA resistors affect flow less on a peristaltic machine (-5% and -35%, respectively) than they did on the venturi machine. This phenomenon is simply a reflection of the different nature of the two pumps. A peristaltic pump is a positive displacement pump (flow pump) which directly acts on the fluid it is pumping, whereas a venturi pump indirectly acts on the fluid by a kinetic effect as well as by creating vacuum in the rigid drainage cassette interface between the pump and the aspiration line.

An easy way to observe the effect of resistors on flow is to look at the bottle drip chamber while using pedal position 2 with test chambers on the IA and phaco handpieces (see Figure 1-24). For a given pump speed/strength setting, the drip chamber activity will be greater with the lower resistance phaco tip; remember that the drip chamber activity mirrors the speed and strength of the anterior chamber current.

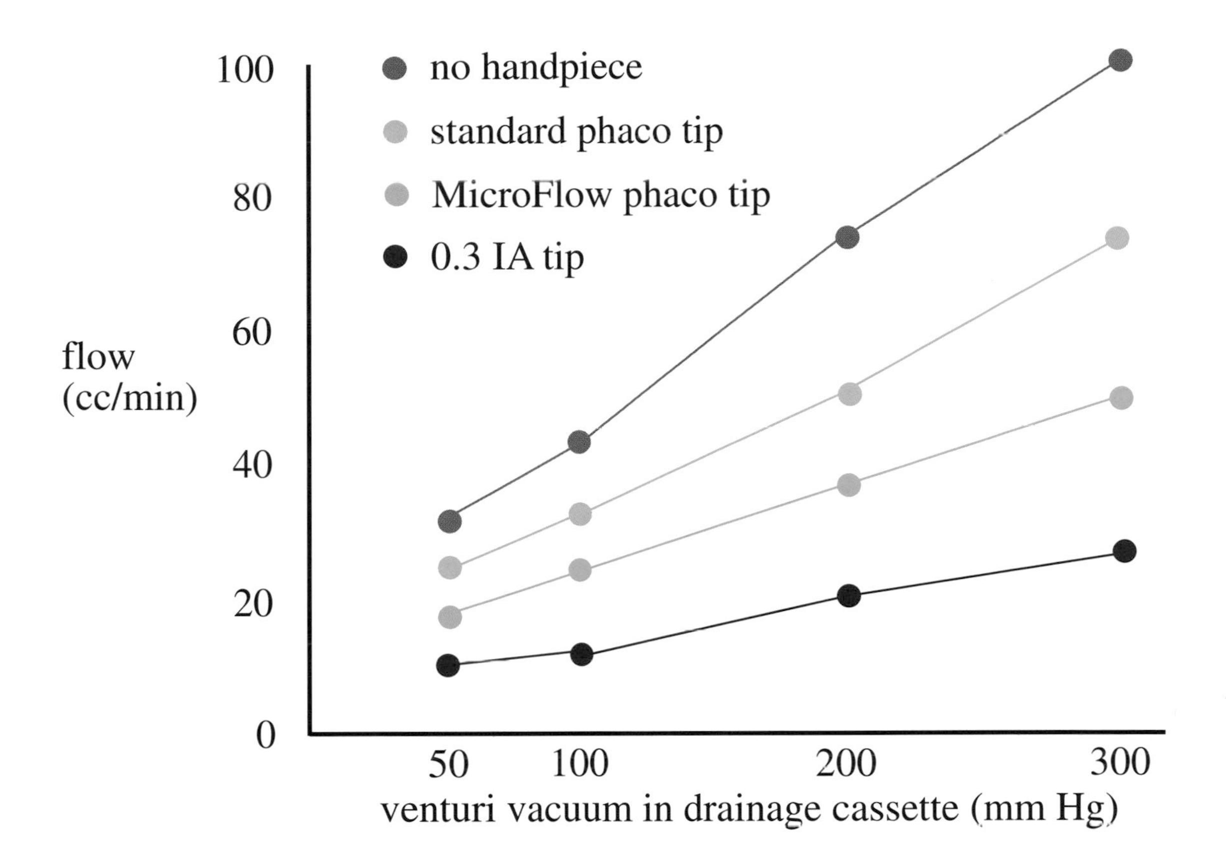

VENTURI 40cc/min (no handpiece) —-25%→ 30 cc/min standard phaco tip

VENTURI 40cc/min (no handpiece) —-70%→ 13 cc/min 0.3 IA tip

PERISTALTIC 40cc/min (no handpiece) —-5%→ 38 cc/min std phaco tip

PERISTALTIC 40cc/min (no handpiece) —-35%→ 27 cc/min 0.3 IA tip

Figure 1-35a

Fluidic Resistors Affecting Vacuum

Whereas Figure 1-35a illustrated the effect of fluidic resistors on flow given a commanded vacuum, Figure 1-35b demonstrates their effect on vacuum at various points in the fluidic circuit given a commanded flow on a flow pump. Bottle height is set to 24 inches above the eye (test chamber where IOP is measured) and the aspiration port in each graph is unoccluded. The machine's vacuum limit is set to 400mm Hg. Zero mm Hg on the graph is calibrated to represent ambient atmospheric pressure. Recall that the commanded flow setting determines the rotational speed of the pump head and that actual flow is less depending on the size of the effective aspiration port (see Figure 1-10). Also, note that a different phaco machine and tube set was used in Figure 1-35b than in Figures 1-21 and 1-22; therefore, the values are somewhat different when comparing the graphs which incorporate a standard phaco tip.

At any given flow rate setting, the pump is pulling much harder in trying to draw fluid through the higher resistance IA tip than the lower resistance standard phaco tip; note the much larger pressure differentials (higher vacuum levels) in the lower graph between the higher IOP and the lower aspiration line pressure at each flow setting. For example, the standard phaco needle at 20cc/min has a pressure differential of approximately 8mm Hg (difference between green and red dots) as opposed to the IA tip's differential of approximately 120mm Hg at the same flow rate. Note also that at any given flow rate, the vacuum in the aspiration line closer to the pump is higher (ie, the pressure is lower) than the vacuum level in the aspiration line where it connects to the phaco or IA handpiece; this is due to vacuum degradation in the line (see Figure 1-39). Another important aspect of a tip's fluidic resistance is the degree to which flow affects IOP (see Figure 1-5). The IOP is seen to be less affected as flow rates increase with the IA tip relative to the standard phaco tip. For example, with the pump speed set for 50cc/min, the IOP measures 6mm Hg with the phaco tip but 22mm Hg with the IA tip (see Figures 1-10 and 1-35b). This difference is explained by the fact that the flow rate setting on the graph refers to the commanded rotational pump head speed, which will in turn produce a lower actual flow in the fluidic circuit with a smaller, higher resistance aspiration port (fluidic resistor).

The lower diagram using the IA tip in Figure 1-35b also determines which combinations of flow and vacuum are effective and which are counterproductive; please see the discussion with Figure 4-1.

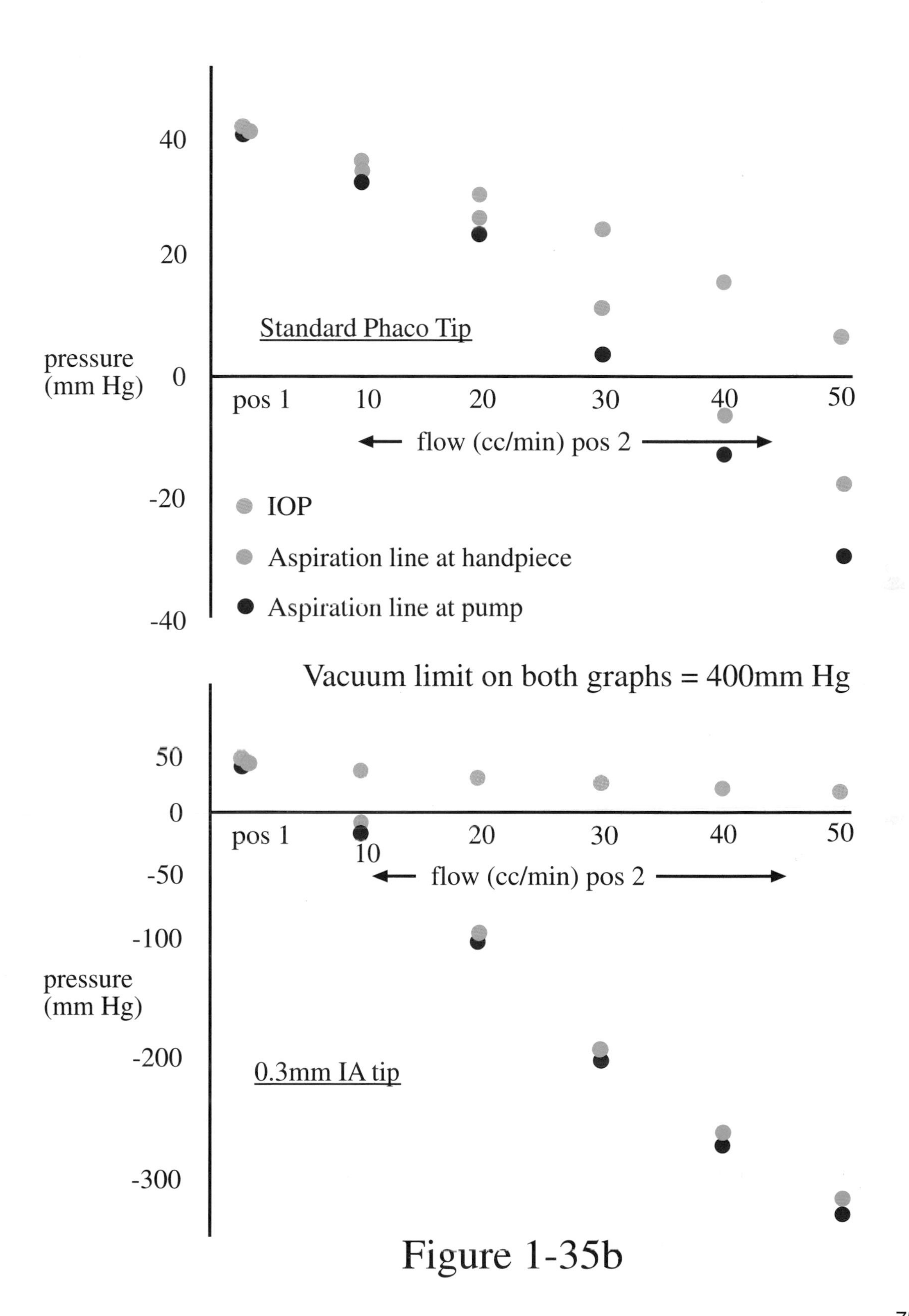
40
20
Standard Phaco Tip
pressure
(mm Hg)
0
pos 1
10
20
30
40
50
flow (cc/min) pos 2
-20
IOP
Aspiration line at handpiece
Aspiration line at pump
-40
Vacuum limit on both graphs = 400mm Hg
50
0
pos 1
10
20
30
40
50
-50
flow (cc/min) pos 2
-100
pressure
(mm Hg)
-200
0.3mm IA tip
-300

Figure 1-35b

Bottle Height: Relationship to Flow

Basically, adjusting the bottle height proportionately adjusts the anterior chamber depth. More specifically, the function of proper bottle height is to produce an adequate IOP which will maintain the anterior chamber despite aspiration outflow as well as any surges or incisional drainage. Higher flow rates require higher bottle heights. Conversely, lower bottle heights (ie, useful for lowering IOP with a small posterior capsule tear) require a correspondingly lower flow rate in order to prevent anterior chamber shallowing and potential collapse. Therefore, bottle height needs to be adjusted dynamically (ie, with an unoccluded aspiration port and active pump function) in foot pedal position 2 or 3. When adjusting bottle height for a given flow rate setting, it is important to know if the height adjustment itself affects flow rate. The effect of bottle height on flow is entirely dependent on the type of pump in question. Because flow is constrained at the point where the aspiration line is first interdigitated by a peristaltic pump roller or a scroll element, changing bottle height has no effect on flow with these machines. In essence, the pump head is acting as a **flow regulator**; despite increased pressure from an increased bottle height, flow cannot proceed any faster than the speed of the pump element traversing the fluid in the aspiration tubing. On a vacuum pump, however, there is open communication without restriction between the irrigation bottle and the drainage chamber in positions 2 and 3. Therefore, increasing bottle height with resultant increased IOP produces higher flow rates by pushing fluid harder through the aspiration line and into the drainage chamber. By corollary, a given increase in bottle height on a vacuum pump will not produce as much of an increase in IOP as with a flow pump because part of the increased pressure head is dissipated in the faster flow rate with the vacuum pump.

In Figure 1-36, both the flow and vacuum machines were set up to produce a measured 30cc/min outflow at 24 inches of bottle height; aspiration and irrigation tubing was simply connected without a handpiece. Outflow was then measured at bottle heights of 12 and 48 inches. It can be seen that the peristaltic machine's flow rate was unaffected by the bottle height changes, whereas the venturi machine's flow rate changed proportionately to the bottle height change. Clinically, it is important to realize when flow rate is being increased so that you can anticipate the resultant faster anterior chamber current and stronger attraction of intraocular material to the aspiration port.

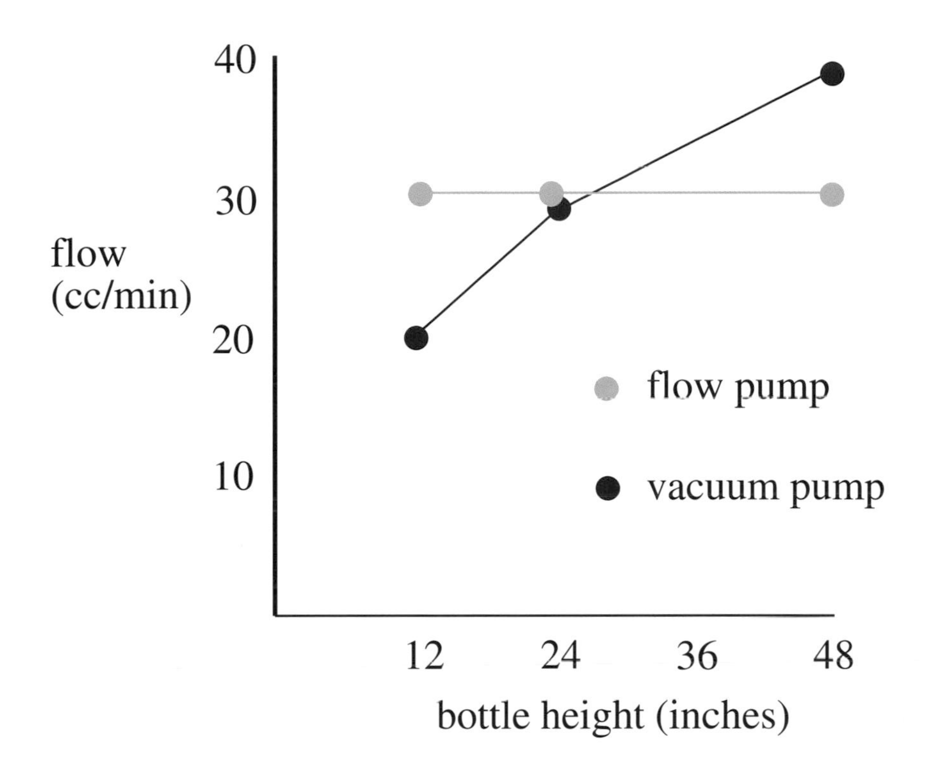
40
30
20
10
flow
(cc/min)
flow pump
vacuum pump
12
24
36
48
bottle height (inches)

Figure 1-36

Baseline Resistance to Flow

In order to further understand the relationship between bottle height and flow with respect to different types of pumps, it is helpful to look at the relation of flow to bottle height without any pump in the fluidic circuit (Figure 1-37). In these cases, the aspiration line is disconnected from the pump and left open to atmospheric pressure at the same height as the phaco handpiece and tip. The pressure head from the elevated irrigating bottle (approximately 11mm Hg above ambient atmospheric pressure for every 6 inches bottle height above the phaco tip) drives fluid through the tube set against the resistances of its various components, including the length and internal diameter (I.D.) of the irrigation line, irrigation sleeve, phaco tip, phaco handpiece, and the aspiration line. The point of greatest resistance in the fluidic circuit is typically the point of minimum I.D., usually found in the phaco (or IA) tip. As expected, flow increases as bottle height increases; a stronger pressure head drives fluid through the circuit more quickly. However, note that for a given bottle height that the flow rate decreases when going from a standard phaco tip (0.9mm I.D.) to a higher resistance MicroFlow tip with its smaller 0.6mm I.D.; this same type of phenomenon was noted in Figure 1-35a.

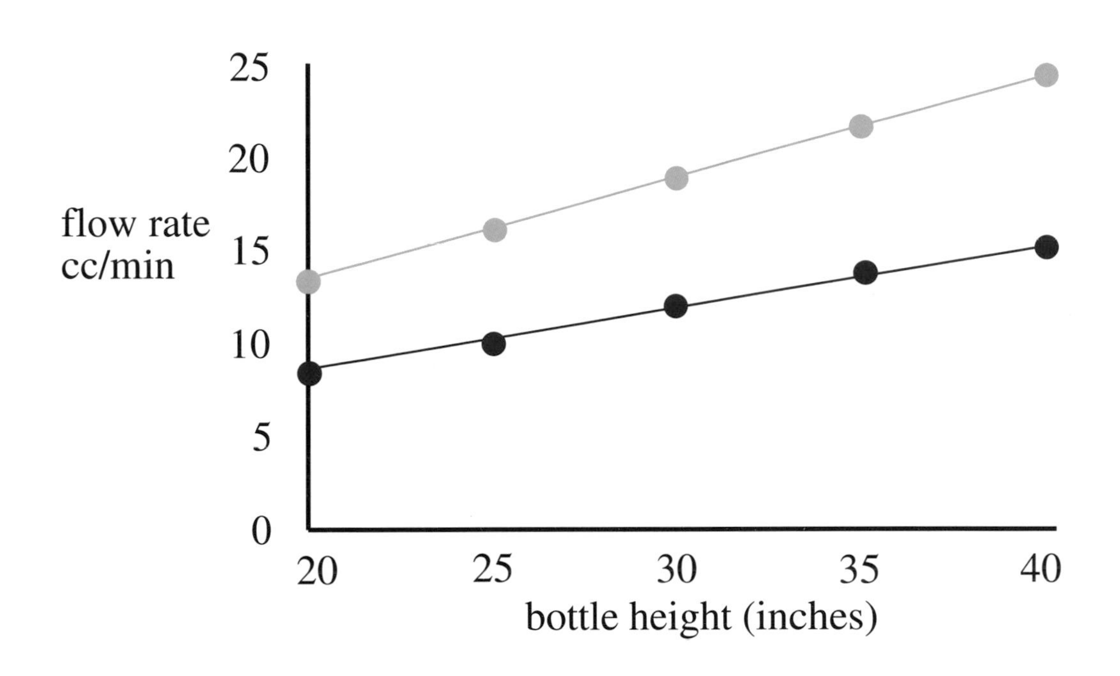
25
20
flow rate
cc/min
15
10
5
0
20
25
30
35
40
bottle height (inches)
standard phaco tip (0.9mm I.D.)
MicroFlow phaco tip (0.6mm I.D.)

Figure 1-37

Flow Control: Vacuum vs Flow Pumps

Figure 1-37 described a fluidic circuit without a pump. If the aspiration line is now reconnected to an active vacuum pump, it will increase the flow rate (in position 2 or 3) for any given bottle height. The reasoning is as follows: the flow vs bottle height graph in Figure 1-37 had the aspiration line disconnected from the pump and left open to atmospheric pressure; this pressure is considered to be zero (ie, neither above or below ambient atmospheric pressure, see Appendix C). The active vacuum pump produces vacuum (negative pressure, below ambient atmospheric) in the drainage cassette. Note that the vacuum is by convention expressed by a positive number in mm Hg even though it represents a negative value relative to atmospheric pressure. When the aspiration line is reconnected to this active drainage cassette, the pressure differential between the irrigating bottle and the fluidic circuit drain is increased, thereby increasing the driving force of the circuit.

Note that because a vacuum pump works by producing vacuum at the end of the fluidic circuit, it can only increase the circuit's pressure differential, thereby increasing flow over the baseline level without the pump (see red arrow in Figure 1-38). However, a flow pump can not only raise but also lower the flow rate at any given bottle height because the interdigitation of the pump element within the fluid circuit allows it to act as a **flow regulator** (see blue arrow in Figure 1-38). The irrigating bottle pressure head cannot drive the fluid any faster than the pump head's rotation; therefore, flow rates below the green baseline (no pump) level can be achieved (see Figures 1-9-3 and 1-38). For flow rates above the baseline level, the flow pump acts exactly the same as a vacuum pump in that it pulls on the fluidic circuit with induced vacuum which increases the pressure differential and thereby increases flow; a given amount of induced vacuum will produce the same incremental increase in flow regardless of whether a flow pump or a vacuum pump produced the vacuum (see also Figure 1-40a).

Note in Figure 1-38 that the relationship of 11mm Hg per 15cm bottle height (Appendix C) has been rounded off to 10mm Hg per 15cm bottle height.

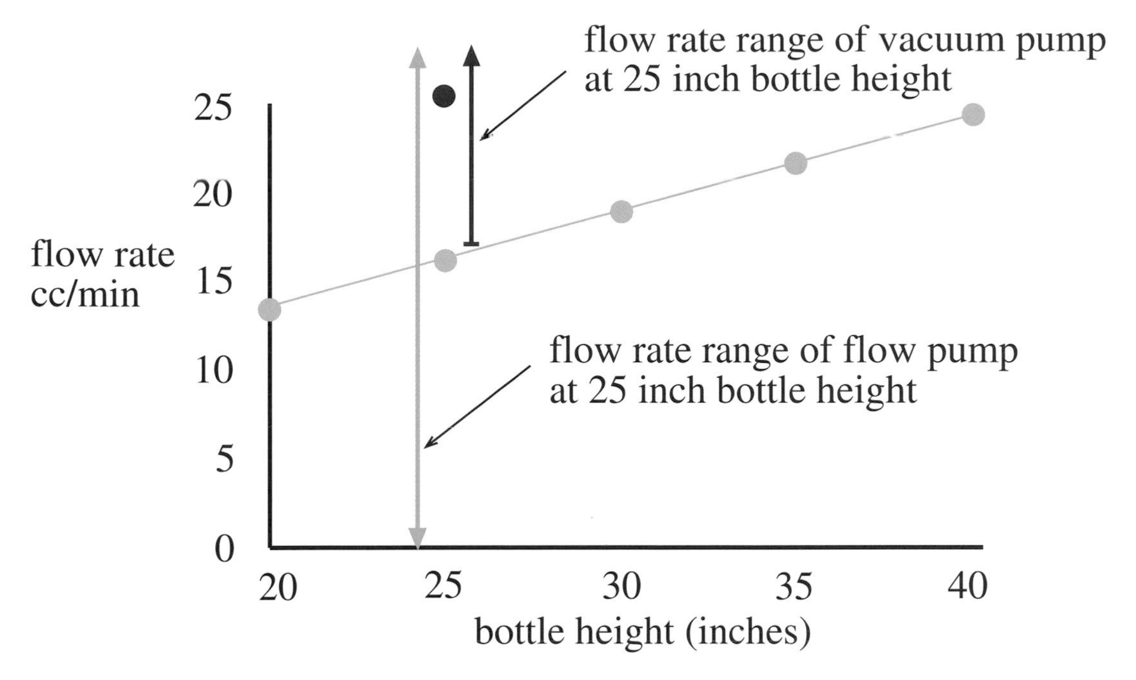

bottle height 25 inches is approximately 60cm

60cm x (10mm Hg / 15cm bottle height) = 40mm Hg

For a fluidic circuit without a pump, the pressure differential within the circuit is the 40mm Hg positive pressure head from the irrigating bottle minus the pressure at the end of the open aspiration line (zero relative to ambient atmospheric pressure).
40mm Hg - 0mm Hg = 40mm Hg

For a fluidic circuit with a pump/drainage cassette vacuum of 50mm Hg (i.e. 50mm Hg below atmospheric), the pressure differential within the circuit is:
40mm Hg - (-50)mm Hg = (40 + 50)mm Hg = 90mm Hg

Figure 1-38

Vacuum Degradation in Aspiration Line

The actual vacuum readout on the phaco machine is derived from the fluidic circuit's pressure transducer, which is located at or near the pump. However, although this is an accurate reading for this location, the vacuum can be noted to degrade as the distance along the aspiration line from the pump to the **unoccluded** aspiration port is increased (Figure 1-39). This figure incorporates either a flow pump operating in vacuum mode (see Figure 1-40a) or a vacuum pump; it illustrates unoccluded flow with a MicroFlow tip at various commanded vacuum levels with additional pressure transducers at locations 1 through 4. Location 1 is measured at the connection between the aspiration line and the drainage cassette. Location 2 is 24 inches away from the cassette, while location 3 is 48 inches away. Location 4 is at the other end of the aspiration line where it connects to the phaco handpiece. The graph illustrates vacuum drop; for example, a commanded vacuum which produces 250mm Hg at the cassette and on the machine readout, but results in only 150mm Hg vacuum measured at location 4, represents a 100mm Hg vacuum drop (-100mm Hg on the graph). Recall that this graph represents unoccluded flow and that upon occlusion, vacuum transfers from the cassette along the aspiration line to the occlusion at the aspiration port so that all locations would have the same vacuum value as the cassette (see Figure 1-25).

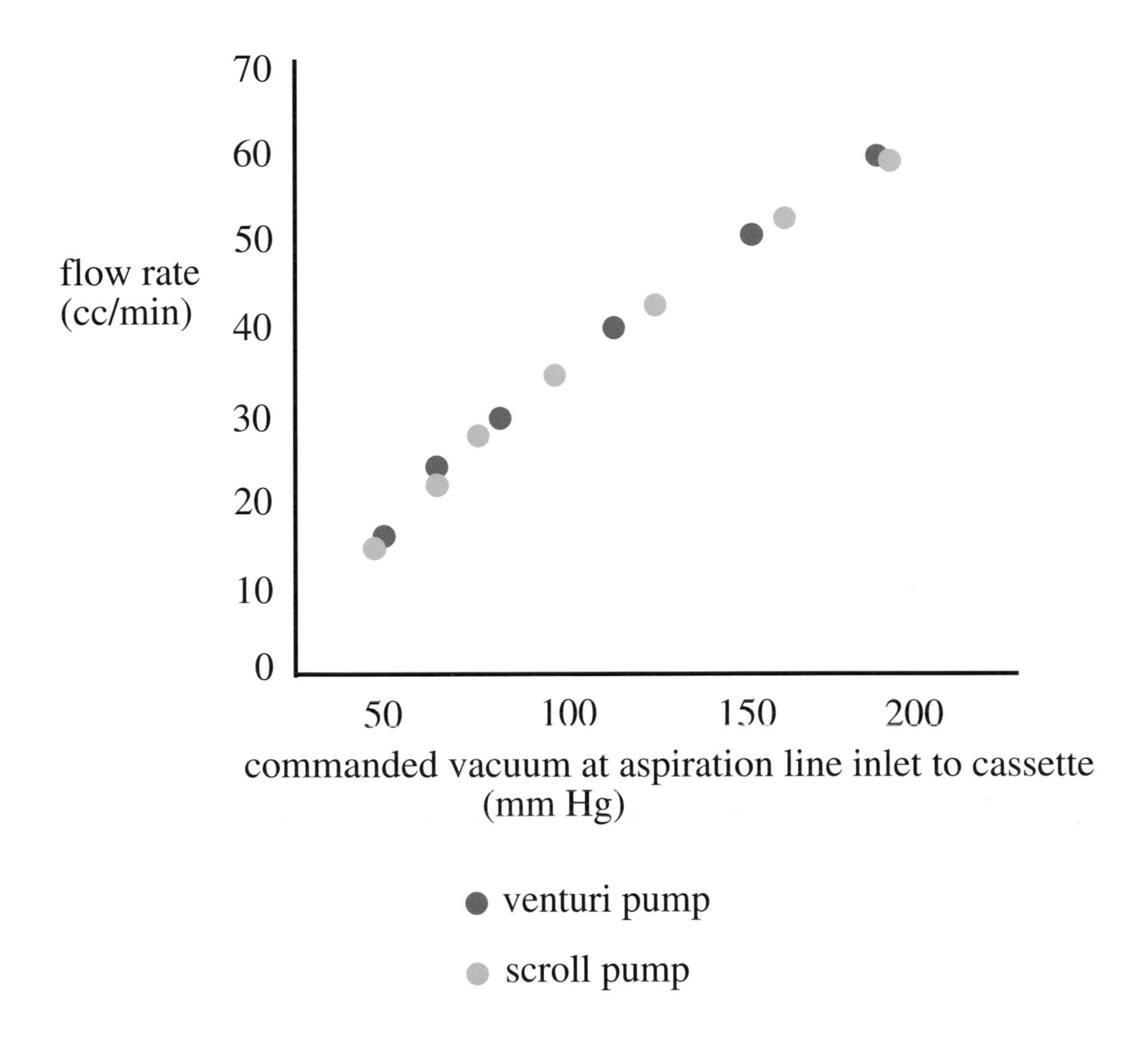
70
60
50
40
30
20
10
0
flow rate
(cc/min)
50
100
150
200
commanded vacuum at aspiration line inlet to cassette
(mm Hg)
venturi pump
scroll pump

Figure 1-40a

Viscosity Relative to Flow Pumps and Vacuum Pumps

When considering a dual function pump as in Figure 1-40a, it is helpful to review the different ways in which a flow pump or a vacuum pump affects a fluidic circuit. For this purpose, viscosity is a useful differentiator. In Figure 1-40b, each pump mode (priority) is tested with two different fluidic circuit viscosities:

1. Normal saline which is equivalent to aqueous humor
2. A higher viscosity mixture of saline plus viscoelastic

Note the upper diagram in Figure 1-40b, which represents a flow priority mode of pump operation; the flow rate is essentially the same even with different viscosity fluidic circuits. However, note the much higher vacuum level in the saline plus viscoelastic section caused by the pump pulling harder against the higher viscosity fluid in order to maintain a commanded flow rate of 17cc/min (which decreases just slightly to 16cc/min as the pump pulls against the higher resistance). Similarly, note the lower diagram representing a vacuum priority pump; the commanded vacuum level of 100mm Hg is the same in the two different viscosities. However, the saline-only circuit has a significantly higher flow rate (21 vs 7) because it offers less resistance to flow for a given vacuum level.

This experimental setup has several clinical corollaries. For example, fluidic circuit viscosity increases during phacoemulsification as the nuclear emulsate accumulates in the aspiration line in proportion to the density of the nucleus and the speed of phacoaspiration. Of course, viscoelastic also increases the fluidic circuit's viscosity. The effect of these different viscosities is usually evident even after the causative material is aspirated from the anterior chamber because it still must traverse the length of the aspiration line before its effect is eliminated from the fluidic circuit. Therefore, bear in mind the effects of Figure 1-40b when using a vacuum pump (or a flow pump in a vacuum priority mode). A decreasing effective flow rate (caused by increased viscosity in the aspiration line) will produce decreased followability as well as less effective ultrasonic tip cooling; the surgeon should appropriately compensate by increasing vacuum level accordingly, preferably with linear control.

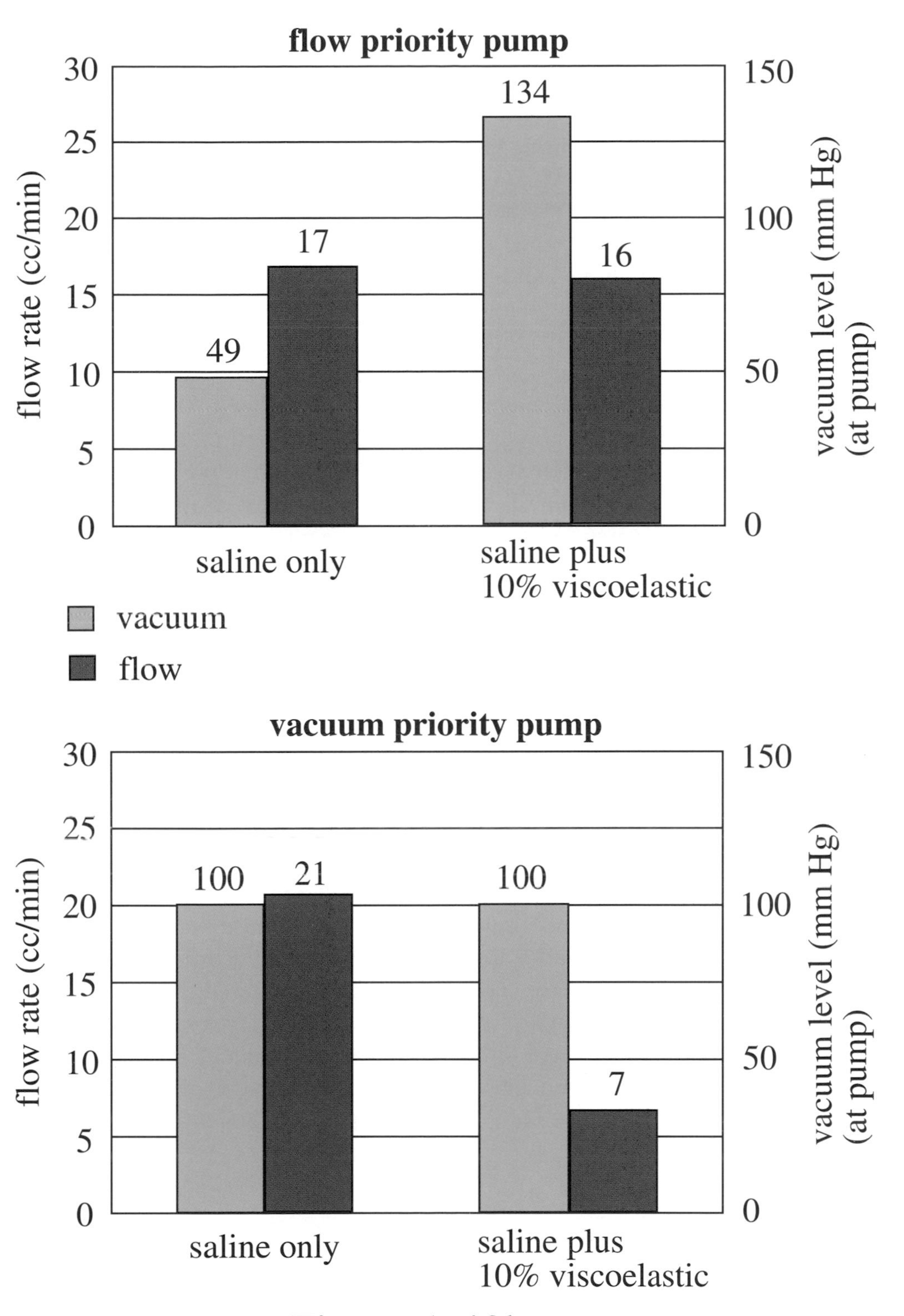
flow priority pump
30
25
20
15
10
5
0
flow rate (cc/min)
150
100
50
0
vacuum level (mm Hg)
(at pump)
49
17
134
16
saline only
saline plus
10% viscoelastic
vacuum
flow
vacuum priority pump
30
25
20
15
10
5
0
flow rate (cc/min)
150
100
50
0
vacuum level (mm Hg)
(at pump)
100
21
100
7
saline only
saline plus
10% viscoelastic

Figure 1-40b

Compliance and Venting 1

Although compliance and venting have previously been discussed separately (see Figures 1-12 and 1-13), it is useful to examine the relationship between them. Recall that venting mechanisms function by neutralizing aspiration line vacuum between the pump (either vacuum or flow pump) and an occlusion at the handpiece; venting also prevents a rotating flow pump from building vacuum past the vacuum limit preset. For example, Figure 1-41-1 shows a large nuclear fragment impaled by the phaco tip up to the silicone sleeve, which prevents further boring into the fragment. The fragment should be released so that it can be reengaged in a more effective carouseling configuration (see Figure 3-31); however, its release is inhibited by vacuum which has built up in the aspiration line between the pump roller pinching off the line at one end and the occlusion at the other end. Even when the foot pedal is released to position 1 or 0 (thereby stopping aspiration flow and pump head rotation), the vacuum will remain unless air or fluid is vented into the aspiration line to equilibrate the pressure with that of the anterior chamber/irrigation line. Therefore, most modern phaco machines automatically engage a venting mechanism when the foot pedal is raised from position 2 into position 1 or 0.

Venting air into the line (ie, venting to atmospheric pressure) can potentially decrease the efficiency of the pump because of air's high compliance. When attempting to rebuild vacuum after reengaging the fragment, the pump must first overcome the air's compliance by stretching it before vacuum effectively builds in the aspiration line fluid, thereby contributing to a rise time lag. Figure 1-41-2 shows the system just after it has reengaged the fragment which was released from its previous position in Figure 1-41-1 by venting air into the aspiration line; note the residual air bubble at the end of the vent tube. As the pump starts to turn, the highly compliant bubble expands its volume with relatively little effort by the pump (note the minimal increase in vacuum between Figures 1-41-2 and 1-41-3). Vacuum starts to significantly build in Figure 1-41-4 only after the air bubble has been fully stretched to the limit of its compliance, and the pump then begins to act on the fluid in the aspiration line; note the effect of the increased vacuum which draws the fragment more strongly onto the tip (aided by light ultrasound power) into a much more favorable tangential engagement as opposed to Figure 1-41-1 (see also Figure 3-31 for a discussion of the importance of tangential engagement of carouseling fragments).

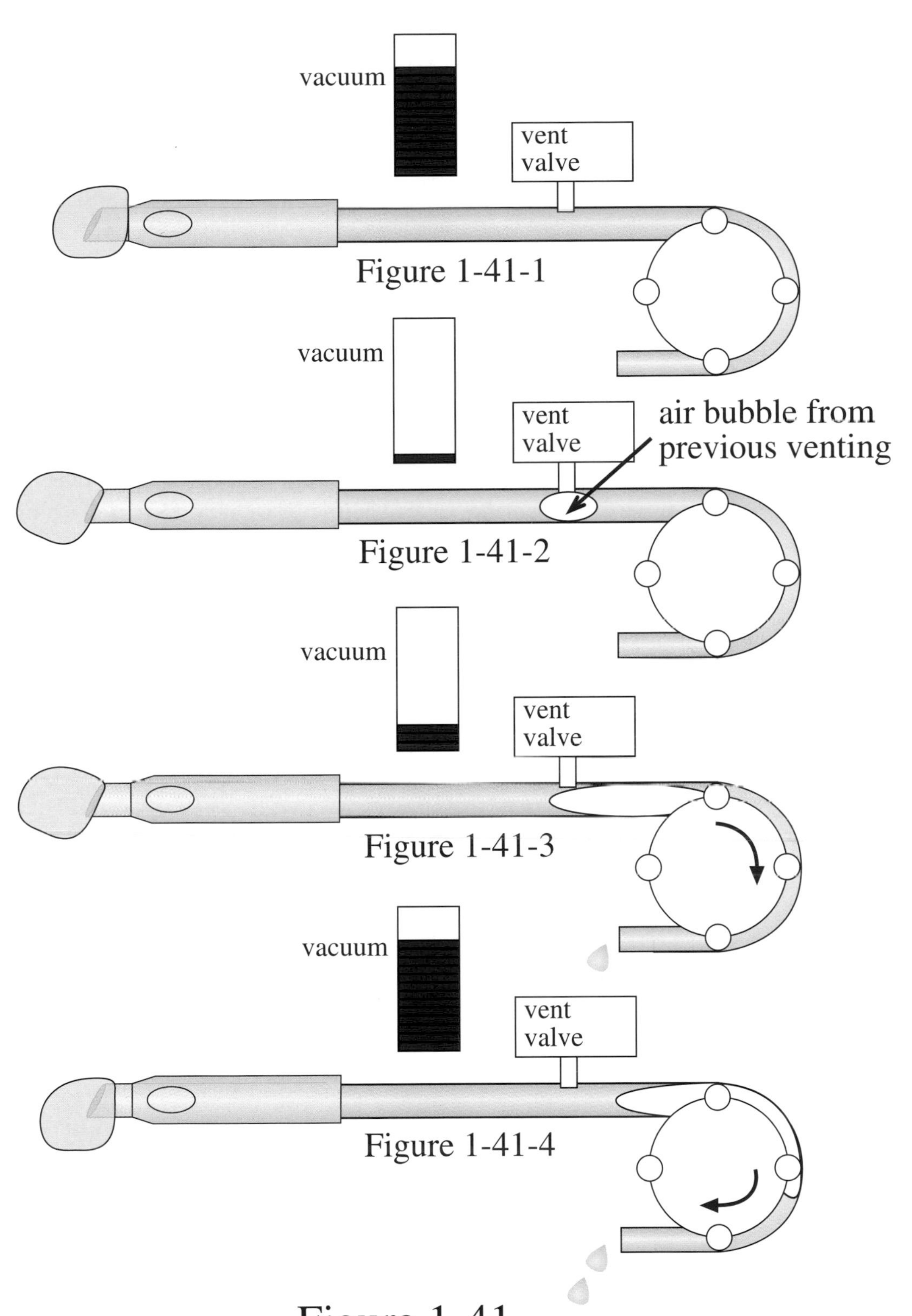
vacuum
vent
valve
Figure 1-41-1
vacuum
vent
valve
air bubble from
previous venting
Figure 1-41-2
vacuum
vent
valve
Figure 1-41-3
vacuum
vent
valve
Figure 1-41-4

Figure 1-41

Compliance and Venting 2

The venting system is not the only determinant of a machine's compliance. For example, if a fluid-vented machine has very compliant tubing, an occlusion will cause the pump to first decrease fluid volume in the partially collapsing line before effectively building vacuum (Figure 1-42); this will lead to longer rise times. Note that the fluid bolus which had previously been vented into this system has not decreased the system's compliance; even though it deforms to conform to the collapsing tubing's dimensions, its volume has not changed (contrast this to the air bolus in Figures 1-41-2 through 1-41-4).

Although a flow pump is used in these illustrations, it should be noted that vacuum pumps also employ venting mechanisms. However, these pumps (along with the scroll pump) can employ less compliant tubing than peristaltic pumps because the latter must be able to completely collapse the tubing with the pump head rollers in order for the pump to function. Also, rise time lags due to air venting in vacuum pumps are typically not as much of a liability because these pumps (especially venturi) inherently build vacuum faster than flow pumps (especially peristaltic); any induced rise time lag is usually minimal and negligible. These inherently fast rise times can be attenuated with some vacuum pumps as desired by the surgeon as discussed in Figure 1-30.

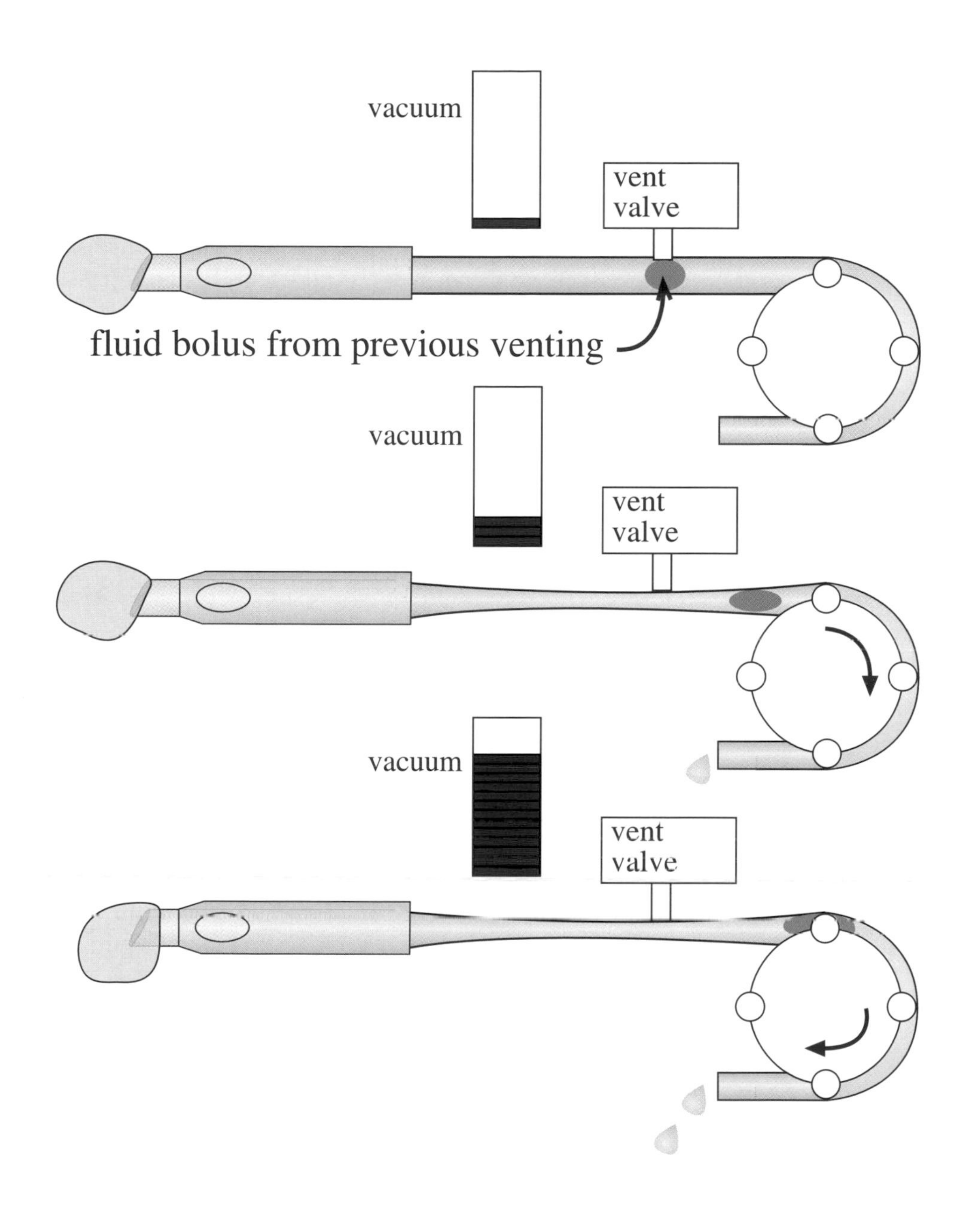
vacuum
vent
valve
fluid bolus from previous venting
vacuum
vent
valve
vacuum
vent
valve

Figure 1-42

Surge

Surge is a phenomenon encountered in pedal position 2 or 3 when an occluded fragment that caused an aspiration line vacuum buildup (Figure 1-43-1) is deformed sufficiently by ultrasound and/or vacuum so that it is abruptly pulled into the tip as the occlusion is broken. At this point the fluid in the higher pressure anterior chamber tends to rush into the lower pressure phaco tip, creating a potential chamber collapse (see Figure 1-43-2) which could cause damage to the cornea or capsule by direct mechanical contact with the phaco needle. The amount of fluid that surges into the aspiration port is a function of the machine's compliance; any fluid circuit component which was changed in volume by vacuum (increased air volume from venting in Figure 1-41 or decreased tubing volume in Figures 1-42 and 1-43-1) needs equilibration. Another source of increased air volume is the production of microbubbles which are pulled out of solution by vacuum (see Figure 1-43-1). In addition to compliance, surge is dependent on the pre-surge vacuum level, as well as the resistance in the irrigation and aspiration portions of the fluid circuit, along with the fluidic circuit's supply pressure head as determined by the irrigating bottle's height.

Surge potential is also influenced by the pump type and setting. For example, a vacuum pump with a level of 200mm Hg will produce a certain amount of gripping force of an occluded fragment (see discussion of Appendix B). Recall that this same vacuum will produce a very rapid flow rate with an unoccluded standard phaco tip (about 50cc/min as in Figure 1-35a). Therefore, at the moment of an occlusion break with this setup, the surge due to compliance equilibration will be intensified by a rapid flow rate corresponding to the high vacuum setting. The surgeon can compensate for this potential problem by titrating vacuum dynamically (with linear pedal control) during the procedure so that high levels are used only when needed during aspiration port occlusion (see also discussion of Figure 2-14b). A flow pump can deal with this issue differently because of the ability to independently set the parameters of vacuum and flow. For example, a flow pump with a vacuum preset of 200mm Hg can grip a fragment with the same force as the vacuum pump with the same setting. However, if the flow rate is set to a low level (eg, 14cc/min), then the pump will not contribute significantly to the surge during an occlusion break relative to the previously mentioned vacuum pump (50cc/min produced on occlusion break with a vacuum setting of 200mm Hg). Unfortunately, this safer, slow flow setting (ie, slow rotational pump head speed) will result in possibly unsatisfactorily slow rise times when dealing with these higher vacuum levels. Furthermore, this theoretical advantage of a flow pump with regard to surge control is offset by its need to use more compliant tubing than is needed by a vacuum pump; increased fluidic circuit compliance tends to lead to more surge potential (see Figure 1-42).

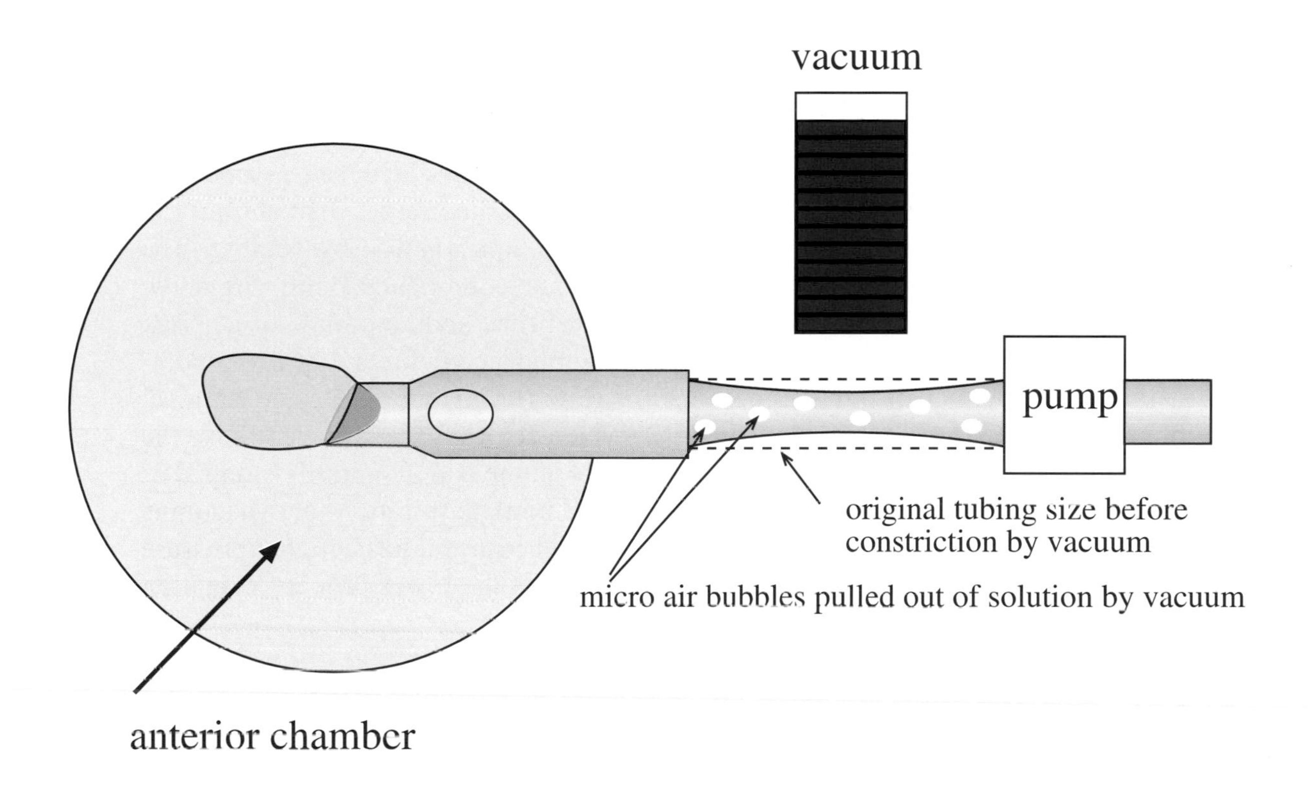
vacuum
pump
original tubing size before
constriction by vacuum
micro air bubbles pulled out of solution by vacuum
anterior chamber

Figure 1-43-1

Surge (continued)

Surge control has been dealt with in a variety of ways by different manufacturers. Fluidic circuits should be engineered with minimal compliance which will still allow adequate ergonomic manipulation of the tubing/handpiece as well as functioning of the pump mechanism, the latter being primarily important for peristaltic pumps. Small bore (internal diameter) aspiration line tubing, utilized by Allergan and Alcon, provides increased fluidic resistance which obtunds surges (see Figure 1-35a for the principle behind this). The AMO Prestige decreases its pump speed as the actual vacuum approaches the maximum vacuum preset. When the pressure transducer senses an occlusion break, the pump speed is increased again over a short time rather than abruptly in order to minimize the amount of vacuum which needs equilibration by venting. The Alcon Legacy utilizes an exceptionally low overall system compliance along with a low resistance irrigation line which minimizes the potential time and amplitude of a surge. The Storz Millennium also achieves a low system compliance via the use of lower compliance tubing with either its vacuum (venturi) or flow (scroll) modules. The Surgical Design machine utilizes a second irrigation bottle which is raised a few inches above the primary irrigation bottle. When a surge is detected, the pump is momentarily stopped as fluid is vented into the aspiration line from the second bottle; aspiration line vacuum is preferentially equilibrated by fluid from this vent bottle because it has a higher pressure than the anterior chamber, which has the same pressure as the lower primary irrigation bottle.

While all of these designs are helpful, it is ultimately up to the surgeon to set parameters which optimize a given machine for a given patient with regard to surge prevention. If mild surge is observed, either the bottle height should be increased or the vacuum level preset and/or flow rate should be decreased. Note that surge is more of a concern when using a standard phaco needle (0.9mm port) with high vacuum and flow settings. It is less of a concern when using the IA handpiece because the smaller 0.3mm port acts as a resistor to flow (see again Figure 1-35a). Similarly, one can decrease the propensity for surge during phaco by utilizing a more resistive needle such as the MicroFlow, MicroSeal, and micro needles (see Figure 1-49).

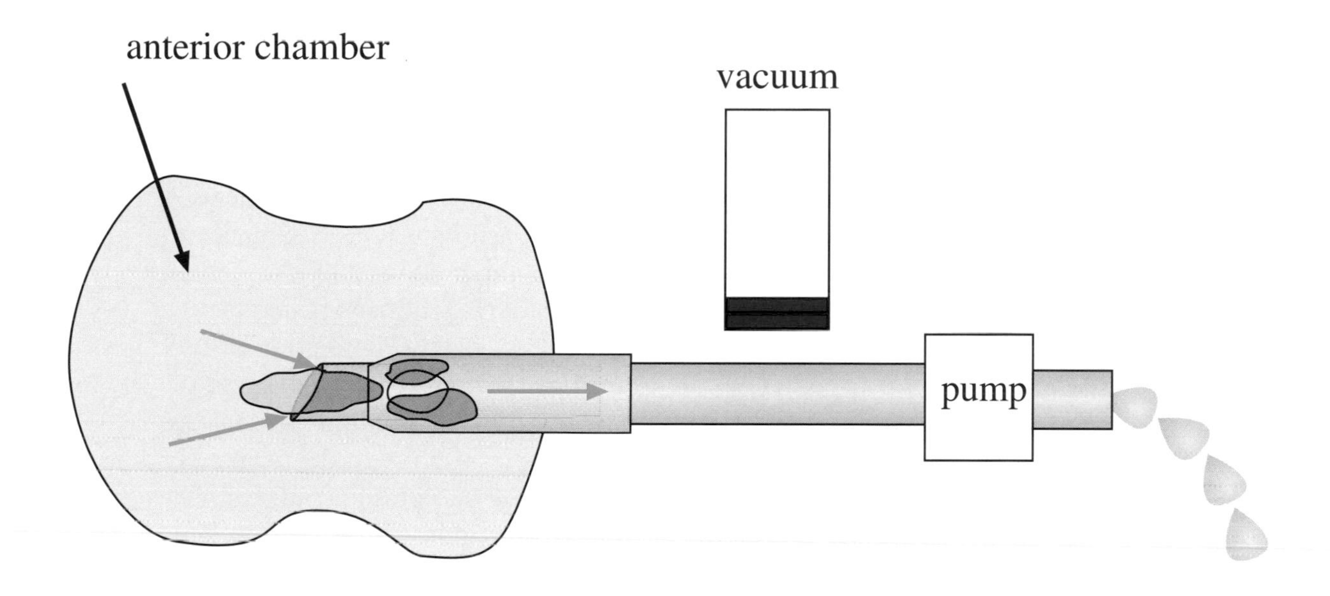
anterior chamber
vacuum
pump

Figure 1-43-2

Surge (continued)

Another way to look at surge is by graphing IOP as shown in Figure 1-43-3. In this setup (utilizing a flow pump machine), the flow rate is 30cc/min, a standard tube set and needle are used, and occlusions are created and released with a stopcock which connects the aspiration line to the phaco handpiece. The bottle height is 30 inches above the test chamber, which was downsized to approximate the volume of the human anterior chamber; this bottle height produces a hydrostatic IOP of 30 inches of water (or approximately 55mm Hg) in foot pedal position 1; recall that these pressures are relative to atmospheric pressure, which is set as zero (either inches H_2O or mm Hg) on the graph. When position 2 is engaged, pump action causes flow through the fluidic circuit which decreases the IOP to a steady state level as long as the pump speed is maintained and the tip is unoccluded (see also Figure 1-5). With sudden occlusion of the aspiration port, the IOP returns to 55mm Hg (see also Figure 1-6, noting the different bottle height and consequently different IOP). However, even though the IOPs are equivalent in segments A and B of the graph, the aspiration line pressure (ALP) is equal to the IOP in segment A, whereas in segment B the ALP reaches the vacuum preset of 50mm Hg vacuum, or -50mm Hg pressure (see also Figure 1-22). Upon occlusion break, surge is produced by the factors discussed in Figure 1-43-1. It is seen in Figure 1-43-3 as a downward deflection of IOP (see shaded area of graph) prior to regaining the IOP associated with steady state flow.

Note the lower diagram of Figure 1-43-3 in which higher vacuum presets are depicted to show the effect on surge of varying this parameter relative to the 50mm Hg preset used in the upper diagram as discussed in the preceding paragraph. A higher vacuum creates a greater change in volume in the aspiration line upon occlusion (eg, larger air bubbles and more tubing constriction) which produces a greater reactive equilibration on occlusion break. As the vacuum preset is increased, the amplitude and time duration of surge proportionately increases (note the progressively larger shaded areas). Correspondingly, the anterior chamber proportionately shallows as surge drives the IOP lower for more time duration. In particular, note that for presets of 160 and 250mm Hg, the surge drives the IOP below zero (atmospheric pressure), with the higher preset value maintaining this pressure for a longer time (larger shaded area below zero pressure). Higher vacuum presets therefore pose a significant danger of anterior chamber collapse. Surgeons must watch for warning signs of momentary anterior chamber shallowing when an occlusion abruptly clears (eg, when chopping or carouseling); if noted, one should compensate by using a higher bottle height, a more restrictive tubing/needle combination, or a lower vacuum preset. Although flow rate could also be lowered, this parameter more directly affects the IOP during steady state unoccluded flow than the amount of transient surge.

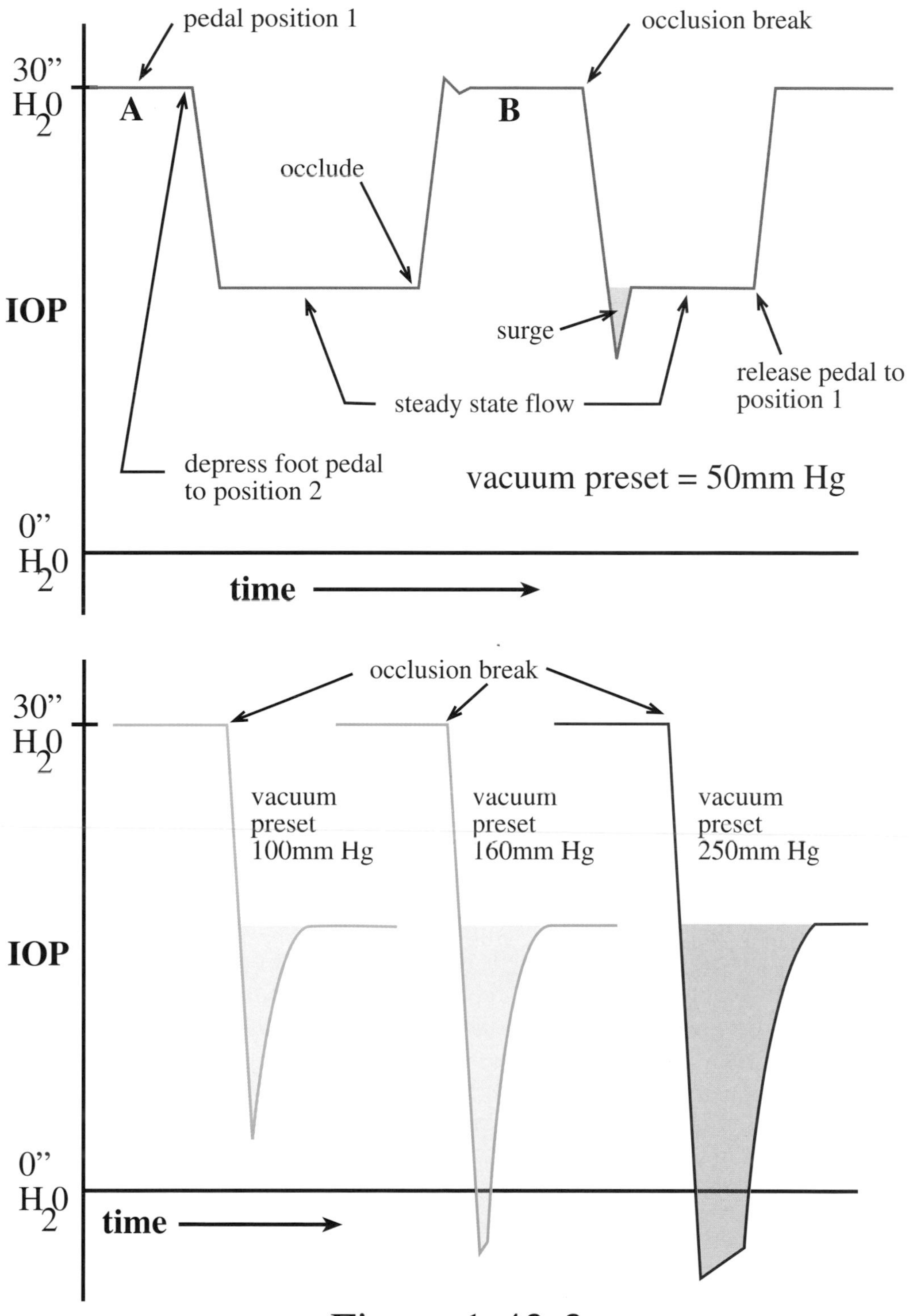
pedal position 1
occlusion break
30"
H_20
A
B
occlude
IOP
surge
steady state flow
release pedal to position 1
depress foot pedal to position 2
vacuum preset = 50mm Hg
0"
H_20
time
occlusion break
30"
H_20
vacuum preset 100mm Hg
vacuum preset 160mm Hg
vacuum preset 250mm Hg
IOP
0"
H_20
time

Figure 1-43-3

Ultrasound Overview

Besides setting fluidic parameters, the surgeon must also decide on the application of ultrasound power, which is produced most often by a piezoelectric crystal oscillating between approximately 25,000 and 60,000 times a second (Hz) for most machines. This frequency is fixed on a given ultrasonic handpiece. This energy is then transmitted along the handpiece into the phaco needle such that the primary oscillation is axial (Figure 1-44). The phaco needle, which is manufactured in various bevel angles as shown, is hollow with the distal opening functioning as the aspiration port. Irrigating fluid flows through two ports located 180° apart on the silicone sleeve. The blue silicone hub threads the sleeve onto the handpiece outer casing. The phaco needle threads directly into the internal mechanism of the handpiece containing the ultrasound generator. Ultrasound power is varied by changing the excitation voltage of the handpiece; increased voltage translates to increased axial stroke length at the phaco needle tip, up to a maximum of about 100 microns (0.004 inches) on most machines. Usually, a maximum ultrasound limit is preset on the machine's front panel, and the surgeon then titrates with linear pedal control the percentage of this preset maximum which is appropriate to a given intraoperative instant. Note that by definition, ultrasonic frequencies are inaudible; the buzzing sound often mistaken for "ultrasound" is actually caused by the sub-harmonic tones of the handpiece and tip.

The actual mechanism of action of ultrasonic phacoemulsification is somewhat controversial. One school of thought centers around the acoustic breakdown of lenticular material as a result of sonic wave propagation through the fluid medium. Another theory concerns the microcavitation bubbles produced at the distal phaco tip; the implosion of these bubbles produces brief instances of intense heat and pressure which are thought to emulsify adjacent lens material. Yet another potential mechanism of action is via the tip's axial oscillations through its stroke length; this resultant jackhammer effect is thought to mechanically break down lens material. This last mechanism also explains the clinical phenomenon of increasing repulsion of free-floating lens material with increasing ultrasound power levels; these levels need appropriate fluidic titration of the attractive parameters of flow and vacuum to counteract this repulsion. Different ultrasonic handpiece frequencies are thought to facilitate different mechanisms of action. A lower frequency (ie, 29kHz) is thought to better facilitate microcavitation bubble formation; furthermore, it is less likely to generate frictional heat. A higher frequency (ie, 40kHz) is thought to cut more smoothly with less repulsion via the mechanical jackhammer effect.

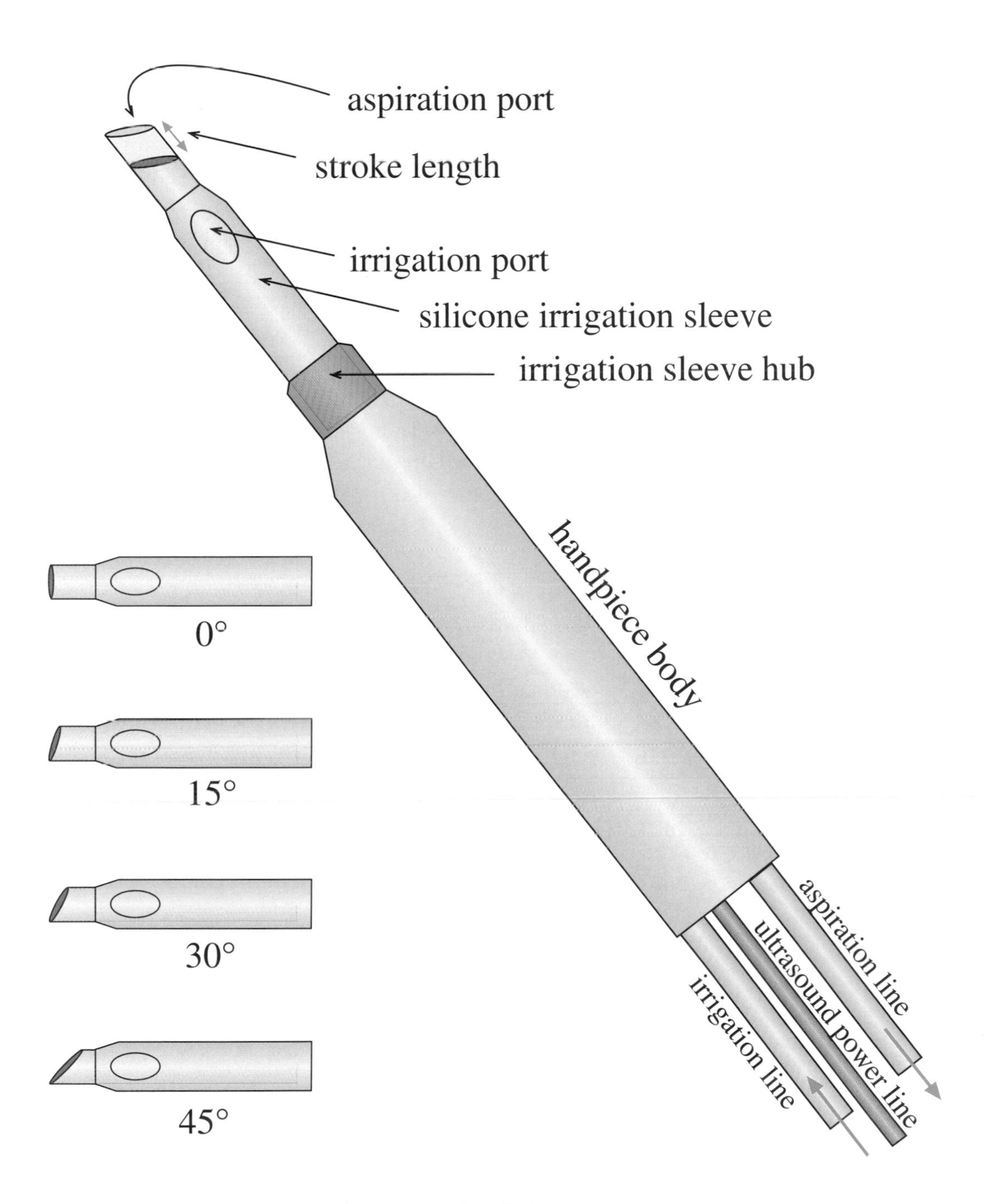
aspiration port
stroke length
irrigation port
silicone irrigation sleeve
irrigation sleeve hub
handpiece body
0°
15°
30°
45°
aspiration line
ultrasound power line
irrigation line

Figure 1-44

Sculpt vs Occlude

By definition, sculpting involves removal of nuclear material by linear excursions of the phaco tip with the aspiration port less than fully occluded (typically one third to one half occluded). It can be seen in Figure 1-45 why sculpting is a less efficient method of phacoemulsification relative to occlusion methods (ie, carouseling fragments into the tip) which typically involve a stationary tip into which nuclear material is fed by vacuum which counteracts the repulsive action of ultrasound. With full occlusion of the tip, vacuum can build up to the maximum preset level; the deformational force provided by the vacuum augments ultrasound in aspirating the occluding fragment into the tip and out of the eye. In contrast, sculpting cannot efficiently build vacuum (due to lack of complete aspiration port occlusion) and therefore relies solely on ultrasonic breakdown of lenticular material as discussed with Figure 1-44. In both illustrations in Figure 1-45, the same ultrasound level is applied for the same amount of time for the same amount of distance (linear excursion). For a given amount of ultrasound power per unit of time, more volume of nuclear material is aspirated with an occlusion method because the entire volume of the needle (as defined by its inner diameter) is utilized as vacuum augments the emulsifying power of the applied ultrasound.

In addition to overcoming the repulsive action of the ultrasonic needle, vacuum also functions to overcome any resistance caused by the possibly large aspirated nuclear plug so that it does not clog the handpiece or aspiration line. Flow functions to drive along nuclear material that was emulsified into smaller particles; it also continues to feed the nuclear fragment into the tip during the intermittent moments when ultrasound breaks down the material so that incomplete occlusion compromises the holding efficiency of vacuum. The combination of attracting fragments to the tip along with feeding them into the tip against the repulsive action of ultrasound using the combined fluidic parameters of vacuum and flow is known as **followability**.

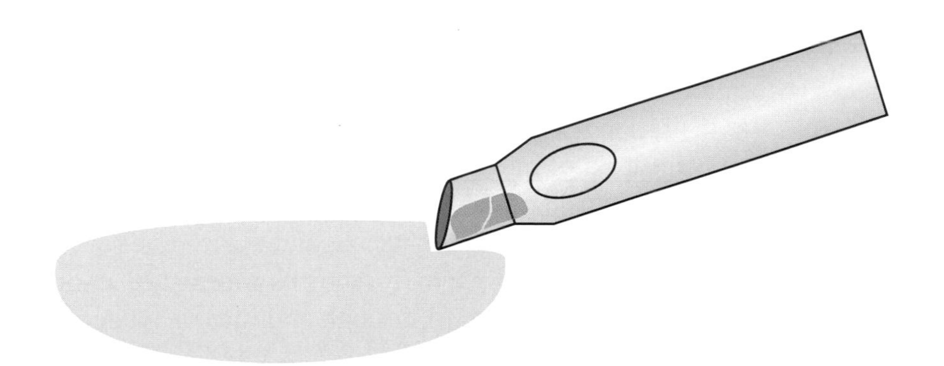

Sculpting

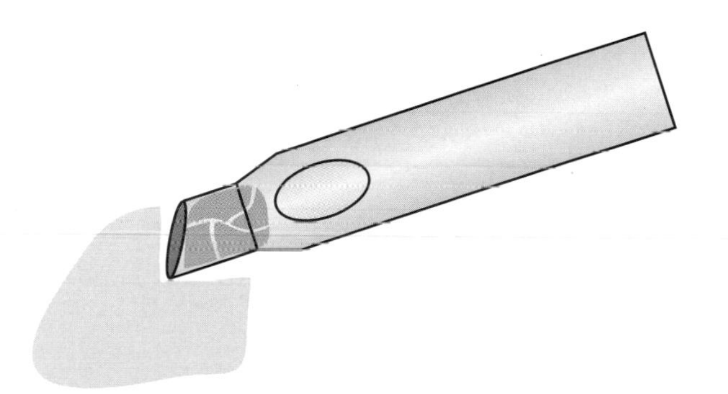

Occlusion

Figure 1-45

Ultrasound: Gel vs Solid

At one extreme, occlusion mode operates to aspirate (remove) aqueous (low viscosity) without the need for any ultrasound power. Similarly, a somewhat higher viscosity gel, such as a viscoelastic, can also be removed by vacuum and flow alone. A still higher viscosity material, such as the semi-solid gel state epinucleus or a softer nucleus, can be aspirated by a still higher vacuum/flow, although the application of **mild** amounts of ultrasound permit aspiration of the material with lower, safer fluidic parameters by aiding in the deformation of the material (Figures 1-46 and 2-12) so that it can extrude through the aspiration port and into the phaco needle and aspiration line. Denser nuclear material is less gel-like and more crystalline, it requires **moderate** amounts of ultrasound in order to trim the occluded portion to fit through and into the phaco tip (see Figure 1-46); correspondingly higher fluidic parameters are needed to overcome the added repulsive force as ultrasound power is increased (see Figure 2-12). Indeed, when encountering difficulty with followability of these dense fragments during carouseling (ie, fragment chattering against the tip rather than being aspirated into it), the parameters of flow and/or vacuum must be increased rather than increasing ultrasound power. These dense nuclei typically require **high** levels of ultrasound when using a less efficient sculpting method; however, sculpting requires only low vacuum and low to moderate flow since the nucleus is typically held stationary in situ by the intact nuclear body and therefore cannot be repulsed by the ultrasonic tip.

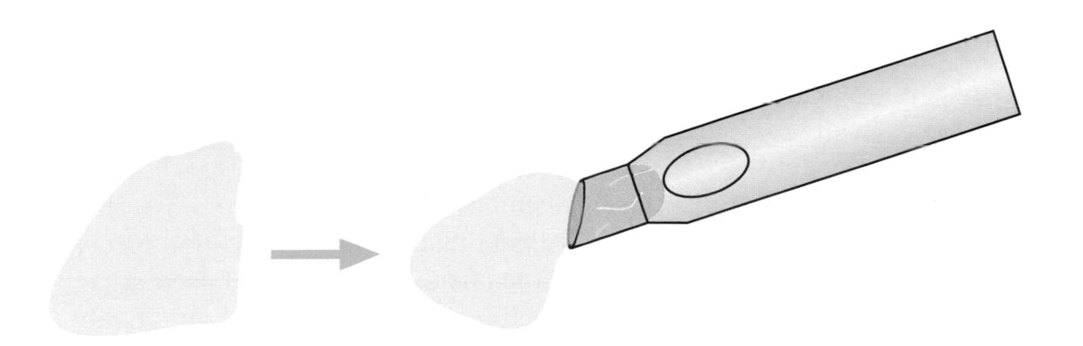

semi-solid gel soft nucleus

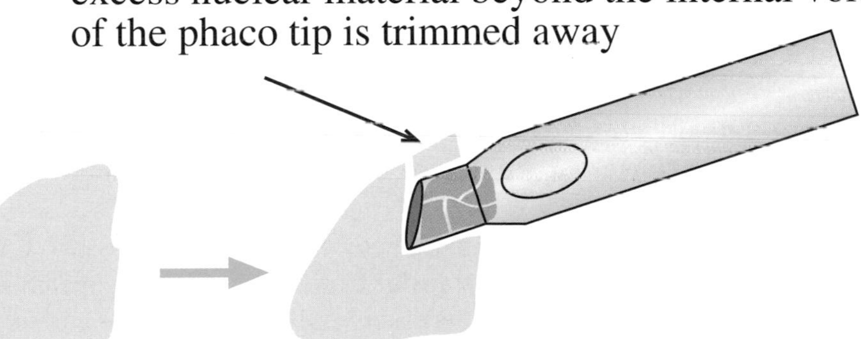
excess nuclear material beyond the internal volume
of the phaco tip is trimmed away

hard crystalline nucleus

Figure 1-46

Phaco Tip Angles 1

Ultrasonic phaco needles are available in a variety of configurations. One basic design parameter is the distal bevel angle, which is most commonly 0°, 15°, 30°, or 45° as shown in Figures 1-44 and 1-47a. The sharper 45° angle is thought to carve dense nuclei more efficiently to the extent that the jackhammer mechanism of action is valid, whereas the 0° tip would be more efficient to the extent that the microcavitation theory is valid (the 0° tip has more frontal surface area perpendicular to the axis of oscillation, thereby producing more cavitation bubbles). In practice, it is difficult to quantitatively compare these efficiencies on a standard density nucleus.

Another traditional teaching regarding tip angulation is that a 0° tip occludes more readily than a 45° tip; this observation is generally inaccurate. A tip occludes readily when the surface to be occluded is parallel to the needle bevel; the surface can and should be manipulated as necessary to achieve this configuration (note Figure 1-47a, which illustrates impaling a heminucleus with mild ultrasound during a stop and chop maneuver). Note that in the upper pair of figures that only a short excursion of the tip into the nucleus is necessary to completely occlude the aspiration port in order to allow vacuum to grip and control the heminucleus in preparation for chopping. Note that in the bottom pair of figures the tip must be buried much deeper prior to complete occlusion of the aspiration port; furthermore, the silicone irrigating sleeve limits how deeply the tip may be embedded, further compromising the effectiveness of the vacuum seal in the lower pair of figures (see also Figure 2-14-1b). Therefore, the bevel angle is arbitrary with regard to ease of occlusion in that the surface to be engaged can easily be manipulated intraoperatively so that its surface is parallel to a given needle's bevel; alternatively, the phaco handpiece can be rotated so that the bevel is parallel to a given surface.

As discussed previously in the book, complete occlusion is necessary for effectively building gripping power and vacuum transfer from the pump to an occluding fragment. However, such gripping is clinically necessary only when dealing with a significantly large fragment which requires further subdivision (ie, chopping) or mobilization centrally for safer emulsification/aspiration further away from the capsule. The only manner in which a 0° tip occludes more easily than a more beveled tip is when dealing with a smaller fragment whose surface area is just enough to cover and occlude the aspiration port of the former, but not the latter; the aspiration port's surface area is greater in a more beveled phaco tip (see Figure 1-48). However, this is a clinically insignificant situation in that such smaller fragments are usually readily attracted centrally to the aspiration port along flow currents whereupon they are aspirated through the larger aspiration port of a larger beveled tip with minimal ultrasound. Using a 0° tip would simply require slightly more ultrasound to deform the fragment to fit into the slightly smaller port (see Figure 1-46).

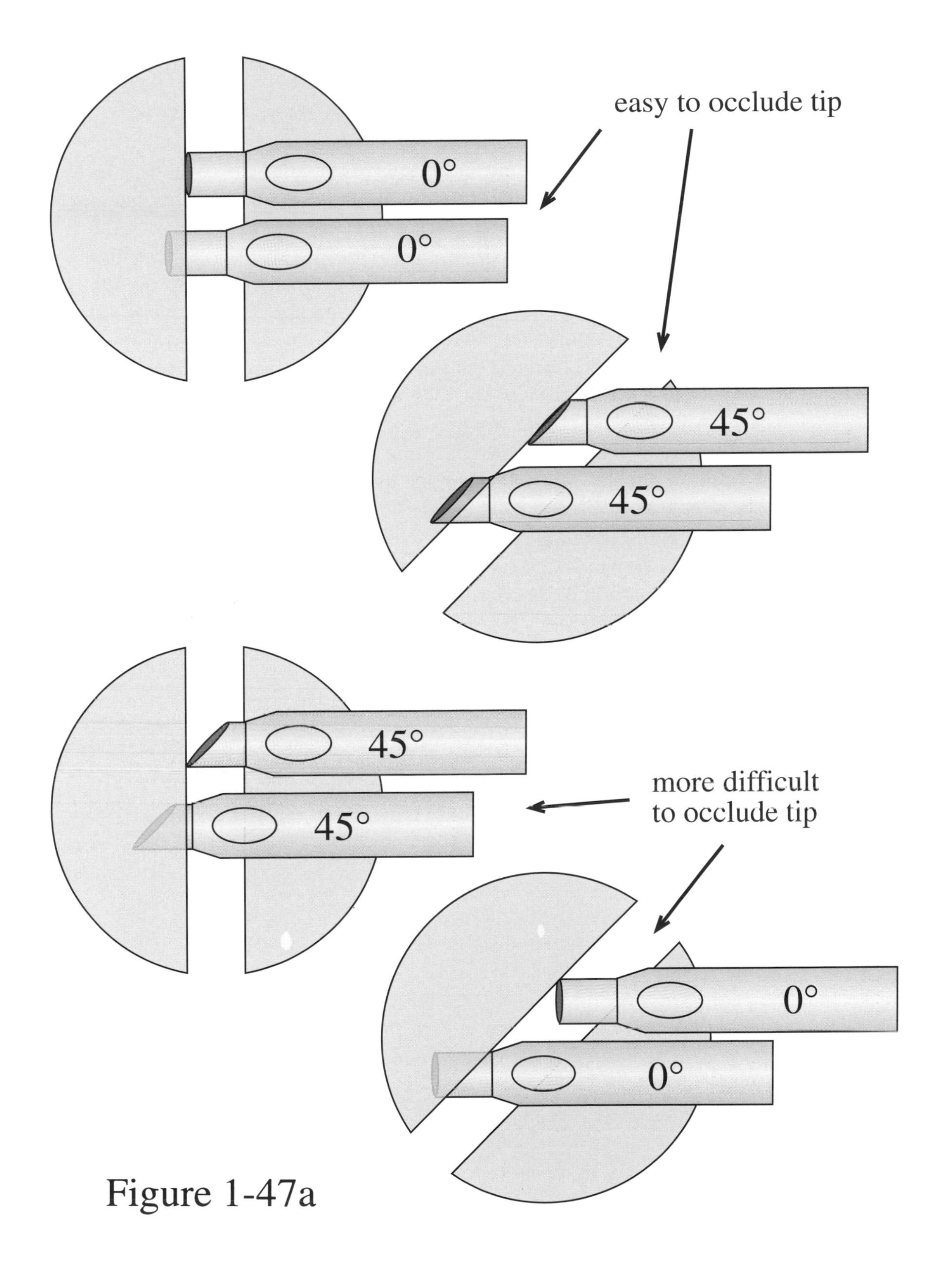
easy to occlude tip
0°
0°
45°
45°
45°
45°
more difficult
to occlude tip
0°
0°

Figure 1-47a

Phaco Tip Angles 2

Theoretically, a 0° tip is easier to occlude because of its smaller surface area relative to a more beveled tip (see Appendix B). Correspondingly, the smaller perimeter (circumference) of the 0° aspiration port is more likely to seal effectively relative to the longer perimeter of a more beveled needle. However, these theoretical considerations have less clinical relevance when carouseling a sufficiently sized fragment into the tip, or when embedding the tip into a fragment whose surface is parallel to the tip's bevel (see discussion of Figure 1-47a). Another relevant clinical example of the arbitrary significance of bevel angle to ease of occlusion is the initial step in the original phaco chop technique. Figure 1-47b-2 illustrates how a 0° tip does occlude during this initial impaling of the nucleus, albeit just barely. The 45° tip in its conventional bevel-up position in Figure 1-47b-1 is seen to occlude poorly in this maneuver relative to the 0° tip. However, by simply rotating the 45° tip by 180° so that its bevel is down (ie, parallel to the surface to be occluded), as in Figure 1-47b-3, the 45° tip is seen to occlude more effectively than the 0° tip. Recall that the silicone sleeve is a physical barrier to further embedding of the tip than is shown in these illustrations; therefore, it is imperative to rotate the bevel as necessary to optimize occlusion when burying the tip in a larger fragment prior to chopping or mobilization.

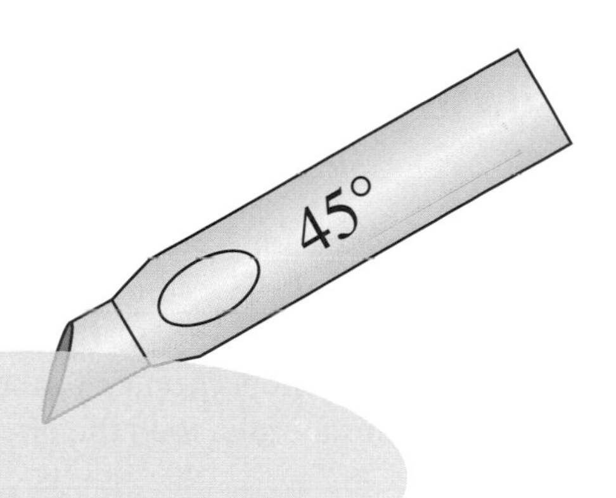

Figure 1-47b-1

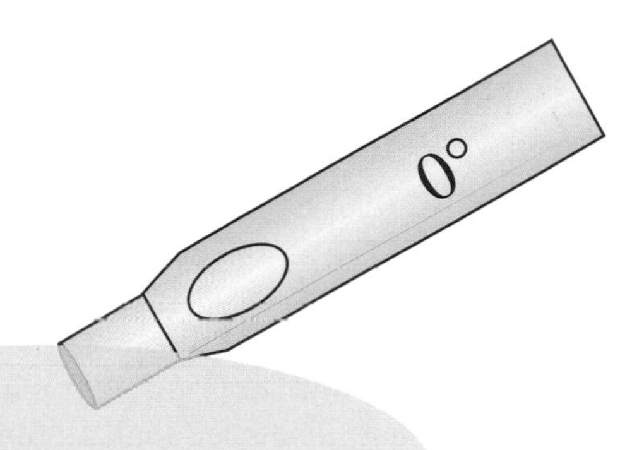

Figure 1-47b-2

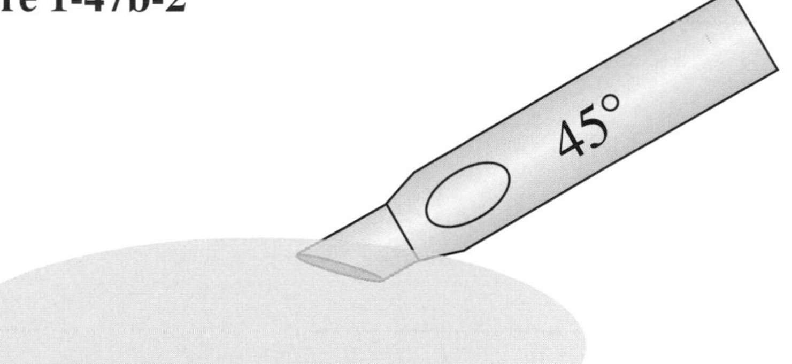

Figure 1-47b-3

Figure 1-47b

Tip Angles and Aspiration Port Surface Area

A 0° tip has the minimum possible surface area for its aspiration port in that the uniform diameter of the circular port is simply that of the cylindrical needle's internal diameter (I.D.). An angled bevel has an oval-shaped aspiration port with its short radius being the same as a 0° tip, but having a longer radius proportionate to the amount of the bevel (Figure 1-48); this oval shape has a larger surface area than the circular shape (see Appendix B).

The holding power of a more beveled tip is greater than that of a less beveled tip because the vacuum (negative pressure) of the pump is exerted over a larger surface area. Pressure is defined as the force per unit area, which is often expressed in units of pounds per square inch (**PSI**). The units of mm Hg have an inherent surface area by definition (see Appendix A), but because the unit of surface area is not expressed, it will be useful to convert mm Hg to PSI for this illustration. Atmospheric pressure (at sea level) is defined as either 760mm Hg or 14.7 PSI, which gives a conversion factor of .019 PSI/mm Hg. Using the derived surface areas of a 0° tip and a 45° tip, assuming a standard I.D. of 0.9mm = .035 inches, the corresponding holding forces per unit vacuum (100mm Hg in this case) can be computed as shown in Appendix B, with the greater bevel having a significantly greater (42%) gripping force. Although this concept is rigorously mathematically proven here, one need look no further than many vacuum cleaner commercials for a clear graphic example in which a small canister model is shown to have enough power to pick up a heavy bowling ball; the key to this performance is linking the small vacuum nozzle to the large bowling ball via a funnel which spreads the vacuum over the large surface area of the ball's hemisphere, thereby providing ample force for lift.

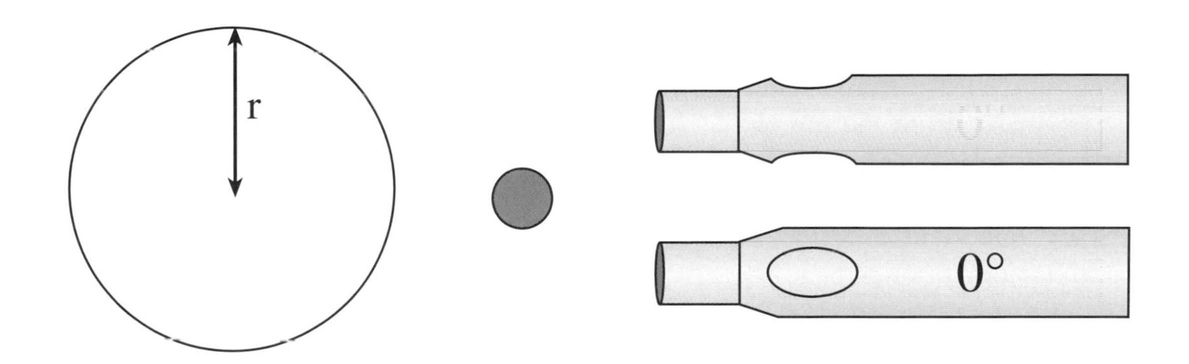

holding force per 100mm Hg = .0019 lbs.

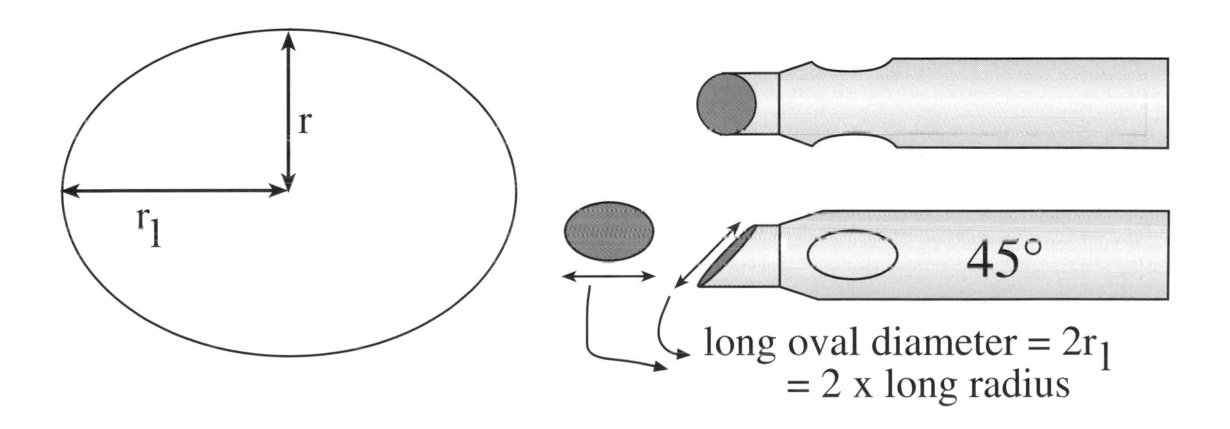

holding force per 100mm Hg = .0027 lbs.

Figure 1-48

Phaco Needle Dimensions

The various inner and outer diameter measurements of a phaco needle affect both its fluidic as well as mechanical performance. The original standard 19-gauge phaco needle is shown toward the top of Figure 1-49 as a reference. By comparison, the 21-gauge micro needle is seen to have both a smaller inner as well as outer diameter. The smaller outer diameter allows it to be used through a smaller incision; this will be an increasingly important attribute as advances in intraocular lens implant technology allow implantation through smaller incisions. The smaller inner diameter works as a fluidic resistor when the tip is not occluded, decreasing the flow rate for a given pump setting relative to a standard needle, especially with vacuum pumps (see Figure 1-35a for discussion of fluidic resistors). When the tip is occluded, the smaller inner tip diameter provides less holding power for a given pump vacuum level because it has less aspiration port surface area relative to a standard tip (see discussion with Figure 1-48). Furthermore, even when using an efficient occlusion mode of phaco, less volume of nuclear material is removed (per unit time and level of ultrasound relative to a standard needle) simply because of the smaller volume that the 21-gauge needle can accommodate.

The MicroFlow and MicroSeal needles have an inner tip diameter identical to that of a standard needle; therefore, they will both have the same holding force for a given pump vacuum level when the tip is occluded. However, the smaller shaft inner diameter provides similar fluidic resistance to that of the micro needle. This is an advantage (especially with vacuum pumps) for the surgeon who desires a high vacuum level for nuclear manipulation and chopping but does not want the attendant dangerously high flow levels which would be present with an unoccluded standard tip. Another advantage of maintaining a standard needle's inner tip diameter is that more volume of nuclear material can be engaged and aspirated per unit time of ultrasound power application relative to a micro needle or any other design with a smaller inner tip diameter; this statement is valid in proportion to the length of the larger inner distal tip diameter prior to the smaller shaft inner diameter.

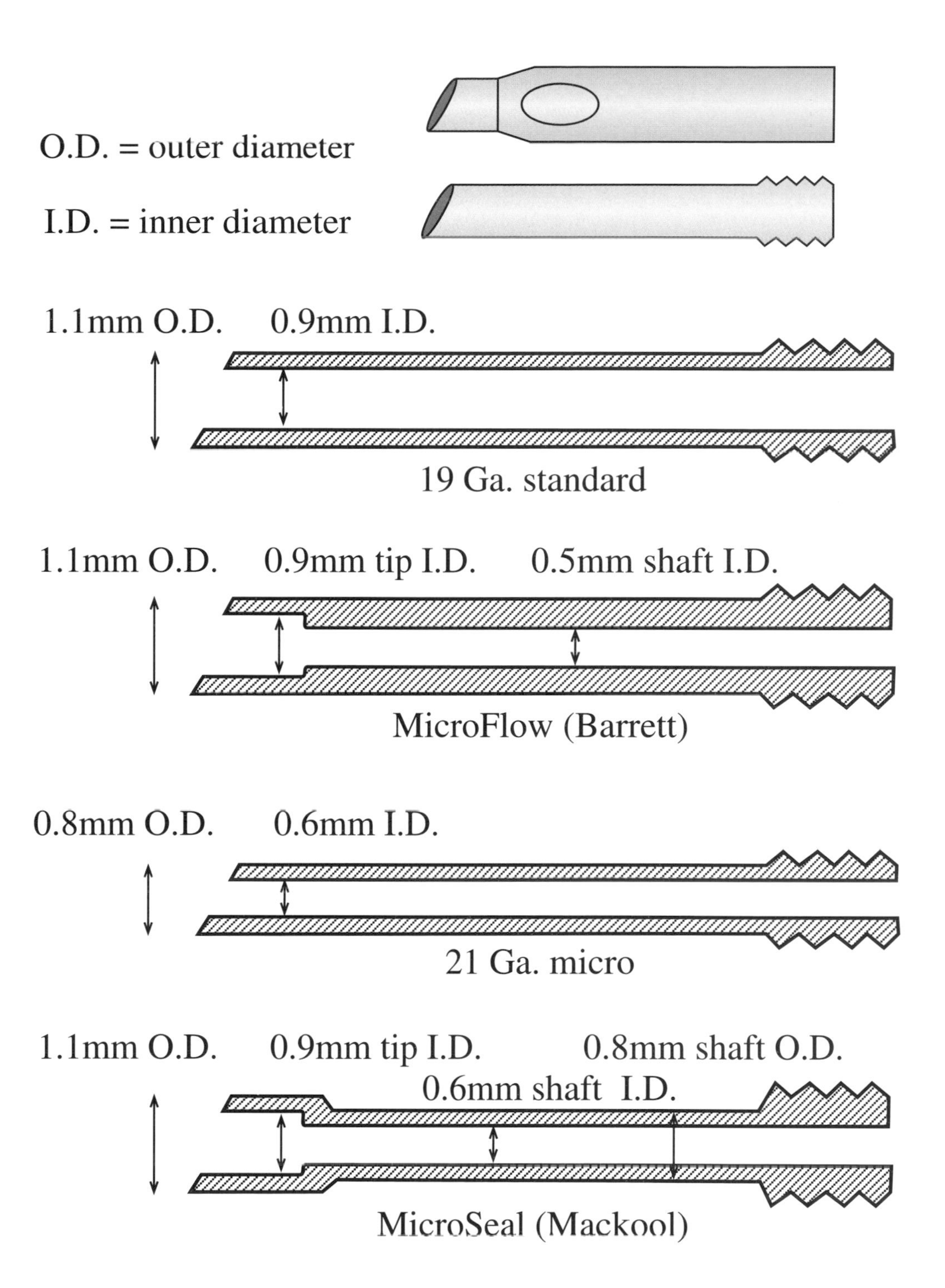
O.D. = outer diameter
I.D. = inner diameter
1.1mm O.D.
0.9mm I.D.
19 Ga. standard
1.1mm O.D.
0.9mm tip I.D.
0.5mm shaft I.D.
MicroFlow (Barrett)
0.8mm O.D.
0.6mm I.D.
21 Ga. micro
1.1mm O.D.
0.9mm tip I.D.
0.8mm shaft O.D.
0.6mm shaft I.D.
MicroSeal (Mackool)

Figure 1-49

Phaco Needle Shapes

The primary direction of ultrasonic oscillation is axial, as shown in Figures 1-44 and 1-50 by the green arrows. Cavitation is usually limited to the area in front of the ring of metal at the end of the needle; the surface of this ring is roughly perpendicular to the long axis of the needle (see top illustration in Figure 1-50). Cavitation bubbles are formed when this surface pulls back from its distal excursion during each oscillation as a vacuum is created by the rapidly retreating surface; implosion of these bubbles is thought to be an important component of ultrasonic breakdown of lenticular material. Note that no cavitation is produced along the external shaft of the standard needle, which is oriented parallel to the direction of vibration and therefore does not encounter the distal ring's resistance to travel within the fluid medium (see dashed green arrow); similarly, no cavitation is produced within the lumen of the standard needle (dashed green arrow).

Cavitation can be augmented by modifications to the needle shape. The distal bend in the Kelman needle adds a nonaxial vibration (red arrow) to the primary oscillation which increases total cavitation at the tip relative to a standard tip with the same amount of ultrasound energy input. The nonaxial vibration further augments the axial vibration by producing an elliptical motion at the cutting tip which enhances mechanical breakdown of nuclear material. By incorporating additional angled surfaces which are roughly perpendicular to the long axis of the needle, the Seibel tip produces additional cavitation along the flat surfaces of the needle which are directed toward the distal tip as shown by the blue arrows. The MicroFlow and MicroSeal needles have an internal ring surface within the tip caused by the decrease from the distal tip's inner diameter to the shaft inner diameter (see Figure 1-49); this inner ring surface is perpendicular to the axial direction of the needle and therefore produces additional cavitation. The Cobra tip has a similar design which produces additional internal cavitation.

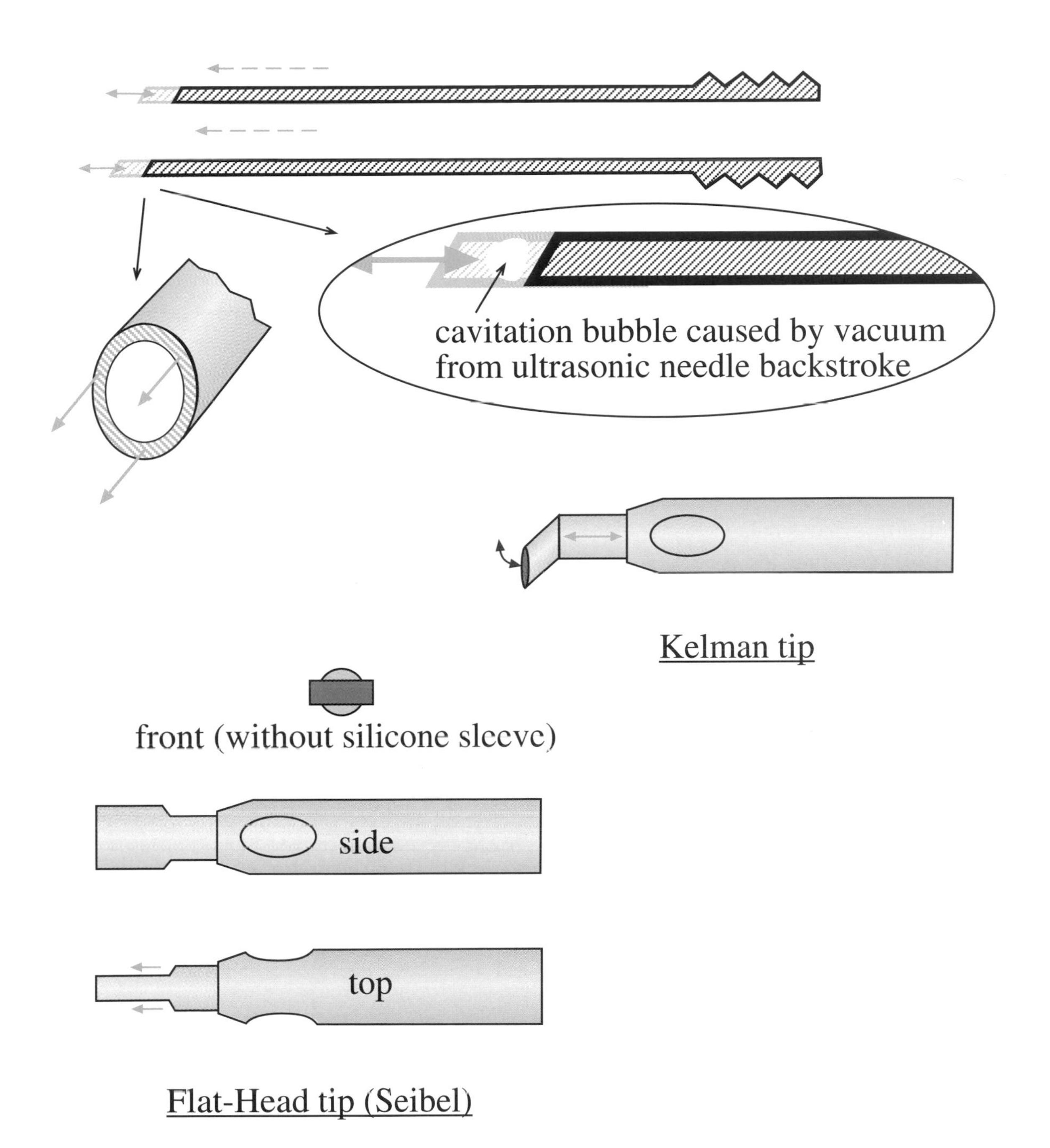
cavitation bubble caused by vacuum
from ultrasonic needle backstroke
Kelman tip
front (without silicone slccvc)
side
top
Flat-Head tip (Seibel)

Figure 1-50

Thermal Implications of Ultrasound

With the needle vibrating at 20 to 60kHz, potentially dangerous heat can build up from two sources in direct proportion to the ultrasound power (stroke length) and the duration for which it is applied. First, friction from the needle shaft's oscillation in aqueous as well as distal cavitation can produce increased temperature, usually at a slow to moderate rate. Second, friction at the point of the silicone sleeve compression by the surgical incision can sometimes rapidly increase temperature to the level of protein denaturation, resulting in a wound burn. Both sources can be influenced by surgical technique. For example, one should avoid maintaining high ultrasound power for long continuous intervals. Unnecessary wound pressure can be prevented by avoiding handpiece positions which result in lifting or extreme angulations at this location.

Fluidic parameters can influence heat production by affecting flow rate; less heat is produced to the extent that more anterior chamber fluid exchange and more fluid flow around the needle shaft provides cooling. Recall that aspiration line fluid becomes more viscous as viscoelastic and dense nuclear emulsate are aspirated, and that flow is consequently diminished, especially with vacuum pumps (see Figure 1-40b); machine parameters should be adjusted accordingly. One should especially avoid maintaining high ultrasound power while the aspiration port is occluded and thus prohibits any cooling flow; however, this caveat does not preclude the use of occlusion phaco methods (see Figure 1-45). For example, some chopping maneuvers require the aspiration port to be fully occluded to effectively build vacuum and gripping power (see Figure 1-25), but this can be accomplished by a brief application of moderate ultrasound to embed the tip, followed quickly by a return to pedal position 2 to titrate vacuum appropriately without any further ultrasound until the chop is completed. Furthermore, occlusion methods of carouseling do not necessarily produce excessive heat even though ultrasound power is maintained for mildly to moderately sustained periods; the reason is two-fold. First, only moderate levels of ultrasound are required because of the greater efficiency of occlusion methods (see Figure 1-46). Second, full occlusion is rapidly and intermittently interspersed with moments of flow which facilitate cooling as well as removal of emulsified material (see Figure 1-45).

Different needle designs have been developed to decrease the likelihood of wound burns as the silicone sleeve is pressed against the vibrating needle by the surgical incision (Figure 1-51). Dr. Graham Barrett designed the MicroFlow needle to incorporate longitudinal grooves along the outer shaft which continue to channel cooling irrigation fluid even when the silicone sleeve is compressed against the outer needle surface. Surgical Design's silicone sleeve applies this principle in reverse, with the sleeve itself having the grooves which maintain irrigation flow even with compression against the needle. Dr. Richard Mackool developed the MicroSeal needle (as well as the similarly designed Mackool System needle) which maintains flow via a rigid polyimide (plastic) sleeve between the needle and the compressed sleeve; the polyimide additionally provides heat insulation via its own material properties.

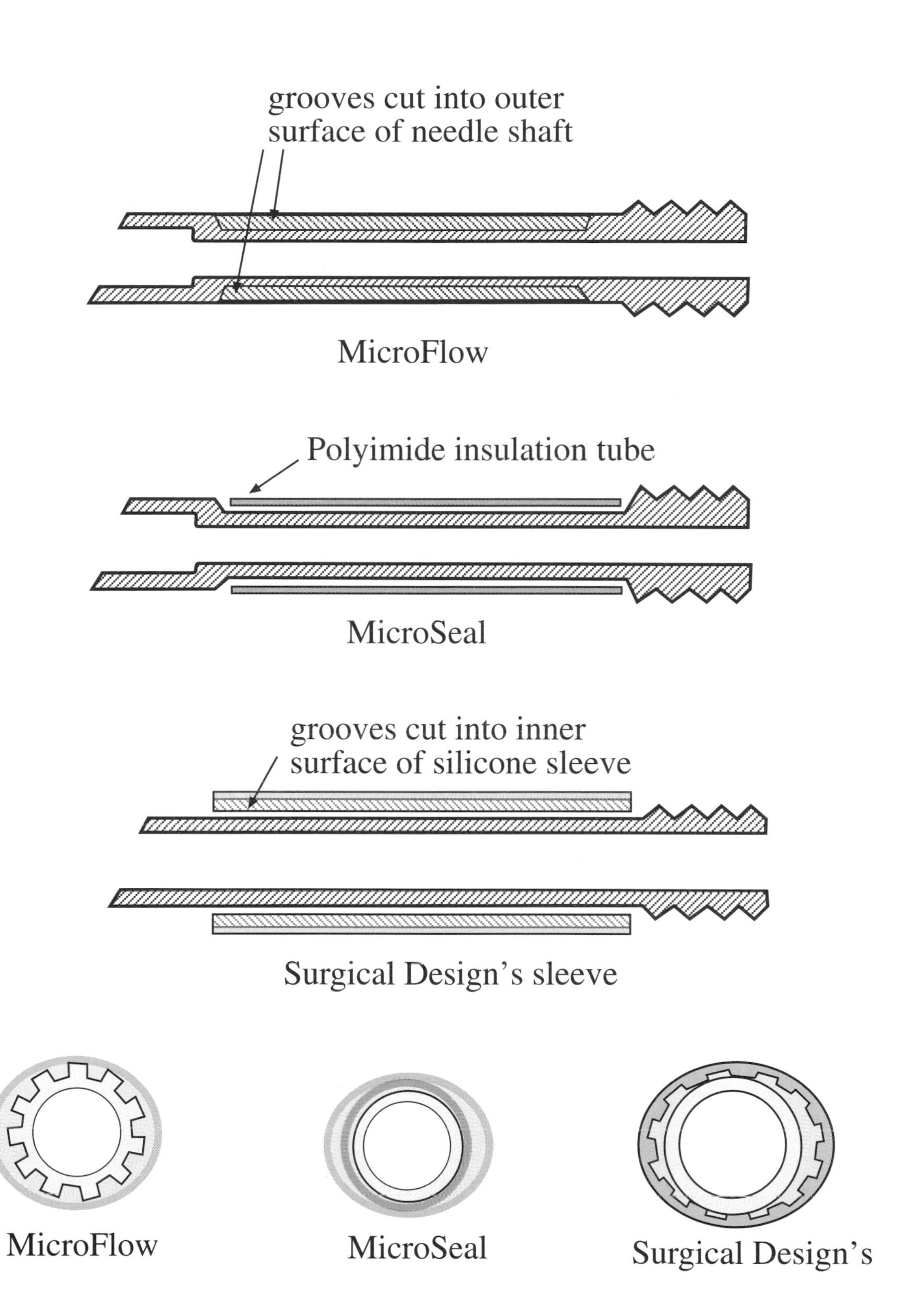
grooves cut into outer
surface of needle shaft
MicroFlow
Polyimide insulation tube
MicroSeal
grooves cut into inner
surface of silicone sleeve
Surgical Design's sleeve
MicroFlow
MicroSeal
Surgical Design's

Figure 1-51

Irrigation and Aspiration Tips

After the ultrasonic handpiece and tip are used to remove the cataractous nucleus and epinucleus, the surgeon usually changes to the slimmer IA handpiece and tip as illustrated in Figure 1-52. The IA tip is ideal for removing the gelatinous or diaphanous cortex as well as any residual viscoelastic. As opposed to the denser and often more crystalline nuclear material, the cortex and any viscoelastic do not require ultrasonic breakdown in order to be aspirated (see also Figure 1-46). The standard IA tip's aspiration port size (diameter) is 0.3mm, which is much better suited than the larger phaco aspiration port to being occluded by the often thin layer of cortex. Even though the high resistance IA port can produce significant vacuum without occlusion (especially with higher flow rates, as in Figure 1-35b), full occlusion allows full transfer of the pump's vacuum to the occluding cortex (see Figure 1-25).

The irrigation sleeve is similar to that of the phaco handpiece, although it is available in metal as well as silicone. The IA tip differs from the phaco tip as illustrated, being smooth and rounded with a single aspiration port usually located on the side of the tip, not at the end. The sleeve may be turned to orient the irrigation ports in any direction, but it is usually most efficient to place them as shown, each 90° away from the aspiration port. If one irrigation port was in the same orientation as the aspiration port, the irrigating fluid would tend to push away the material to be aspirated.

In addition to the straight tip, 45°, 90°, and 180° tips are available to allow more versatility in accessing difficult areas of cortex (ie, sub-incisionally). One handpiece design allows the tips to be quickly interchanged using an O-ring/twist-lock attachment.

A fascinating IA tip has been developed by Ed Zaleski of AMO; a similar version of the tip was conceived by Dr. Charles Kelman and is under development by Alcon. The tip is made of silicone instead of metal, and its transparency allows visualization of cortex as aspiration is taking place, thus providing valuable additional visual feedback, especially at times when the aspiration port is not optimally visible. However, the most remarkable advantage of the design is that it allows you to readily transform the tip from a straight configuration through an entire range of curved configurations by sliding the sleeve controller as illustrated in Figure 1-52.

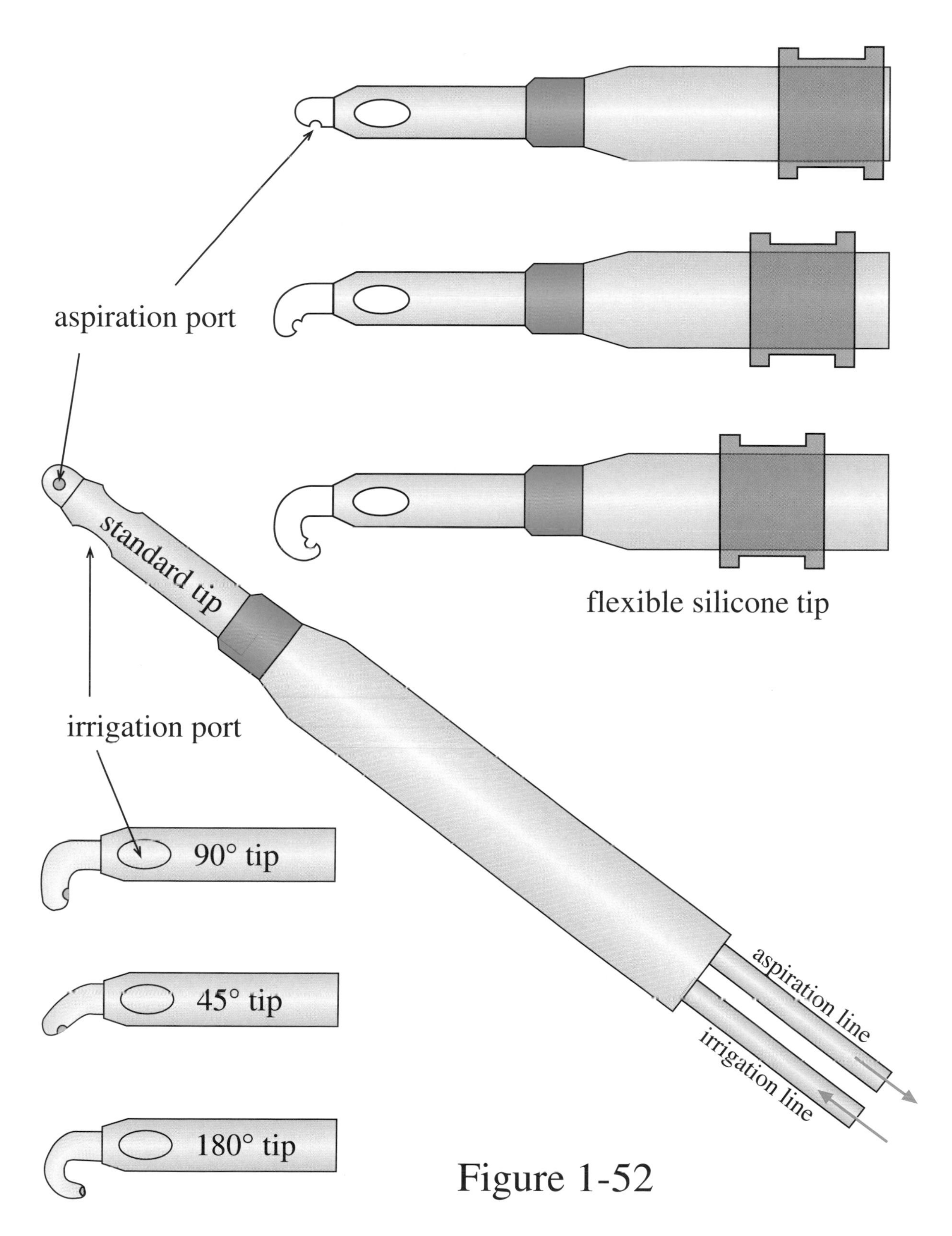
aspiration port
standard tip
flexible silicone tip
irrigation port
90° tip
45° tip
180° tip
aspiration line
irrigation line

Figure 1-52

Individual Machine Characteristics

Know your machine! Although this book describes the fundamental characteristics shared by many phaco machines, each particular company's machine has unique features. You must be aware of all features of a given machine to maximize your surgical options and to take full advantage of the machine's capabilities. Company representatives can often provide very comprehensive information on their products. The machine's operational manual is also a valuable resource and should be considered required reading.

All machines give audible feedback during their operation; it is important to understand and be aware of these sounds during surgery. Many sounds are secondary to the mechanical operation necessary for a given function. For example, the sound of releasing compressed gas is present on venturi machines in position 2 or 3; furthermore, it is noted to become more intense as vacuum is increased by progressively depressing the foot pedal with linear control. A peristaltic pump will hum as its electric motor turns the pump head. A faster pump flow results in a louder and/or higher pitched sound as the pump head turns faster. Occlusion during aspiration on a peristaltic machine will often give an intermittently irregular cessation to the humming sound as the machine vents to keep the vacuum at the level selected by the combination of foot pedal position and vacuum preset; a surgeon hearing this noise, for example, might elect to increase the vacuum preset if the pedal was fully depressed and cortical/epinuclear material was engaged but not aspirating. Another example would be if you hear the machine venting while engaged in position 2 even though the aspiration port is not visibly occluded; this usually indicates an obstruction somewhere in the aspiration line which will require checking the line for kinks and perhaps trying to dislodge any occult material by refluxing into a test chamber. Entering irrigation mode almost always produces a metallic click as the plunger that was pinching the irrigation tubing is snapped into the open position. Engaging ultrasound power always produces a buzzing sound, the intensity of which increases with increasing power. Recall that this sound is not ultrasound but rather the sub-harmonic tones of the handpiece and needle; the increasing intensity is secondary to the increasing amplitude of the stroke length caused by increasing power. Tactile feedback during ultrasound power application is present in the form of subtle vibration in the handpiece, which also increases with increasing power.

Many machines supplement their audible mechanical feedback with various electronic sounds. A particular machine may have a beeping sound for IA, which increases in frequency as vacuum increases. It may utilize a steady tone to designate ultrasound application. Some machines produce a tone to indicate occlusion of the aspiration port, often sensed by the machine's actual vacuum reaching the preset limit. Some machines allow user modification of these electronic feedbacks with regard to type and intensity of sound for a given function.

The foot pedal offers valuable tactile feedback. Some simple mechanical units feel identical in both phaco and IA modes, giving detents between positions 1, 2, and 3. More elaborate electromechanical models override a detent in IA mode so as to combine positions 2 and 3 into a single larger pedal excursion in position 2. Some models may not have any detents; some of these may have uniform resistance for their entire travel, while others may have progressively increasing resistance with increasing depression of the pedal. Several AMO units allow the surgeon to opt for the pedal to vibrate in between positions. You should note the actual machine readings for a given pedal position by putting a test chamber on the phaco handpiece while observing the machine panel during pedal operation. For example, with a phaco preset maximum of 100% and linear pedal control, one machine might yield 50% actual power with the pedal depressed halfway into position 3, whereas another machine might produce 75% actual power with its pedal halfway into position 3. Linearity and responsiveness of the foot pedal during vacuum and flow changes may also be observed in the same manner.

When reading your machine's manual, pay attention to the section on setup. It is the surgeon's responsibility to know more about the equipment than anyone else in the operating room. If your regular scrub technician is unavailable one day, your patients must not be compromised because of a substitute scrub tech's lack of familiarity with your machine. Knowledge of proper machine setup also proves invaluable when intraoperative troubleshooting is necessary. Many problems may be traced to kinked or improperly connected tubing.

SECTION TWO

Logic of Setting Machine Parameters

Overview of Logic Behind Setting Machine Parameters

In order to appropriately adjust the machine parameters for various stages of surgery, it is necessary to analyze the function of those parameters for a given stage. For example, sculpting requires proper titration of ultrasound power so that the phaco needle carves the nucleus without excessively displacing it and stressing zonules. Furthermore, sculpting requires only enough flow to clear the anterior chamber of the emulsate produced by ultrasound as well as sufficient flow to cool the phaco tip. There is little need for vacuum during sculpting; there are not yet any fragments which need to be occluded and gripped. Furthermore, vacuum is not needed to counteract the repulsive action of ultrasound since the nucleus is held stationary by the capsule, zonules, and its intact structure at this point. However, a modest level of vacuum does help to prevent clogging of the aspiration line when sculpting dense cataracts.

Once the nucleus is debulked or grooved by sculpting, it then needs manipulation such as rotation or cracking. These maneuvers should be performed in pedal position 1 so that the chamber will be pressurized but without any pump action which might inadvertently aspirate unwanted material. Once the nucleus is debulked or cracked into fragments, machine parameters need to adapt to the needs of emulsifying these fragments. Ultrasound power requirements are lower at this stage relative to sculpting because of the increased efficiency of phacoaspiration with complete or almost complete tip occlusion (see Figure 1-45). However, flow rate and vacuum usually must be increased from their sculpting levels in order to overcome the repulsive action of ultrasound at the axially vibrating needle tip. These parameters should ideally be linearly titrated intraoperatively to a given ultrasound level and nuclear density. This level of control has only recently been available to the surgeon with the advent of Dual Linear pedal control as previously described.

Chopping maneuvers often require further manipulation of parameters. The actual chop may require only moderate vacuum because the nucleus is mechanically fixated between the phaco tip and the chopper. However, higher vacuum levels can be used advantageously to grip and manipulate the nucleus. For example, the gripped nucleus can be displaced so that the chopper is more centrally located when engaging the nuclear periphery. This maneuver is especially effective if the nucleus was previously grooved and hemisected as has been described by Drs. Paul Koch and Ronald Stasiuk (see Figure 2-13). Higher vacuum levels are also useful when gripping and manipulating quadrants in preparation for emulsification. The higher vacuum levels require appropriate caution in order to prevent surge problems; Figures 1-43-1 through 1-43-3 address this issue.

Although specific parameter values will be given in this section of the book, it is crucial to remember that these are only a baseline guide. Recall from Section One that the panel setting on a given phaco machine can produce variable results depending on numerous factors. For example, vacuum degrades in the aspiration line when the aspiration port is not completely occluded (see Figure 1-39); therefore, for a given panel preset vacuum level, the actual attractive force at the phaco tip will vary according to the aspiration line length as well as the degree to which the aspiration port is occluded. Similarly, flow can be set directly on a flow pump (by choosing a panel preset pump speed) or indirectly with a vacuum pump (by choosing a panel preset vacuum level); however, the actual flow through the aspiration port will vary according to the degree of aspiration port occlusion as well as the size of the aspiration port and the inner diameter of the phaco needle (see Figures 1-10, 1-24, and 1-35a). Actual flow will also vary intraoperatively secondary to changing viscosity in the aspiration line as variable amounts of viscoelastic and emulsified nucleus are aspirated; recall that vacuum pumps are more sensitive to fluidic resistance (see Figure 1-35a). Because actual values of flow and vacuum can therefore vary considerably on different machines with similar settings, the baseline setting suggestions in this section must be adjusted according to clinical intraoperative feedback as will be described.

Anterior Chamber Currents

A conceptual framework of anterior chamber fluid dynamics is necessary in order to apply the principles outlined in Section One. At the most basic level, the intraocular current is simply a function of the location of the irrigation and aspiration ports as depicted in Figures 2-1-1 and 2-1-2. Intraocular fluid as well as free-floating particles are drawn along the current lines toward the unoccluded aspiration port when in foot position 2 or 3. A faster flow rate will produce a stronger current (see Figure 2-1-2) than a slower flow rate (see Figure 2-1-1). Current strength can be increased with a flow pump by simply increasing the flow rate parameter. Because there is no independent flow rate adjustment on vacuum pumps, current strength is increased by increasing the commanded vacuum. Changing the vacuum preset on a flow pump will generally not affect the flow rate; an exception would be setting a low vacuum preset with a high resistance 0.3mm IA tip. In this instance, most peristaltic machines would be incapable of high flow rates because of intermittent pump cessation and/or venting when the vacuum preset was reached at low to moderate flow rates (see discussions with Figures 1-10, 1-19, 1-35b, and 4-1). These schematic currents of course represent an ideal laminar flow environment. In reality, some turbulence and eddy currents are produced because of incisional leakage as well as variable anterior chamber fluid viscosity due to suspended particles, air bubbles, and viscoelastics.

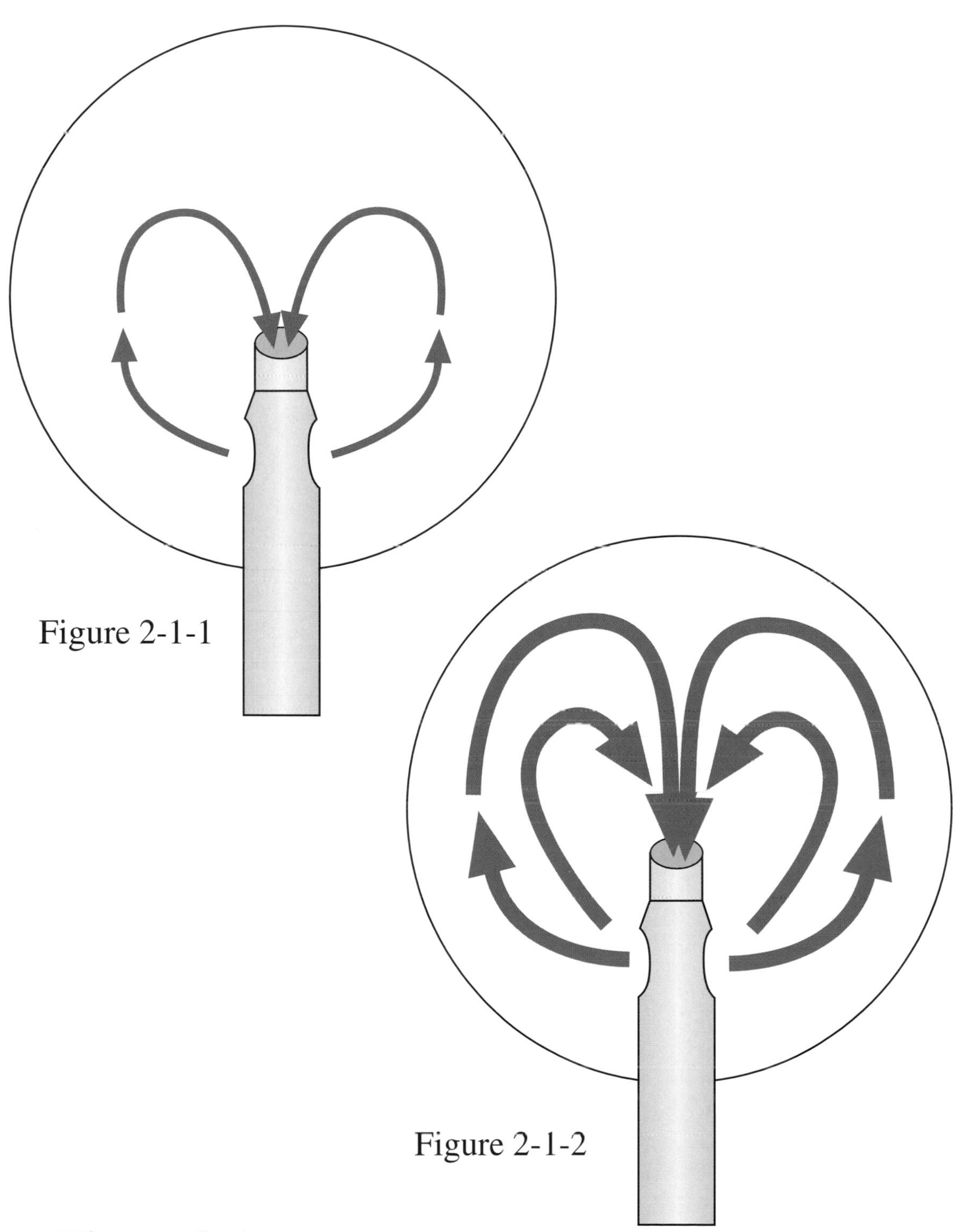

Figure 2-1

Flow Rates and Currents

These illustrations attempt to quantify anterior chamber currents with regard to flow rate. For example, Figure 2-2-1 shows three purple dots per row flowing through the phaco tip per unit time, which is represented as the distance between the rows of dots. Each dot may be thought of as a quantum or unit volume of fluid. Therefore, you can think of this schematic as representing a flow rate of three quanta per unit time, or perhaps 30cc/min. Correspondingly, Figure 2-2-2 represents 50cc/min (five dots or quanta per row). Note that as the distance from the tip increases, the density and speed of the current diminishes because the three or five quanta per row are drawn from an increasing area or volume of intraocular fluid. This phenomenon is analogous to a river in which a wider, deeper section has a slower, gentler current than does a narrower, shallow section which must transfer the same volume as the larger section in the same amount of time, thus producing the stronger current.

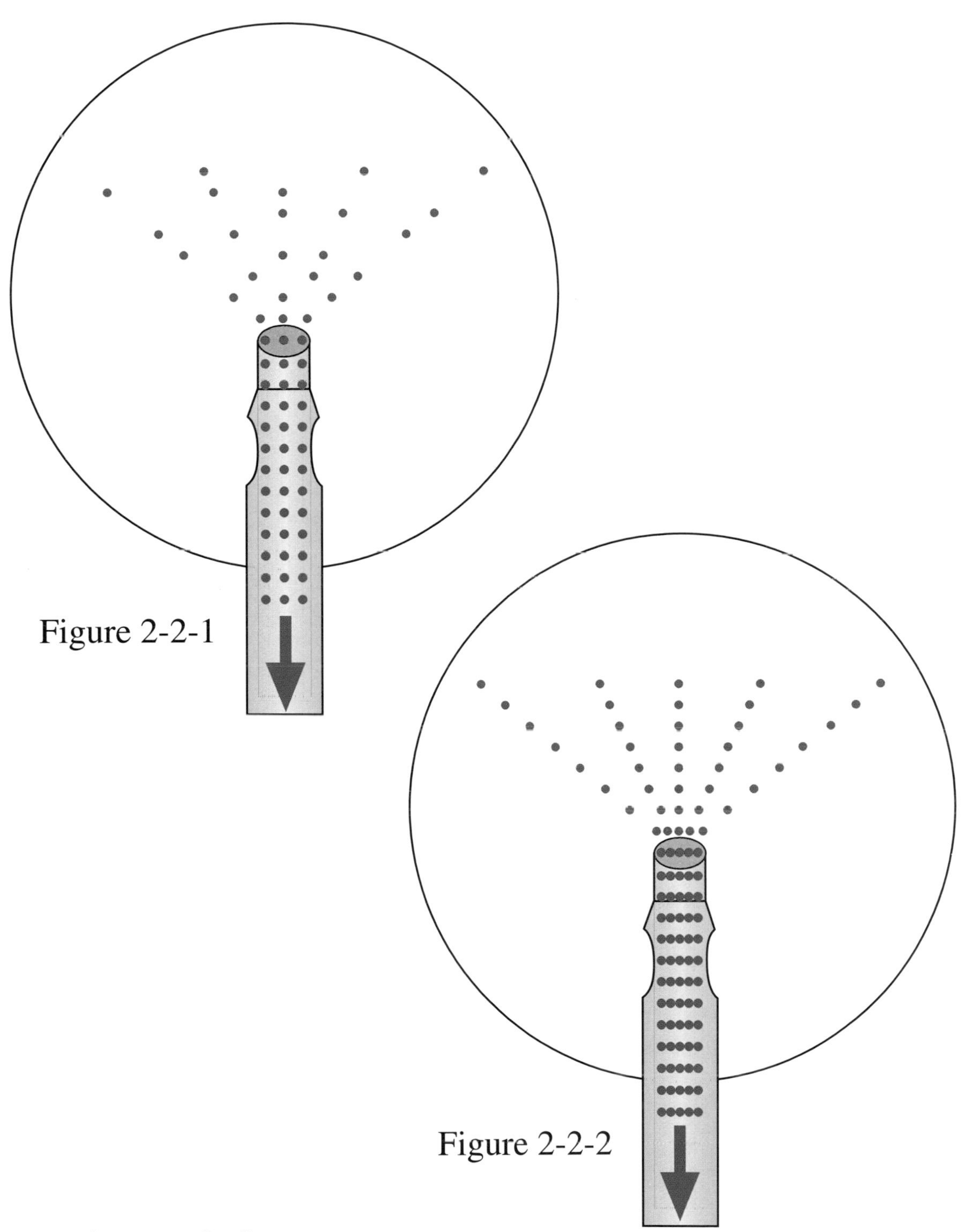

Figure 2-2

Force and Currents

The anterior chamber current, which is directly proportional to the aspiration flow rate, is the force which draws intraocular fluid and any suspended particles or fragments into the aspiration port. The current is propagated on a microscopic level by the moving water molecules pulling adjacent molecules by intermolecular attraction and friction while pushing adjacent molecules by collision and friction. These forces can be schematically represented by the quanta of fluid (purple dots) exerting a pushing force on a suspended fragment (red bar) as they travel into the aspiration port. In Figure 2-3-2 (50cc/min), the fragment when located right at the tip has five quanta of fluid/force pushing it into the tip. Contrast this with only three quanta of force pushing the corresponding fragment into the tip in Figure 2-3-1 (30cc/min). Therefore, increasing the flow from 30cc/min to 50cc/min increases the force pushing (drawing) the fragment into the port by almost 70% (three quanta increasing to five quanta). When the fragment is 1.5mm from the tip, the higher flow rate still draws the fragment more strongly than the lower flow rate (three quanta of pushing force as opposed to two quanta). However, the differential between flow rates is less at this distance from the tip (50% increase from two to three quanta) than when the fragment is right at the tip; this is due to the decreasing speed and strength of the current with increasing distance from the tip. This effect is especially prominent when the fragment is 3mm from the tip, where in these two schematics an identical one quantum of force is exerted despite the different flow rates.

Several important clinical corollaries can be drawn from this information. First, more attraction or followability can be exerted on intraocular fragments by increasing the flow rate; this effect is more prominent closer to the tip. Second, to exert more attraction farther away from the tip, especially 3mm or more, flow rate has to be raised considerably. However, recall that very fast flow rates can decrease your safety margin by quickly drawing in potentially unwanted material (iris and capsule) as well as allowing less reaction time for reflux because of the corresponding rapid rise time. Furthermore, this attractive force will be exerted in all directions following the circular currents (see Figure 2-1) and the conical distribution of the schematic quanta. Therefore, much greater control can be achieved by using more moderate flow rates and working in the area closer to the tip.

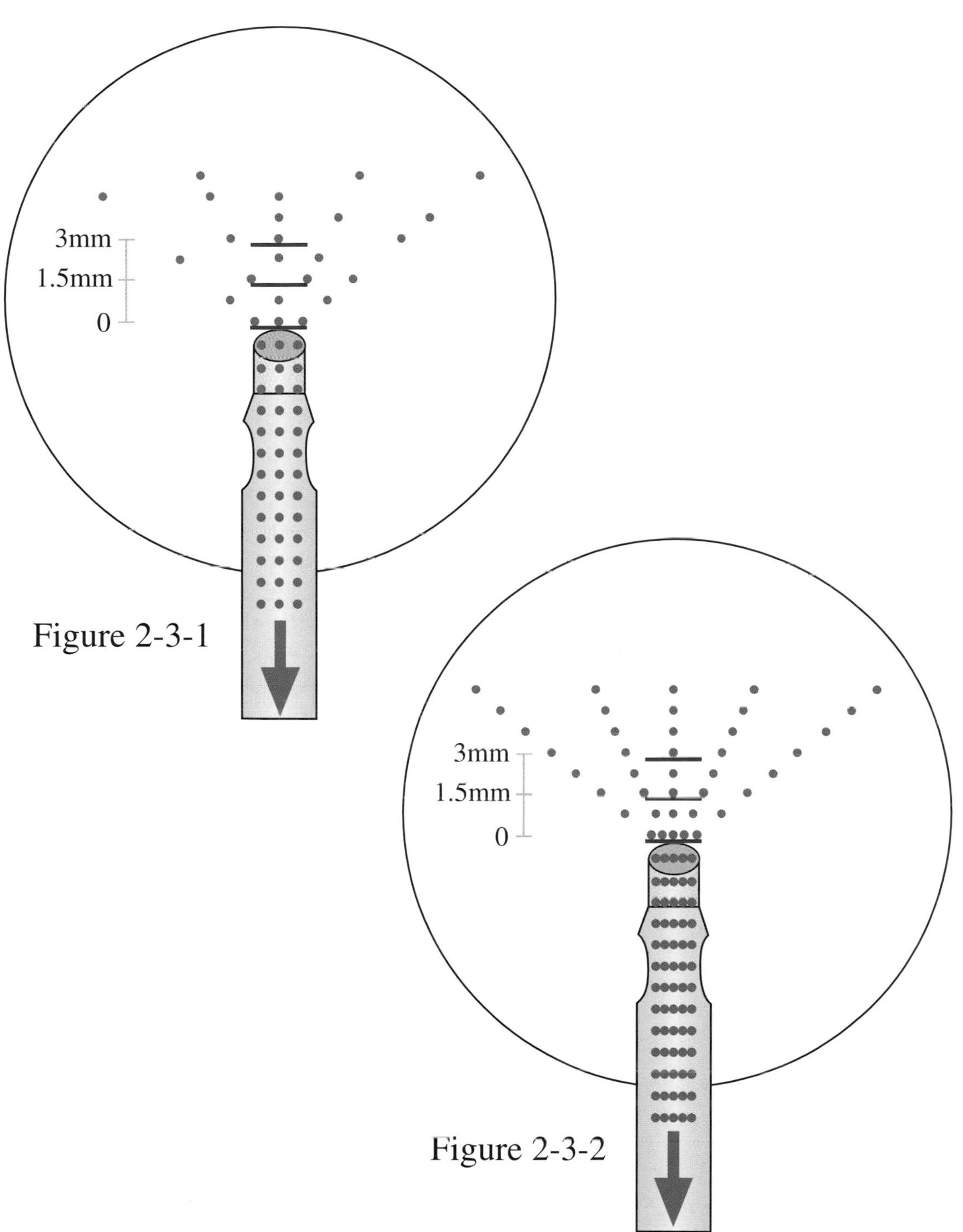

Figure 2-3-1

Figure 2-3-2

Figure 2-3

Flow and Vacuum Settings 1

In order to place the foregoing schematics in a more clinical perspective, we will now look at a scenario in which we wish to attract the final nuclear segment after a chopping procedure. Moreover, we will determine when flow and vacuum are relevant parameters at various intraoperative stages. **Aspiration flow rate** (cc/min) determines how strongly fluid and fragments are attracted toward the tip. Once a fragment occludes the aspiration port, **vacuum** (mm Hg) determines how strongly it is held to the tip.

For example, in Figure 2-4, let's assume a flow pump machine with a flow rate of 16cc/min and a vacuum preset of 100mm Hg. If the quadrant were entirely free-floating, this low flow rate would probably be sufficient to attract it to the tip. However, if the quadrant were not moving toward the tip (ie, because of residual epinuclear adhesions), then an appropriate adjustment would be to increase flow rate in order to produce a stronger current and therefore a stronger attraction (a surgeon using a vacuum pump could at this point increase commanded vacuum in the drainage cassette, which would increase flow through the unoccluded tip as in Figure 1-23). Alternatively, you could simply move the tip closer to the quadrant, recalling that the current is stronger closer to the tip (see Figure 2-3). Note that even though the vacuum limit preset is 100mm Hg, the actual vacuum just inside the tip is minimal because of the negligible resistance to flow from the large bore phaco needle (see Figures 1-23 and 1-35b). Therefore, increasing the panel vacuum setting in this scenario (ie, Figure 2-4 with a flow pump) would not enhance attraction; it would simply change the vacuum preset reading on the panel (green bar) without affecting the fluidics. Recall that a flow pump's vacuum preset limit only determines the level to which actual aspiration line vacuum will rise given sufficient resistance to flow, usually with occlusion of the aspiration port (see Figure 1-10).

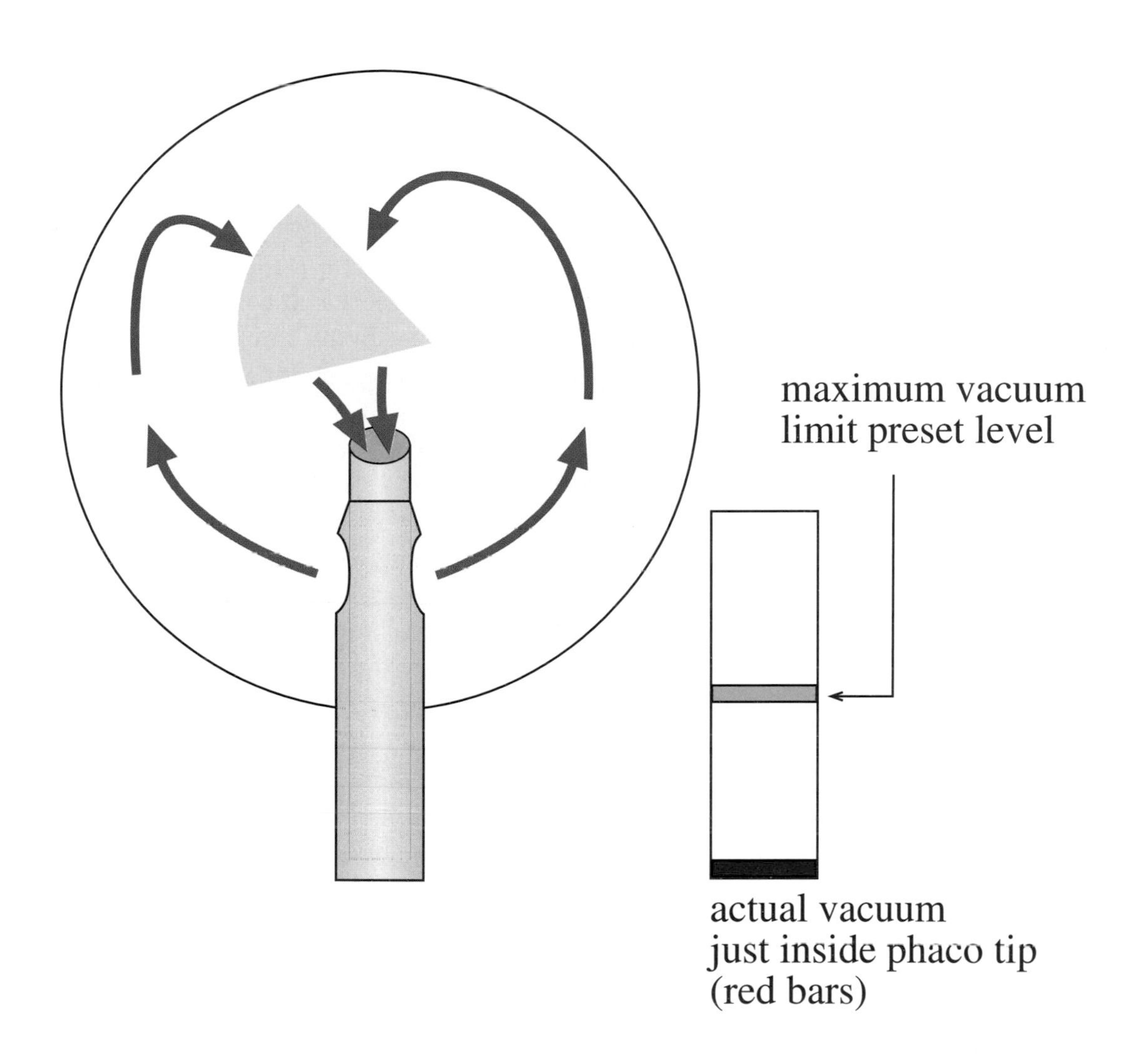
maximum vacuum
limit preset level
actual vacuum
just inside phaco tip
(red bars)

Figure 2-4

Flow and Vacuum Settings 2

In Figure 2-5, ultrasound energy (pedal position 3) has been used to embed the tip into the nuclear fragment such that approximately two thirds of the aspiration port is occluded. Flow still exists through the unoccluded portion of the port, albeit at a reduced rate (see Figure 1-10). This flow still functions to pull the fragment onto the tip although with less force than the higher flow in Figure 2-4. To the extent that the pump's force is not directed into flow production, it builds vacuum as it pulls fluid through the increased resistance of the smaller effective surface area of the aspiration port; the vacuum (holding force) is applied to the portion of the nuclear fragment that occludes the aspiration port (see Figures 1-10 and 1-35b). However, vacuum cannot build up to the full preset limit of 100mm Hg in the absence of complete occlusion. The combination of vacuum and flow contribute to the overall attraction (**followability**) of the fragment to the tip, especially against any applied ultrasound which tends to push fragments away from the tip (see discussion with Figure 1-45).

This is a typical configuration (see Figure 2-5) when carouseling a fragment into the tip while vacuum and flow as described above feed the particle into the aspiration port against the repulsive action of ultrasound. During the carouseling process, the port rapidly alternates between complete and partial occlusion, with vacuum or a vacuum/flow combination contributing to followability, respectively. These fluidic forces must be appropriately titrated to the amount of applied ultrasound as well as to the nuclear density. For example, if the nuclear fragment in this illustration was dense and chattering without being progressively fed into the tip, then the machine parameters would need to be adjusted so that either the repulsive force was decreased (ie, decreasing ultrasound power) or the attractive forces (flow and vacuum) were increased. If a flow pump is used, then both the flow rate and the vacuum limit preset could be increased to enhance followability. With a vacuum pump, only the commanded vacuum could be increased, although this effectively increases flow as well during the instances of partial occlusion as the fragment carousels into the tip. Indeed, this **autoregulation** of vacuum and flow (according to the degree of port occlusion) is a relative advantage of a vacuum pump (or mode) over a flow pump with regard to optimizing followability.

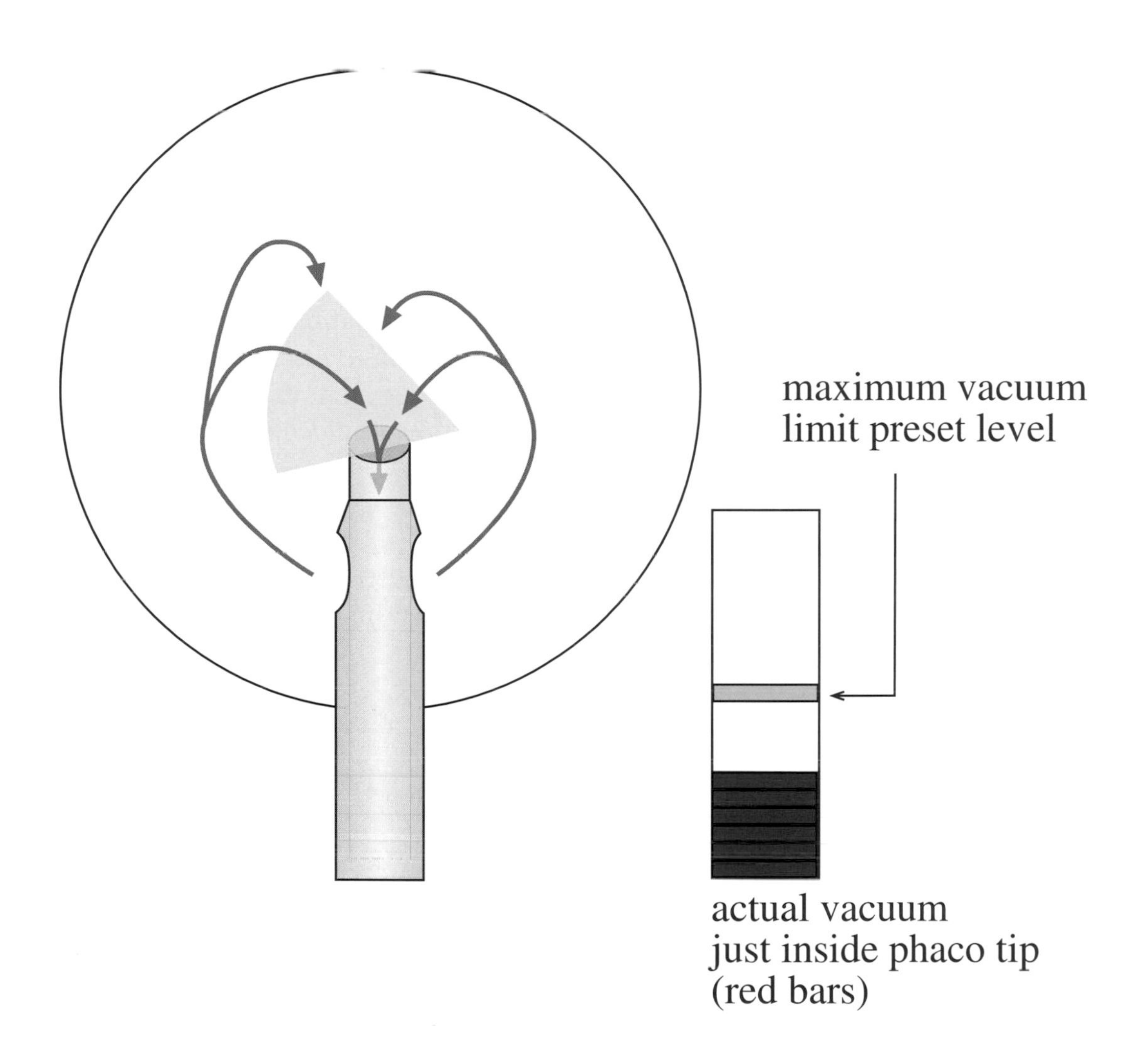
maximum vacuum
limit preset level
actual vacuum
just inside phaco tip
(red bars)

Figure 2-5

Flow and Vacuum Settings 3

The state of partial occlusion shown in Figure 2-5 might also be encountered by a surgeon who has engaged the fragment in order to manipulate it further (ie, to chop it into smaller pieces for easier carouseling). In this case, the pedal would be in position 2 after having used ultrasound only briefly to embed the tip. However, because the tip is incompletely embedded with the aspiration port partially unoccluded, vacuum cannot build efficiently up to the preset level. If the surgeon attempts to chop the fragment at this point and finds that the chopper dislodges the fragment from the tip prior to completing the chop, then it can be determined that insufficient holding force is present. However, the solution in this case is not to increase the vacuum limit preset; this would serve only to raise the green bar on the meter without changing at all the actual vacuum just inside the tip, a value that was determined by the degree of tip occlusion. The solution would be to completely embed the tip (Figure 2-6) so as to completely occlude the aspiration port, thus interrupting flow and transferring all of the pump's force into producing vacuum and holding power at the occluding fragment up to the limit established by the vacuum limit preset (see Figure 1-25). If the holding force were still insufficient at this point, then it would be appropriate to raise the vacuum limit preset further.

The complete occlusion of the aspiration port interrupts the fluidic circuit and stops intraocular flow; note the lack of purple flow arrows in Figure 2-6. Therefore, adjusting the flow rate on a flow pump will not affect either holding force in position 2 or followability in position 3; it will only change the speed with which the vacuum limit is reached (rise time) by changing the rotational speed of the pump head (see Figure 1-11). **In summation, flow is the relevant parameter when the aspiration port is unoccluded, while vacuum is the relevant parameter with complete tip occlusion; both parameters work together to enhance followability with partial tip occlusion.**

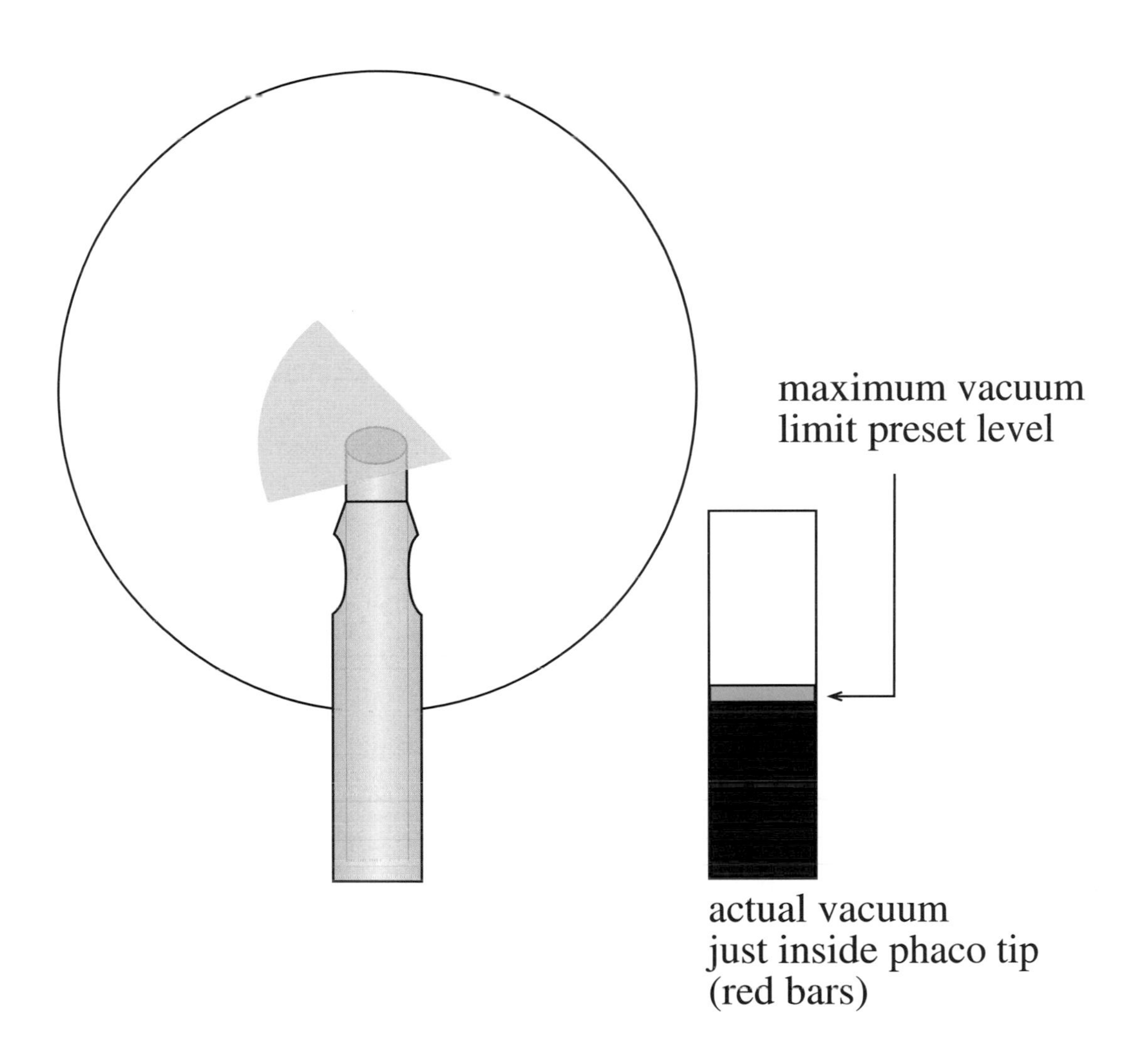

maximum vacuum
limit preset level
actual vacuum
just inside phaco tip
(red bars)

Figure 2-6

Sculpting Settings: Vacuum and Flow

Whereas the previous illustrations established the relevancy of flow and vacuum parameter adjustment according to the amount of aspiration port occlusion, the following diagrams will examine the logic behind setting these parameters with regard to their function during specific surgical techniques. Although sculpting is a relatively inefficient mode of phacoemulsification (see Figure 1-45), it can nonetheless be a useful prelude in preparing the nucleus for various segmentation methods including cracking and chopping; Figure 2-7 illustrates the sculpting of a central groove in preparation for cracking the cataract into two heminuclei. Vacuum is not needed at this stage because there are not yet any large fragments which need to be occluded and gripped, and the particulate emulsate produced by ultrasonic tip action does not typically provide any appreciable resistance which would need vacuum to overcome. Indeed, even with a high vacuum preset, actual vacuum would not necessarily reach the preset level because the tip is usually not occluded more than halfway during sculpting (see Figures 1-10 and 2-5). Furthermore, vacuum is not needed to counteract the repulsive action of ultrasound since the nucleus is held stationary by its intact structure at this point along with the surrounding capsule and zonules. Therefore, low vacuum settings of 20 to 30mm Hg are usually adequate for sculpting while still providing a reasonable safety margin in case of inadvertent contra-incisional peripheral epinuclear, capsular, or iris incarceration. Levels lower than 20mm Hg increase the likelihood of aspiration line clogging when sculpting a dense nucleus which produces larger particles when emulsified; this potential problem of course varies according to the particular machine being used, especially with regard to the inner diameter of the aspiration line and the phaco needle.

Flow rates can be relatively low for sculpting since the only surgical function of flow at this stage is to remove the emulsified lens material without allowing it to fill the anterior chamber. If lens particles are observed in the anterior chamber and the aspiration port appears unoccluded, you should assume the handpiece and/or aspiration line is clogged and take appropriate steps (remove the tip from the eye, inspect the aspiration line for kinks, increase vacuum with a test chamber to reestablish flow as observed in the bottle drip chamber, etc). Again, with a well-designed machine that guards against clogging, you can use the lowest flow rate the manufacturer recommends; recall that a minimum flow is required for ultrasonic tip cooling (see Figure 1-51). A typical low flow range is 12 to 20cc/min. Recall that this flow rate can be either set directly on a flow pump machine or achieved indirectly on a vacuum pump machine by an appropriate commanded vacuum level with the partially occluded sculpting tip (see discussion with Figure 1-35a).

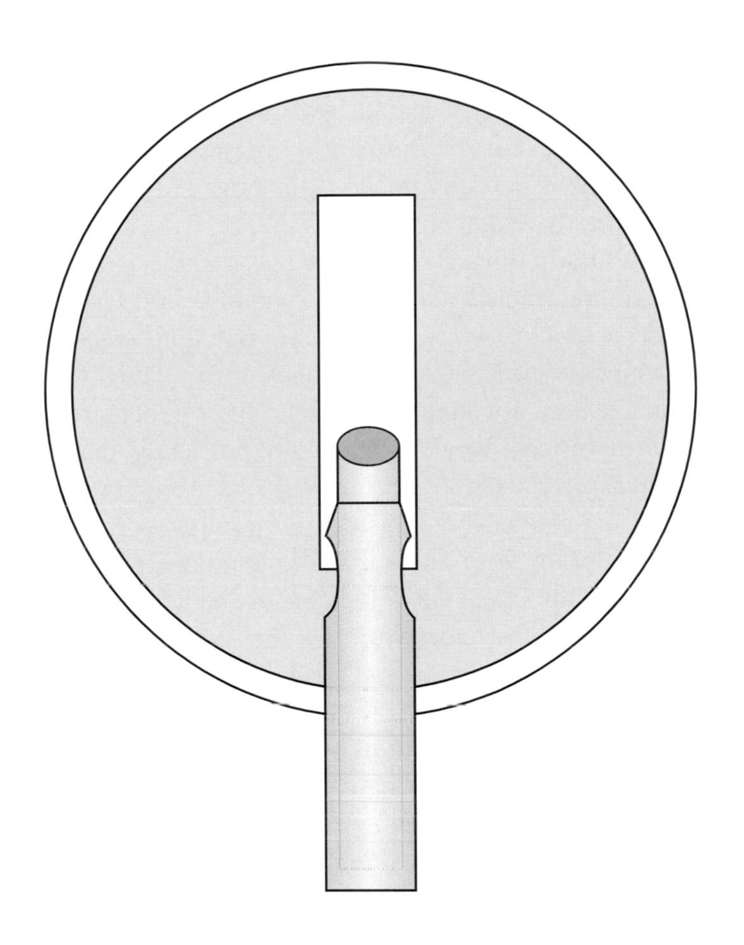

Figure 2-7

Sculpting Settings: Ultrasound

The parameter of ultrasound power during sculpting is set to achieve smooth sculpting without pushing the nucleus (too little power) or delivering excessive intraocular energy with increased potential for complications, such as a wound burn or suddenly piercing the nucleus and possibly capsule (too much power). The appropriate phaco power for a given surgical case is determined by three variables:

1. The density of the nucleus where the phaco tip is engaged
2. The amount of the tip that is engaged
3. The linear velocity of the tip during sculpting

In Figure 2-8-2, the phaco tip sculpts from point A to point B in 2 sec (linear velocity). The nuclear density is 2+ and is homogeneous. With the tip one third engaged, 30% phaco power (on this particular machine) is sufficient to accomplish the sculpting. Using less power would cause zonular stress as the needle would push the nucleus without smoothly sculpting through it. Using more power in this case would deliver more potentially damaging intraocular energy without any beneficial effect.

In Figure 2-8-1, the tip is engaged twice as deeply compared to Figure 2-8-2. In order to preserve smooth sculpting with this two-fold increase in resistance, either power must be doubled (60%) or the linear tip velocity must be halved (4 sec from point A to point B). A more experienced surgeon may opt for the former solution to minimize surgical time and amount of intraocular irrigating fluid. The important point to realize is that there is no predetermined "correct" power setting for a given category of patients; instead, proper power delivery is determined intraoperatively and is dependent on other variables as listed above. The optimum power changes as these variables change from moment to moment in the operation; linear phaco power control is invaluable in making smooth transitions to adapt to these changes. I often use a high maximum phaco power preset (85%) and titrate power as needed with linear pedal control.

A common error for the beginning phaco surgeon is to use far too little power, the rationale being that less power is inherently safer than high power. However, as explained above, too little power can lead to numerous pitfalls by pushing (rather than carving through) the nucleus with potential zonular stress/disruption as well as extension of any pre-existing tears in the capsulotomy. The safest phaco is performed not with low power but rather with **appropriate** power for the variables as listed above. Your microscopic view should be of the phaco needle smoothly carving through a relatively immobile nucleus; if the nucleus is moving significantly, you must increase power, decrease the linear velocity of sculpting, or decrease the amount of the tip engaged. Also, remember that ultrasound energy should be engaged only on each forward sculpting stroke; the pedal should be raised to position 2 or 1 to disengage ultrasound on each backstroke. Otherwise, twice as much ultrasound energy would be expended in the anterior chamber than is necessary.

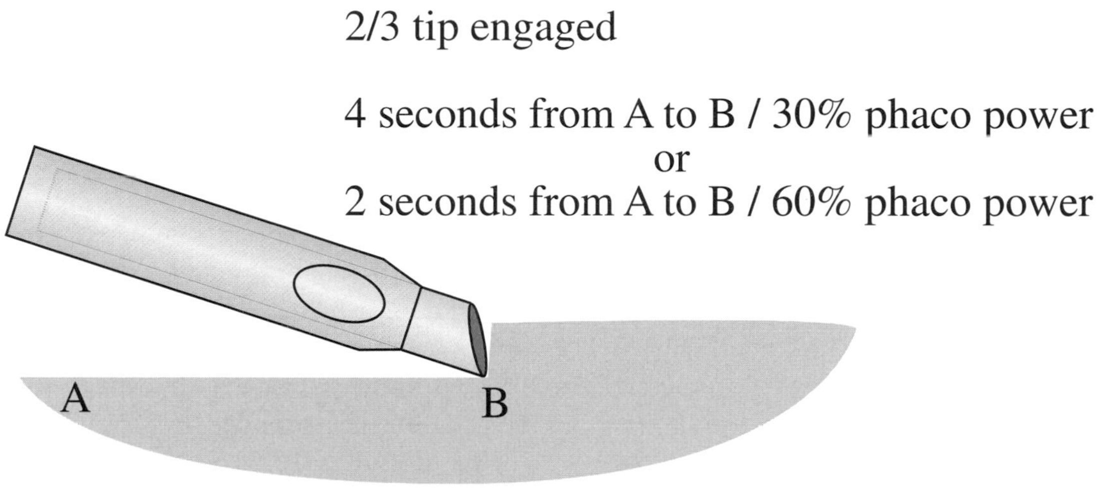

2/3 tip engaged

4 seconds from A to B / 30% phaco power
or
2 seconds from A to B / 60% phaco power

A

B

Figure 2-8-1

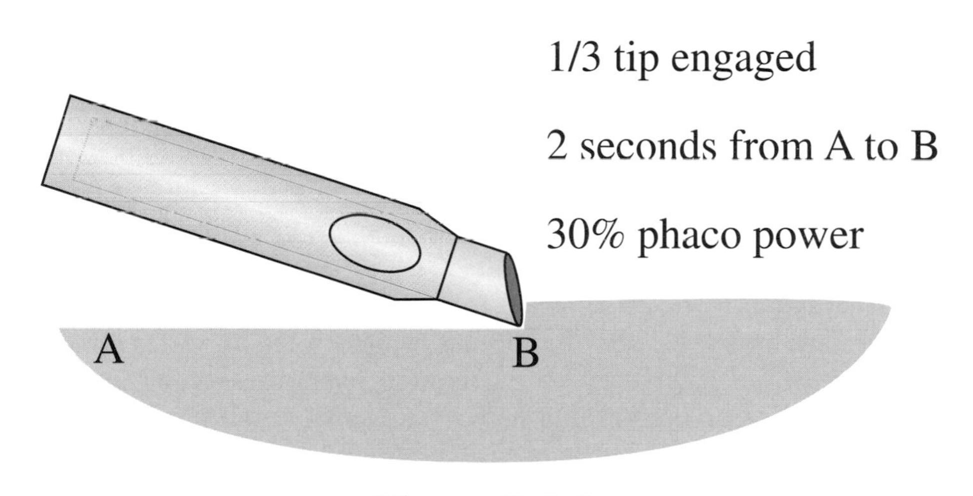

Figure 2-8-2

Figure 2-8

Linear Phaco Sculpting

Figure 2-8 utilized a homogeneous nuclear density to illustrate various concepts. However, most nuclei have variable density with the central portion being most dense. Some nuclei have a smooth transition of density, while others have a more abrupt "lens within a lens" configuration which is readily apparent on preoperative slit-lamp examination. If the amount of tip engaged and the linear velocity of sculpting remain constant, the phaco power must be varied while sculpting through these nuclei with variable density. The following illustrations (Figure 2-9) assume a very dense central nucleus and a maximum phaco power preset of 100%. Thirty percent linear power may be sufficient to begin sculpting in the periphery. Depressing the pedal further provides 60% and then 90% as sculpting proceeds through progressively denser portions of the nucleus. Note that the pedal is let up to decrease the power as the center is passed and less dense material is again encountered; this concept is particularly important as the sculpting tip approaches the contra-incisional epinucleus, where excessive power may lead to abrupt engagement of the epinucleus and juxtaposed capsule. Keeping the power at 90% at this phase would decrease your safety margin as well as needlessly deliver excessive intraocular ultrasound energy. Another important rule for limiting intraocular ultrasound (as mentioned with Figure 2-8) is remembering to relax the foot pedal into position 2 or 1 when retracting the phaco tip to prepare another sculpting excursion.

Note that the above scenario describes how to vary power while maintaining a constant degree of tip engagement and linear velocity of sculpting. However, the principles from Figure 2-8 could also be applied to vary different parameters in Figure 2-9. For example, ultrasound power and the degree of tip engagement could be held constant while the linear velocity of sculpting is progressively slowed as the central densest nucleus is approached and then progressively accelerated as it is passed. However, safety might be compromised as the more vulnerable peripheral nucleus and capsule are approached at an accelerating linear velocity of sculpting, which would allow less time for the surgeon to react in case of inadvertent peripheral epinuclear or capsular incarceration. Alternatively, the ultrasound power and linear velocity of sculpting could be held constant while the degree of tip engagement was progressively decreased when approaching the central densest nucleus and progressively increased after passing through it. However, this latter solution would be counterproductive in that it would sculpt less deeply in the central nucleus, which is the thickest area that requires the most sculpting (see Figure 3-4).

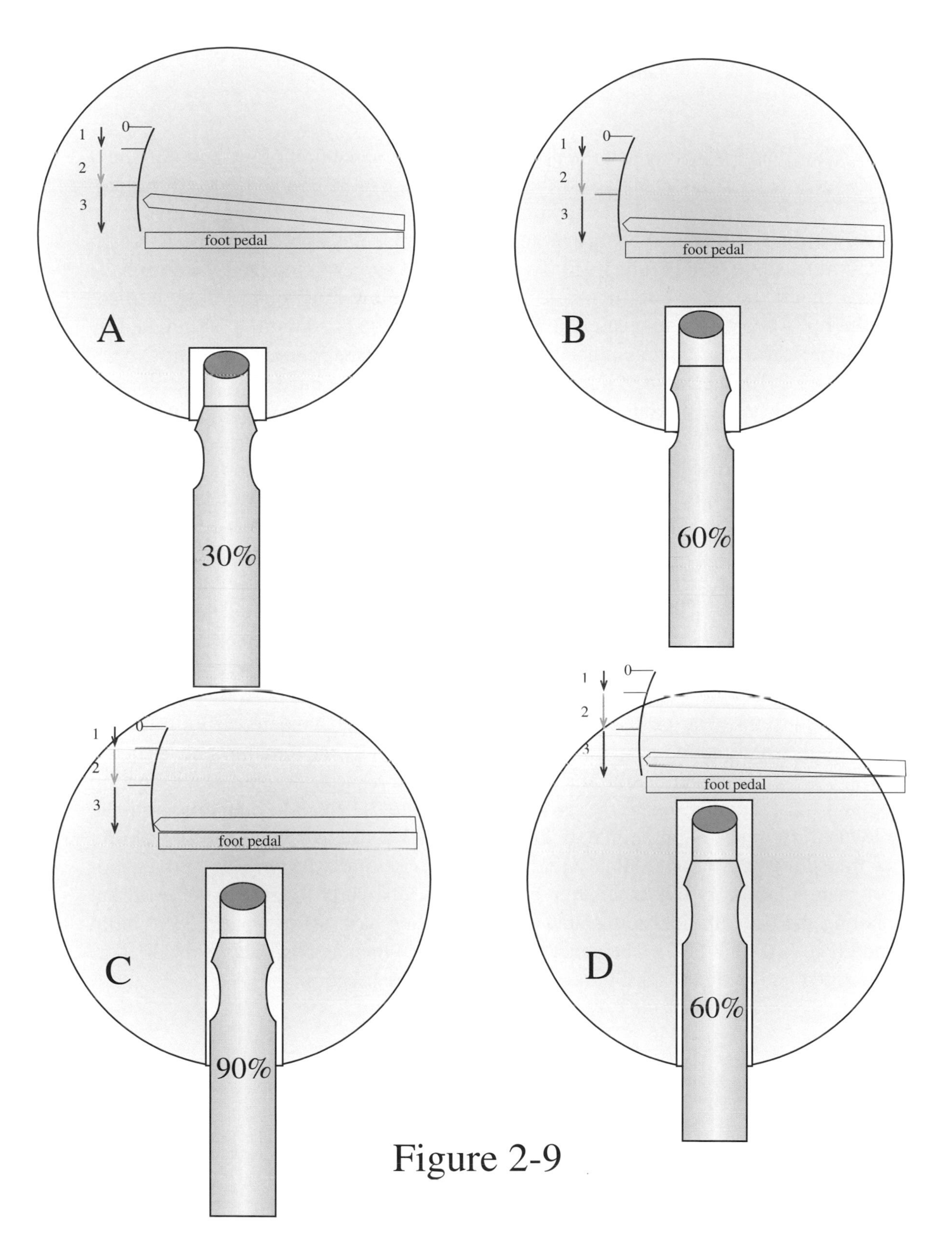
A
1
2
3
0
foot pedal
30%
B
1
2
3
0
foot pedal
60%
C
1
2
3
0
foot pedal
90%
D
1
2
3
0
foot pedal
60%

Figure 2-9

Quadrant Settings 1

Dr. John Shepherd originated the popular quadranting method of phacoemulsification, in which grooves are sculpted so that the nucleus can be cracked into four quadrants. Each quadrant is then individually emulsified in a carouseling fashion which more effectively utilizes ultrasound energy in an occlusion mode as opposed to the less efficient sculpting mode (see Figure 1-45). At this stage of surgery, flow and vacuum have additional functions relative to their role in sculpting. Flow functions to draw a quadrant to the tip, whereas vacuum can allow manipulation of a quadrant that is impaled by the tip. Both flow and vacuum contribute to followability (see Figures 1-45 and 2-5).

In Figure 2-10, the grooves have been completed and the quadrants have all been cracked posteriorly. A reasonable starting point for the vacuum limit preset would be 80mm Hg, although you may have to increase to 120mm Hg, 150mm Hg, or higher if dense nuclear chatter disengages the quadrant during carouseling in position 3 after it had been significantly engaged by the tip (see Figure 2-5). Another reason to increase vacuum would be insufficient holding power after completely impaling the quadrant (see Figure 2-6) when attempting to pull it centrally for carouseling; in particular, the first quadrant often requires a higher vacuum (grip) because of the difficulty in disengaging it from its interlocked position caused by the other three quadrants and the capsule.

There are some options for flow rate setting at this point. If the tip remains stationary in the center as shown, a higher flow rate (30cc/min or higher) may be required to disengage and attract the first quadrant from the other three as well as from any residual epinuclear adhesions. The posterior capsule is relatively well protected from quadrant tumbling by the interlocking posterior nuclear plate formed by the remaining three quadrants which are cracked but in situ; the sharp point of the aspirated quadrant will tend to ride up and over the other quadrants as shown in Figure 2-10-2. Alternatively, you can use a lower flow rate of approximately 25cc/min which will contribute to followability when carouseling as well as produce a reasonably fast rise time when engaging the quadrant for manipulation; in this case, simply move the tip slightly to engage the quadrant by impaling the tip with light ultrasound power and then back off to position 2 to build vacuum (as in Figure 2-11-2). The engaged quadrant can then be positively controlled as it is dislodged and pulled toward the center for safe emulsification.

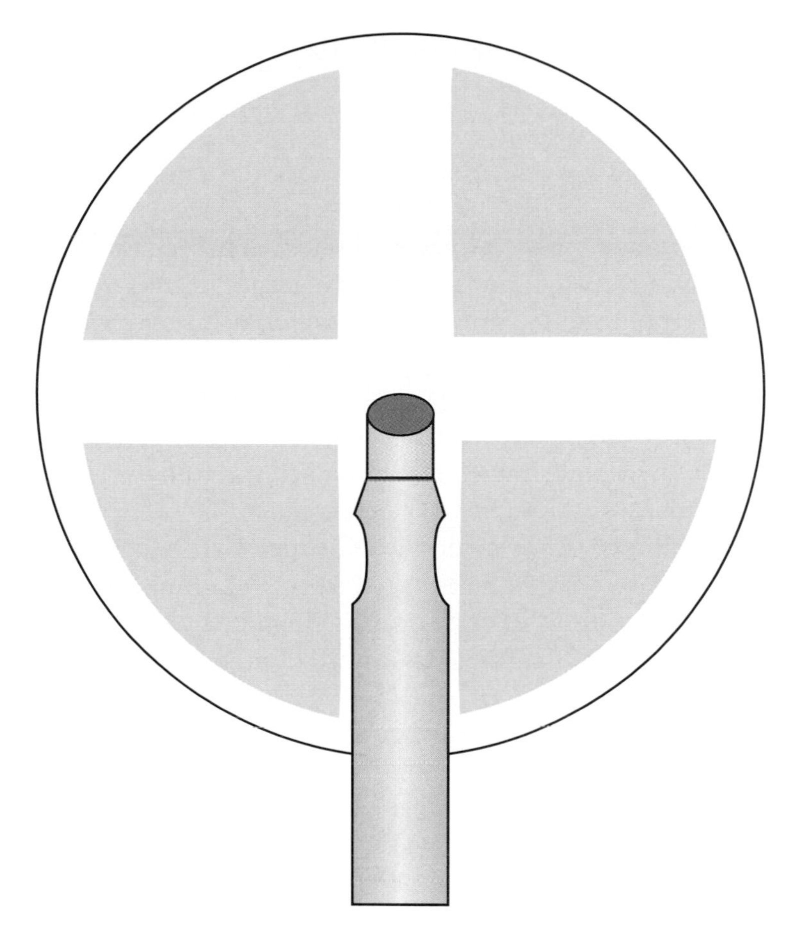

Figure 2-10-1

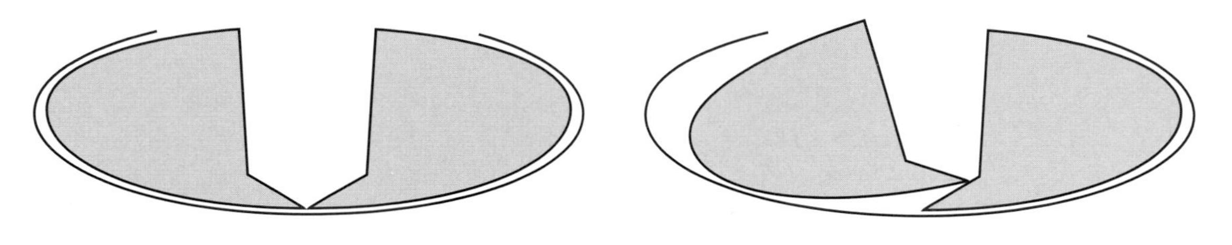

Figure 2-10-2

Figure 2-10

Quadrant Settings 2

With only one or two remaining quadrants, there is not as much latitude with flow rate as there was in Figure 2-10. If a high flow rate was used in Figure 2-11-1, the quadrant is likely to tumble on its way to the aspiration port. It is just as likely to tumble its sharp tip posteriorly as anteriorly with potentially dangerous results for the posterior capsule, especially when dealing with hard cataracts which offer correspondingly little epinuclear and cortical protection for the capsule. By using a low flow rate and positively engaging the quadrant (first with light ultrasound and then with pump vacuum only) as shown in Figure 2-11-2, positive control is maintained and the potential for random tumbling is minimized; the quadrant can then be maneuvered away from the capsule toward the center of the posterior chamber or iris plane for safe phacoemulsification with a carouseling technique. The vacuum level is ideally titrated to provide sufficient holding force to positively control the engaged fragment; too little vacuum is present if the surgeon attempts to draw the fragment in Figure 2-11-2 centrally only to observe the phaco tip pulling out of the fragment instead of drawing the fragment with it.

With regard to the above concept of adjusting machine parameters and surgical technique in order to protect the posterior capsule from sharp nuclear edges, I must acknowledge Dr. Robert Osher's award-winning video from the 1997 ASCRS Film Festival. This video innovatively illustrated that sharp nuclear edges probably do not pose a threat to the posterior capsule. Nevertheless, the preceding paragraph is a useful exercise in the application of phacodynamic principles, and it may in fact be useful when dealing with difficult cases such as positive vitreous pressure or possibly abnormal posterior capsules (eg, posterior polar cataracts, pseudoexfoliation syndrome, small posterior capsular tear).

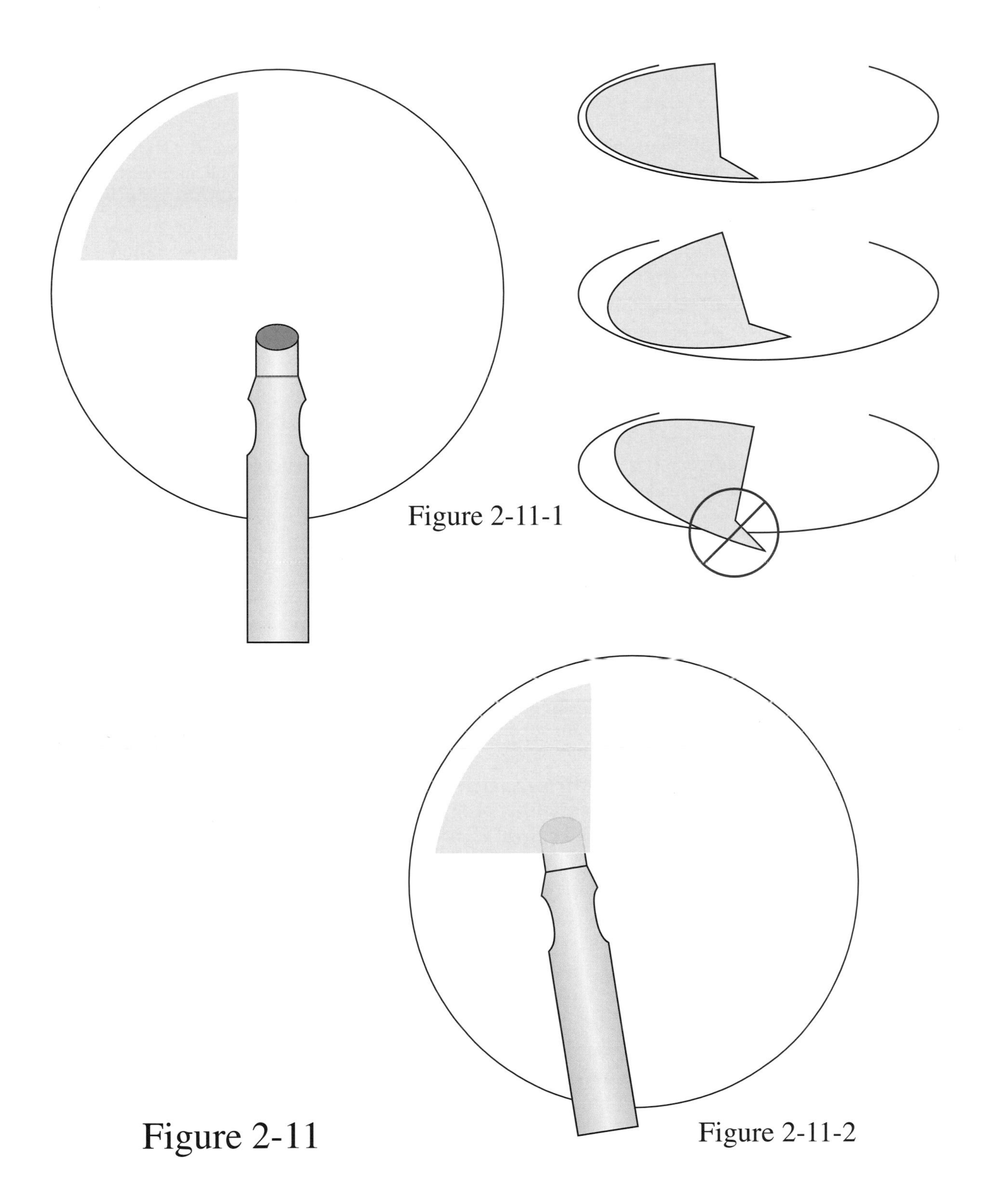
Figure 2-11-1
Figure 2-11-2

Figure 2-11

Settings for Quadrant/Fragment Emulsification

Ultrasound power (repulsive) is titrated along with fluidic parameters (flow and vacuum, which are attractive) to nuclear density as discussed with Figures 1-46 and 2-5; this applies to quadrants as well as smaller fragments resulting from chopping. In order to better visualize the relationship among machine parameters during this stage, Figure 2-12 includes inset graphs which represent a Dual Linear pedal seen from in front (these inset graphs are patterned after illustrations from Dr. Paul Koch). Vacuum is seen to linearly increase as the pedal is further depressed in pitch, while ultrasound linearly increases as the pedal is moved in a yaw (lateral) direction. The light blue shaded area represents an appropriate range of optimal positions for the pedal (gray bar) for a given nuclear density and a given machine. For example, note that the **soft gel-like nucleus** can be aspirated with either a combination of 50mm Hg and 20% power (top of blue shaded area) or a combination of 120mm Hg and 10% power (bottom of blue shaded area). In this case, the nucleus **deforms into the aspiration port with increasing force from either vacuum <u>or</u> ultrasound; therefore, if one parameter is increased, then the other can be correspondingly decreased.** Positions outside of the shaded area represent overuse of a given parameter (ie, more than is required for aspiration of the nuclear material). For example, the red bar has the pedal using 50% more vacuum than is required (180 instead of 120mm Hg) for an ultrasound setting of 10%. Similarly, the green bar is using much more ultrasound than is necessary (40% instead of 10%) for the vacuum of 120mm Hg. Using such unnecessarily high parameters compromises the operation's safety margin without yielding any benefit.

A moderate to hard nucleus requires different logic in choosing a combination of machine parameters for aspiration/emulsification. These **harder nuclei** require more ultrasound power (minimum 25% in this case) to trim the fragment sufficiently to fit into the aspiration port because even relatively high vacuum levels cannot deform the crystalline structure appreciably as with the softer cataracts. However, as the cataract's density and hardness become greater, it is more likely to be repelled by the axially vibrating ultrasonic needle, especially at higher power settings. Therefore, **increasing power requires a proportional increase in vacuum and/or flow; note the opposite slope of the shaded area in the Figure 2-12-2 relative to Figure 2-12-1.** Any pedal position within this blue shaded area will result in the fragment progressively aspirating into the phaco needle in a carouseling fashion as indicated by the curved arrow. If the pedal is put in the position of the red bar (180mm Hg, 25% ultrasound power), the fragment will still be aspirated but with a compromised safety margin due to the higher than necessary vacuum. A pedal at the purple bar's position (Figures 2-12-1 and 2-12-2) will cause the nuclear fragment to be gripped but not aspirated. If the pedal is placed in the position of the green bar (100mm Hg, 50% ultrasound power), the ultrasound power will be too great for the amount of vacuum; the fragment will not be aspirated but will instead chatter against the tip as it rapidly alternates between repulsion from ultrasound and attraction by vacuum/flow. If the surgeon wishes to maintain 50% ultrasound power, then the pedal must be depressed further in pitch until it is within the blue shaded area so that attractive fluidic forces will overcome the repulsive ultrasonic forces so that the fragment can be aspirated as shown in the lower part of Figure 2-12-2.

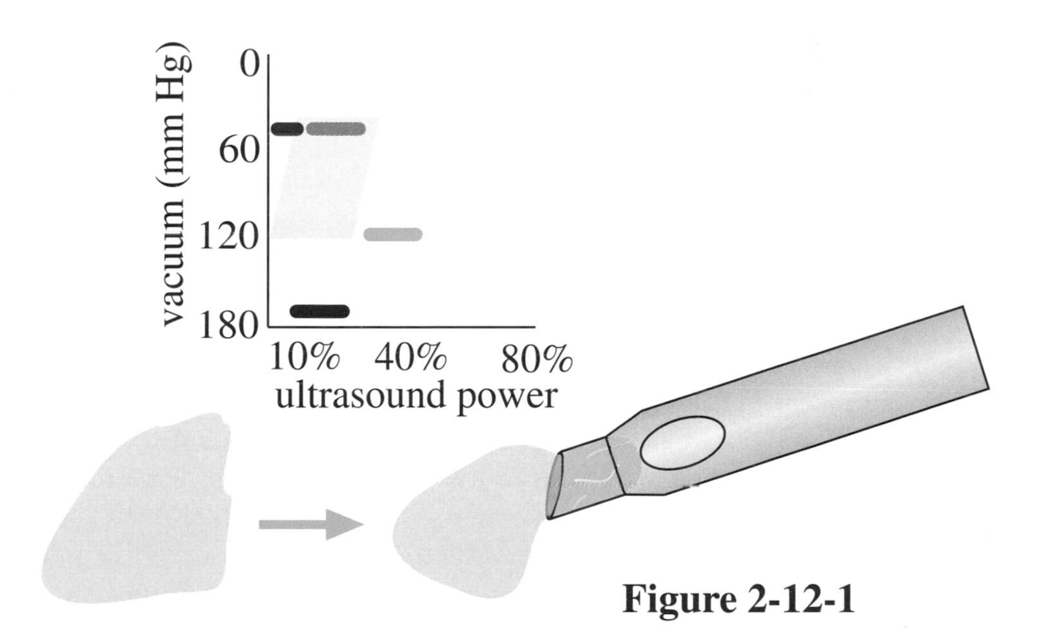
vacuum (mm Hg)
0
60
120
180
10% 40% 80%
ultrasound power
Figure 2-12-1
semi-solid gel soft nucleus

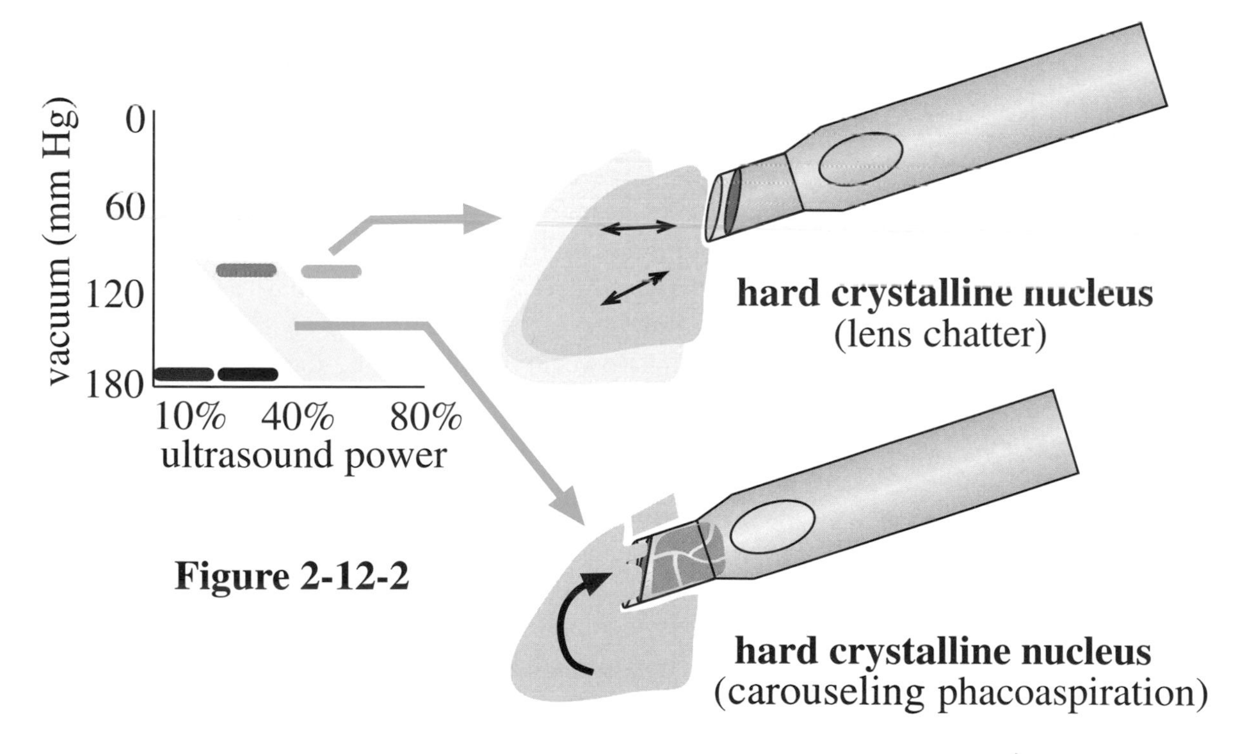
vacuum (mm Hg)
0
60
120
180
10% 40% 80%
ultrasound power
hard crystalline nucleus
(lens chatter)
Figure 2-12-2
hard crystalline nucleus
(carouseling phacoaspiration)

Figure 2-12

Phaco Chop Settings

The phaco chop method, originated by Dr. Kunihiro Nagahara, involves impaling the nucleus with the phaco tip either as a first step or, as shown in Figure 2-13, after first sculpting a small bowl to allow access to the denser central nucleus which will give the best vacuum seal. Then, after allowing for rise time to build vacuum to the panel preset level, the phaco chop instrument (inserted through the side-port incision) is embedded in the nucleus toward or at the periphery and drawn toward the phaco tip, splitting the nucleus as it advances (green and blue arrows). The nucleus is then rotated and the process is repeated to produce multiple nuclear fragments which are then safely emulsified in the center of the posterior chamber or iris plane. Because the aspiration port is completely occluded during chopping, flow rate is not an important parameter other than its effect on rise time. If a flow pump is used, 26cc/min is a useful compromise between a reasonably rapid rise time and a reasonable safety margin against surge. If a vacuum pump is used at 200 to 250mm Hg, the surge potential is especially high. When the chop is completed and the occlusion breaks, the subsequent induced flow with a standard needle would be over 60cc/min. A MicroFlow or similar needle with a reduced inner diameter (therefore increased fluidic resistance) significantly reduces this flow to a safer level (see Figure 1-35a). Additionally, the surgical technique should be optimized to use the high vacuum level during the actual manipulation and chop when gripping the nucleus, and then to dynamically decrease the vacuum with linear pedal control just as the chop is completed to minimize the surge potential.

The most important setting for chopping is vacuum, which needs to be sufficient to stabilize the nucleus while the phaco chop instrument is splitting it, notwithstanding the degree to which the nucleus is mechanically fixated between the chopper and the phaco tip. For many cases, 120mm Hg may be adequate, but this level may need to be increased (in some cases to 200mm Hg or higher) if the action of the phaco chopper is dislodging the vacuum seal on the phaco tip. However, before raising the vacuum level, make sure the chopping instrument is being drawn directly toward the phaco tip (green arrow). If it is being drawn at a slightly different vector (ie, red arrow), a torque will be induced which can dislodge the nucleus from the phaco tip prior to chop completion. Therefore, make sure your technique is optimized before unnecessarily raising vacuum and thereby lowering your safety margin. It should be noted that once the chopper is drawn completely up to the phaco tip, an alternate vector (red arrow) may then be used to further extend the nuclear crack. If this technique is employed, then vacuum may have to be raised accordingly to maintain a firm hold on the nucleus by the phaco tip.

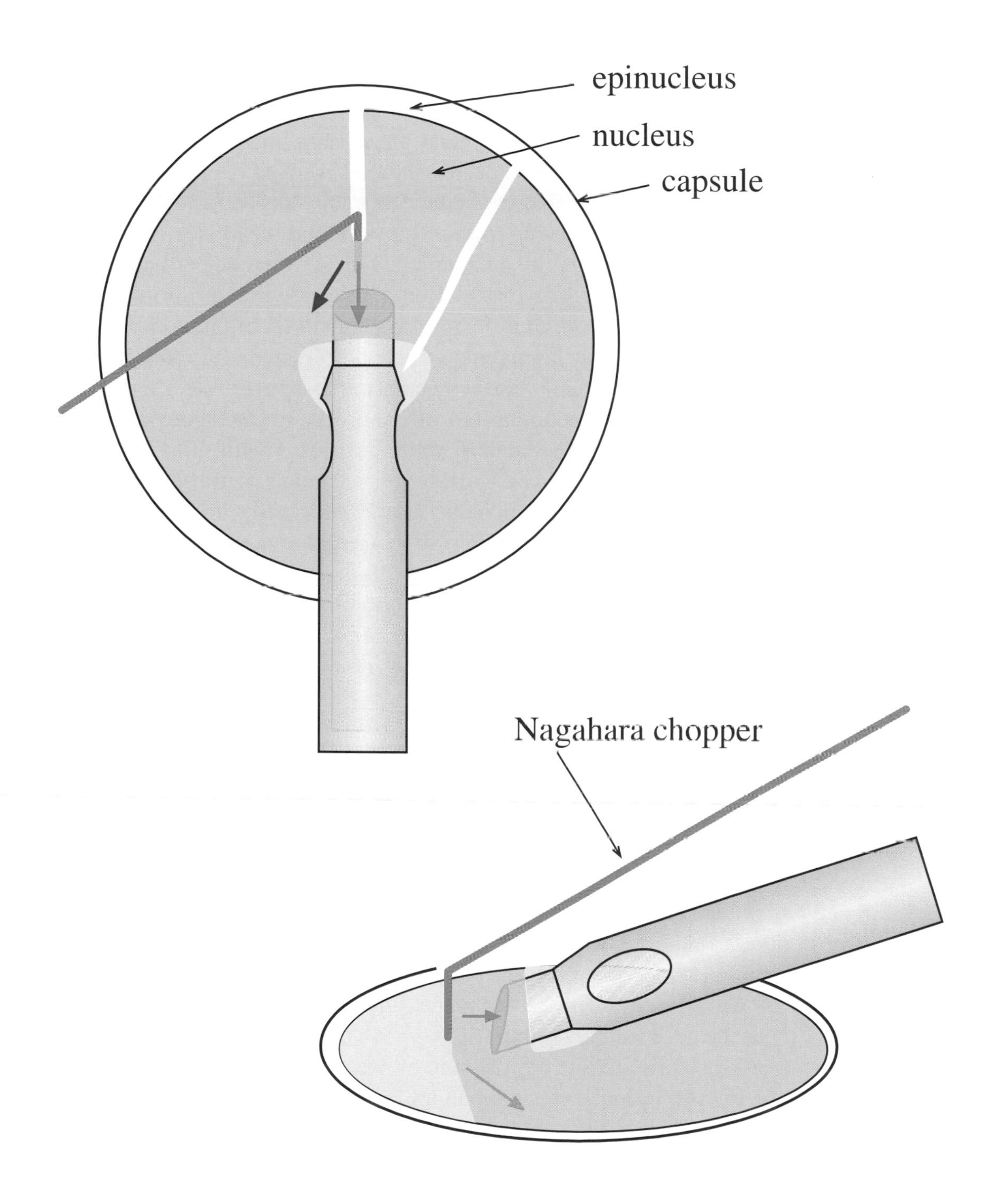

Figure 2-13

Modified Chop

When operating on denser nuclei with the original phaco chop method, it can be difficult to remove the initial chopped segments because they are wedged in place by the surrounding intact nucleus. To overcome this problem, Dr. Paul Koch developed the stop and chop method, which begins by carving a central groove and then bisecting the nucleus. Dr. Koch then utilizes the chopping technique to subdivide the nuclear halves. This technique was independently developed by Dr. Ronald Stasiuk as the mini-chop technique. The nuclear debulking by the initial groove formation allows ample room for dislodging and manipulating the nuclear fragments which are created by chopping. Settings for the initial groove are the same as for any sculpting maneuver (see Figures 2-7 through 2-9). In order to begin the chopping part of the procedure in Figure 2-14-1a, the phaco tip enters the heminucleus in standard pedal position 3 with mild linear ultrasound; the pedal is then raised to position 2 in order for vacuum to build up without any accompanying ultrasound. Sufficient vacuum is required in order to allow the engaged heminucleus to be drawn away from the periphery (see blue double arrow) so that the chopping instrument is less likely to engage capsule as it is inserted into the nucleus; this maneuver is facilitated by the initial groove formation which creates space for the central heminuclear displacement. A typical vacuum range for this step is 160 to 240mm Hg with a standard phaco needle; correspondingly more vacuum is needed if using a needle with a smaller distal surface area (see Figure 1-49). Vacuum should be increased if the phaco tip pulls out of the heminucleus when attempting to draw it centrally, assuming that techinique was optimized in ensuring complete initial occlusion of the aspiration port as well as discontinuation of ultrasound as soon as the tip was embedded to an adequate depth; **ultrasonic vibration of the phaco needle dramatically decreases its ability to grip and pull impaled fragments.** If residual posterior adhesions prevent complete separation of the chopped fragment, the phaco tip and the chopper can be separated as shown by the red arrows in Figure 2-14-2, resulting in the ready-to-carousel positioning of the fragment as shown in Figure 2-14-3. Note that the chopped fragment is smaller than a quadrant. It is usually easier and more efficient to handle smaller segments when dealing with harder nuclei; the chopping technique readily facilitates this without the need for carving multiple grooves. Also note that the chop has been directed so that it is completed just to the side of the phaco tip, thereby maintaining the occlusion of the aspiration port (ie, vacuum seal); positive control of the fragment is maintained, allowing it to be manipulated into optimal position in preparation for carouseling emulsification.

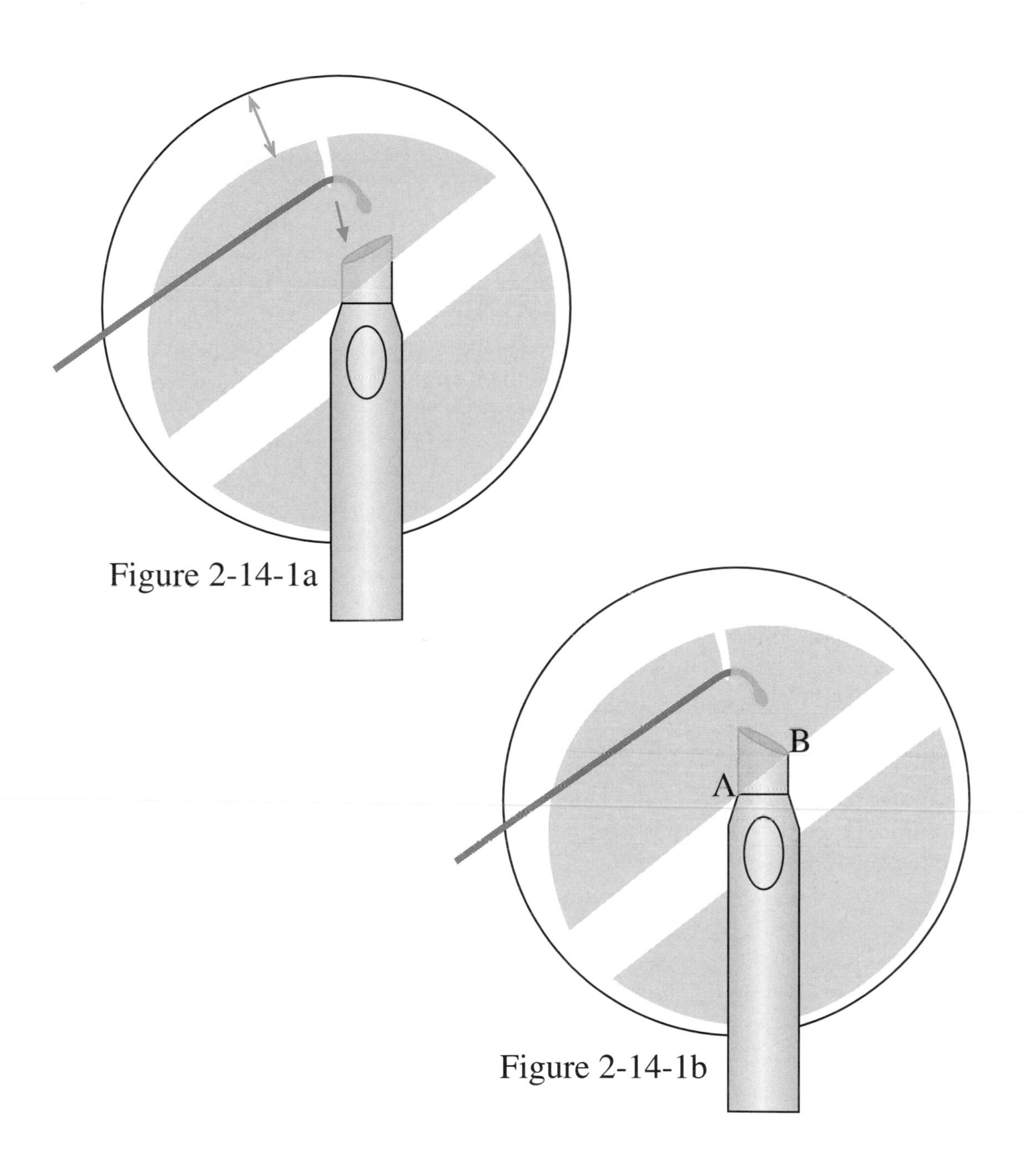

Figure 2-14-1a

Figure 2-14-1b

Figure 2-14a

Modified Chop (continued)

Recall that the vacuum range (160 to 240mm Hg) in the preceding paragraph is required for gripping and mobilizing the relatively large heminucleus centrally so that the chopper can safely engage the heminuclear periphery. However, once the heminucleus is mechanically fixated between the chopper and the phaco tip, the need for vacuum fixation is diminished. Furthermore, typically less vacuum is required for carouseling the fragment once the chop is completed (see Figure 2-12) relative to the higher vacuum required for mobilizing the heminucleus. Linear pedal control will allow dynamic reduction of vacuum as the chop is propagated and completed so as to maintain the appropriate vacuum level for each moment of the operation; this will maximize safety by reducing the propensity for surge during carouseling as well as when the chop happens to break the vacuum seal (tip occlusion). For example, a stop and chop procedure using Dual Linear pedal control (see Figure 1-4) would begin with the phaco tip being placed against the face of the heminucleus, and the pedal being depressed slightly in pitch so that a proportionate amount of vacuum will be generated in anticipation of the next step, which is to yaw the pedal into just enough ultrasound so that the tip will be embedded in the epinucleus. At this point, the pedal is yawed back to its central position (zero ultrasound) while the pitch is depressed fully to achieve maximum vacuum and gripping power. The gripped heminucleus can then be pulled centrally so that the chopping instrument is less likely to engage the peripheral capsule when it is placed at the perimeter of the heminucleus. The pitch of the pedal is then raised as the chop is completed so that the vacuum level will be appropriately lower for the subsequent task of emulsifying the chopped fragment as ultrasound is again engaged by a yaw motion while maintaining the new pitch position.

Note the suboptimal needle configuration in Figure 2-14-1b, in which the bevel has been rotated 180° relative to the needle bevel in Figure 2-14-1a. Further penetration is inhibited by the silicone sleeve at point A, yet at this configuration the aspiration port is very close to the surface of the engaged half at point B (see also Figures 1-47a and 3-28). The vacuum seal is likely to be compromised at this point as the tip is used to pull the heminucleus centrally; furthermore, the action of the chopper will create a counterclockwise torque on the heminucleus which will induce a pivoting around the tip and a break in the vacuum seal at point B. When the vacuum seal is broken, vacuum can no longer be effectively transferred from the pump to grip the engaged fragment; optimal control is therefore compromised. This situation can be avoided by proper orientation of the needle bevel as shown in Figure 2-14-1a, in which the bevel of the phaco tip is roughly parallel with the surface which it engaged, thus allowing sufficient and uniform penetration to ensure a good vacuum seal (see also Figure 3-28).

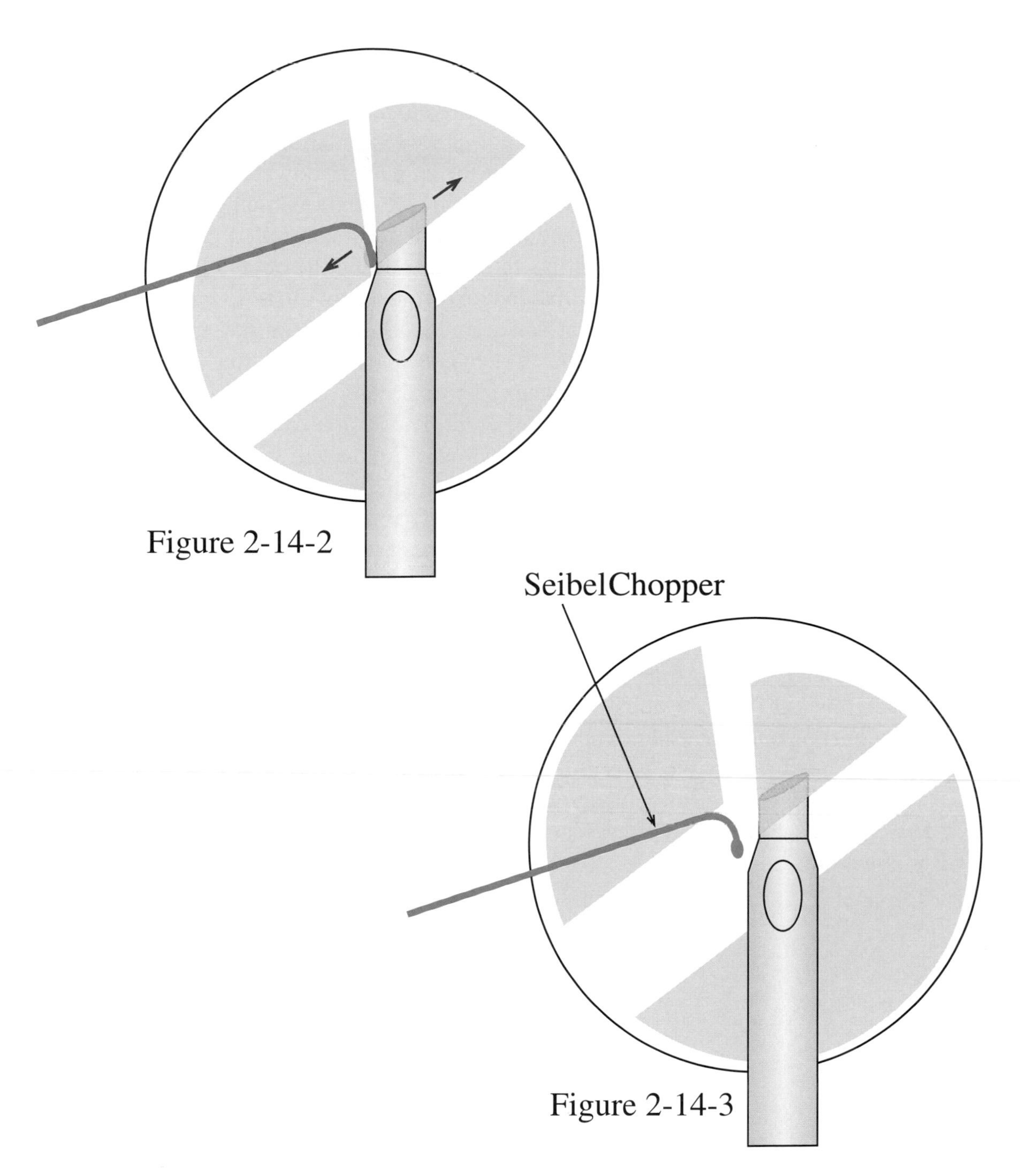

Figure 2-14-2

Figure 2-14-3

Figure 2-14b

Epinucleus Settings 1

Optimal flow and vacuum settings for epinuclear removal are often similar to those used for quadrants. Figure 2-15-1 shows the initial phaco tip positioning just prior to engaging the posterior surface of the anterior rim of the epinuclear bowl. Given the fact that the capsule is adjacent to the epinucleus at this point, it would be inappropriate to use high flow rates because of the potential for abrupt, uncontrolled aspiration. However, because of the angle between the in situ epinucleus and the bevel of the aspiration port (blue lines), very low flow rates may not exert sufficient attraction to the tip. A flow rate of 18 to 24cc/min is usually effective and safe for this initial epinuclear engagement. Once the epinucleus has been attracted to and occludes the phaco tip (Figure 2-15-2), a sufficient force must be exerted to maintain the occlusion during tip/epinuclear manipulation. Because flow ceases with tip occlusion, vacuum is now the correct parameter to adjust. Low vacuum is obviously inappropriate at this point because it would not exert enough gripping force to maintain the occlusion. However, you must also avoid too high a vacuum, which would abruptly aspirate the occluding epinucleus, allowing the tip to penetrate the bowl and threaten the capsule (Figure 2-15-3); this scenario would also fail in the goal of maintaining a positive hold on the epinuclear bowl. A moderate vacuum level of 60 to 120mm Hg is often effective, but do not hesitate to increase the vacuum preset if you are unable to maintain a positive hold on the bowl after allowing for rise time to build vacuum after occlusion. Linear vacuum control in phaco mode is ideal for epinuclear removal.

A primary goal in epinuclear removal is to free it from the surrounding capsule and cortex as an intact bowl if possible, thus eliminating the need for chasing after multiple pieces. Once the phaco tip is firmly engaging the epinucleus, the bowl is rotated as in Figure 2-15-4 in order to break any residual adhesions which sometimes remain even after hydrodissection.

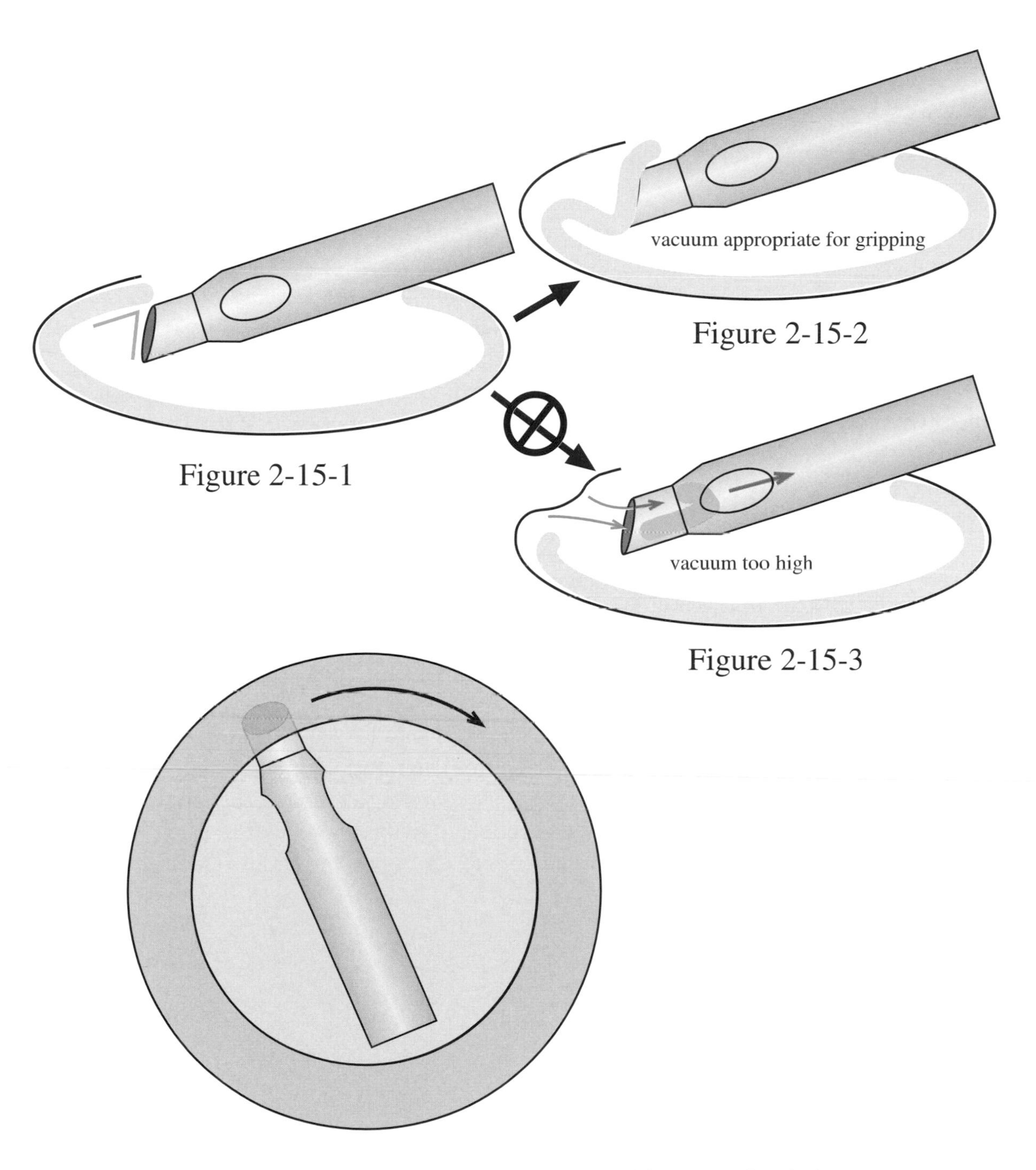

Figure 2-15-4

Figure 2-15

Epinucleus Settings 2

Once the bowl's perimeter and posterior surface have been freed by rotation as in Figure 2-15-4, the bowl is "flipped" (per Dr. I. Howard Fine) so that aspiration and emulsification (often pulsed either manually or automatically) can take place at the iris plane or the middle of the posterior chamber. This increases your safety margin by avoiding aspiration or emulsification of the epinucleus when it is adjacent to the capsule. In Figure 2-16-1, the contra-incisional bowl has been pulled away from the capsule with the phaco tip. A second instrument inserted through the side-port can then be used as a fulcrum and handle as shown to pull the sub-incisional bowl inferiorly and flip the epinucleus over. This instrument (a Seibel Chopper in this case) should engage the epi-nucleus over a sufficiently large surface area (see blue arrows in Figure 2-16-1) such that the instrument's force pushes and manipulates the epinuclear bowl rather than penetrates it (see Figure 3-16). Once you have obtained the configuration in Figure 2-16-2, you can increase vacuum at this point to deform and aspirate the engaged epinucleus; this is especially convenient if the machine has linear foot pedal control of vacuum in position 2 of phaco mode. Alternatively, you can augment the original (gripping) vacuum level with light ultrasound energy to emulsify the part of the bowl engaged by the tip (recall the light blue shaded range of appropriate pedal positions in Figure 2-12-1, which are appropriate for epinucleus as well as a soft gel-like nucleus). Choosing the latter strategy achieves a safer, slower flow rate with a vacuum pump and decreases the likelihood of a surge with any pump. The remaining epinucleus is then reengaged to repeat the process as necessary as shown in Figure 2-16-3. Just as quadrant/fragment control and aspiration depended on precise and appropriate titration of the vacuum level, epinuclear removal is also very dependent on proper vacuum to allow proper control of the epinuclear bowl by the phaco tip for the purposes of gripping as well as aspirating; linear control of vacuum in phaco mode is therefore an important feature on a phaco machine.

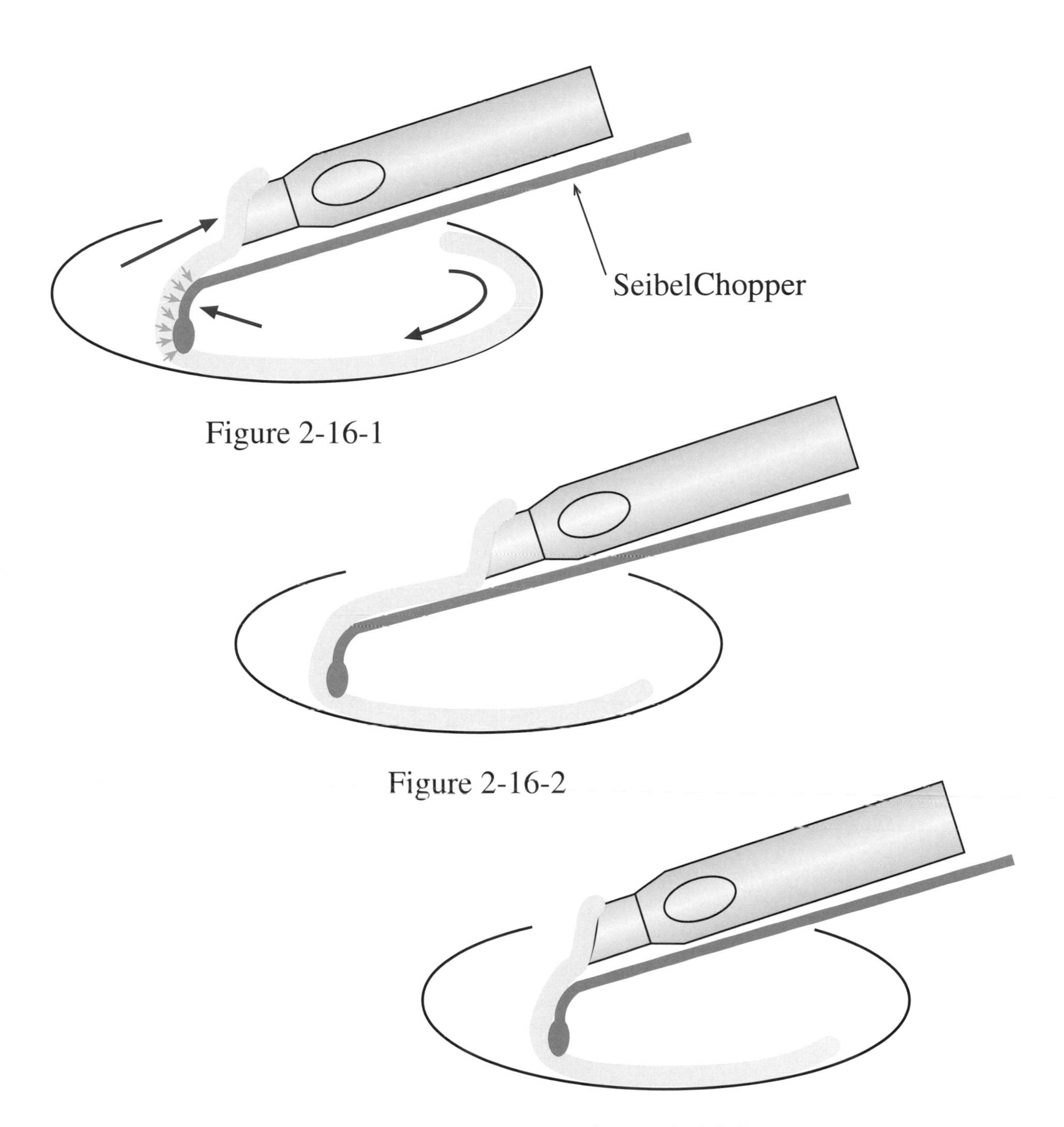

Figure 2-16-1

Figure 2-16-2

Figure 2-16-3

Figure 2-16

SECTION THREE

Overview of Phacoemulsification Techniques

Overview of Phaco Methods

The following method descriptions are relatively brief synopses; refer to the Bibliography for complete descriptions by the methods' originators and proponents.

Nuclear Segmentation

Also known as a cracking or splitting technique, the basic idea behind this method is to fracture the cataract into two or more pieces which can be more easily manipulated and attracted to the phaco tip as opposed to a single whole nucleus. Moreover, safety is enhanced because the nuclear segments can therefore be emulsified in a carouseling fashion in the posterior chamber or iris plane as opposed to emulsifying the nucleus completely by sculpting in its in vivo position juxtaposed to the capsule. Dr. Howard Gimbel originally described bisecting the nucleus; Dr. John Shepherd extended the technique to quadranting, a version of which is described here. Begin with a capsulorhexis; then use hydrodissection and hydrodemarcation to facilitate nuclear rotation. Begin phaco by sculpting a deep groove. Rotating the nucleus 180° is often necessary to complete this groove. The nucleus is then split into halves at the base of the groove. Rotate the two halves 90° to carve a groove into the middle of one of them. Perform a second fracture here and then phaco the two quadrants separately after drawing them safely to the middle of the posterior chamber or the iris plane. Repeat this procedure on the remaining nuclear half. The epinucleus is then removed, if possible, as an intact bowl utilizing the phaco tip as discussed in Section Two.

Fault-line phaco is a technique which I developed to exploit the design attributes of the Flat-Head Phaco tip. It differs from the classic quadrant procedure in that the "grooves" are actually channels within the body of the nucleus which are created by a more efficient occlusion mode boring as opposed to sculpting. The channels can also be used as a precursor to chopping.

Dr. Kunihiro Nagahara developed the phaco chop technique. As described in Figure 2-12, the nucleus is impaled by the phaco tip while a phaco chop instrument is used to split the nucleus into multiple fragments, which are then safely emulsified in the center of the posterior capsule or iris plane. This procedure readily facilitates making multiple nuclear segments which are smaller than full quadrants; the smaller segments are easier to handle and are more readily emulsified in a carouseling motion with fewer manipulations by a second instrument, especially with denser nuclei. Furthermore, chopping and its variations discussed below minimize sculpting and instead utilize the more efficient occlusion mode phacoemulsification (see Figure 1-45).

Sometimes it can be difficult to dislodge the first nuclear fragment because it is wedged into place by the surrounding nucleus. To overcome this problem, Dr. Paul Koch developed his stop and chop method, which is described in Figure 2-13 (independently developed by Dr. Ronald Stasiuk as the mini-chop method). The initial groove formation allows sufficient room for dislodging and manipulating the nuclear halves as well as the fragments that were created by chopping.

Some generalizations can be made when comparing chopping techniques to cracking techniques. For example, chopping tends to stabilize the nucleus between the tip and the chopping instrument. Furthermore, mechanical force is directed centripetally as the chopping instrument cleaves the nucleus. Therefore, minimal force is directed outward against the capsule periphery. Contrast this to cracking methods, during which the nuclear periphery is pushed outward against the capsule by the cracking instruments; any defect in the capsulorhexis is therefore at greater risk for peripheral and posterior extension with cracking as opposed to chopping. Chopping is also a more efficient method than cracking with respect to ultrasound power expenditure because chopping uses mechanical force for nuclear segmentation as opposed to sculpting grooves; furthermore, ultrasound during chopping is most often applied in the more efficient occlusion mode (see Figure 1-45). Finally, chopping is a more time efficient method than cracking in that a segmenting chop can be made with a single instrument movement as opposed to multiple ultrasonic sculpting passes required for a groove; also, the smaller chopped fragments are more readily emulsified in a carouseling fashion with less repositioning required relative to larger quadrants (see Figure 3-31).

Two-Handed Technique

This designation actually applies to several methods, including most of the nuclear segmentation techniques. One hand manipulates the phaco handpiece while the other hand manipulates a second instrument, such as a cyclodialysis spatula, nucleus rotator, nucleus cracker, or chopping instrument. This second instrument is inserted through a side-port incision and is used to move the nucleus into optimum position for phacoemulsification. Although a two-handed technique is a virtual necessity for nuclear subdivision methods, it is often associated with Dr. Richard Kratz's method (popularized by Dr. William Maloney) of central sculpting followed by removal of the nuclear rim; this is followed by pushing inferiorly at the contra-incisional nuclear rim so that the sub-incisional rim can be prolapsed anteriorly and emulsified. The nucleus is then rotated and more rim is removed until only a nuclear plate remains. This plate is often free-floating and is emulsified by allowing it to carousel into the phaco tip. This sculpting-intensive method typically requires significantly more ultrasound energy for a given cataract than the occlusion-intensive methods such as chopping.

This method was originally described utilizing a can-opener type capsulotomy, which facilitated nuclear prolapse. However, this type of capsulotomy has several disadvantages. The loose tags of capsule often interfere with cortical removal by clogging the aspiration port. More importantly, it can lead to posterior capsular tears via extension along one of the anterior capsular can-opener tears. These difficulties can be eliminated by employing a continuous tear capsulotomy, or capsulorhexis, as described originally by Dr. Howard Gimbel and Dr. Thomas Neuhann. Although it is possible to perform a two-handed nuclear prolapse technique with a capsulorhexis, it is not generally recommended because of the inherent difficulty of prolapsing the nucleus through the capsulorhexis. However, in some cases involving a relatively large capsulorhexis, a thick epinucleus, and a distinct, smaller, inner nucleus, you can employ hydrodemarcation to prolapse the inner nucleus into the anterior chamber or iris plane. In these cases, this small inner nucleus can be emulsified by carouseling without rim removal or other manipulations. This is essentially Dr. Howard Fine's chip and flip method in which emulsification of the hydrodemarcated inner nucleus (the chip) is followed by removal of the epinuclear bowl by engaging the 6 o'clock anterior rim and pulling superiorly so as to flip it upside down in preparation for emulsification.

One-Handed Technique

Dr. Robert Sinskey originally developed this technique; it has been popularized by Dr. Marc Michelson and Dr. Richard Livernois. The method's name is a misnomer in that both hands are usually used to manipulate the phaco handpiece. Because there is no side-port incision or second instrument, all nuclear manipulations are performed with the phaco tip. Deep central sculpting is followed by nuclear rim removal and rotation, and ultimately by nuclear plate removal. Although the theoretical advantage of this method is additional control of the phaco handpiece, I feel that it is outweighed by the disadvantage of losing the additional nuclear manipulating capability afforded by a second instrument. However, one-handed techniques are sometimes useful on soft nuclei which are often difficult to rotate and crack with a second instrument.

Applying Fundamentals to All Methods

Sections One and Two have stressed the importance of appropriate machine parameter settings. Surgical technique is not only just as important, but is moreover integrally related. Smooth sculpting which avoids nuclear movement and zonular stress is critical to all methods. Well-controlled deep and peripheral sculpting facilitates cracking in segmentation methods and rim removal in one- and two-handed methods. By using just enough ultrasound power to embed the phaco tip and then backing off to the IA position (standard pedal position 2), the nucleus can be positively engaged for rotation, manipulation, etc; this extra versatility of the phaco tip is especially important for one-handed techniques as well as chopping techniques. The principles of mechanical advantage apply to all methods; safety is maximized by using the minimum force and movement required to accomplish a given task. Many of the examples and illustrations that follow depict a segmentation method, but each example is not so much a step in a phaco method as it is an illustration of a fundamental concept which is applicable to all methods. By understanding these concepts, the surgeon will be able to transpose as necessary between methods, improvise new methods, and adapt to virtually any surgical situation.

Sculpting Angle of Attack

As discussed previously, the ultrasonic needle operates like a jackhammer with oscillations occurring in an axial fashion as indicated by the green arrows. If the long axis of the needle were placed parallel to the surface to be sculpted as in Figure 3-1-1, the needle would simply vibrate back and forth over the surface without sculpting. Figure 3-1-2 shows how introducing an angle of attack takes advantage of the axial direction of needle vibration so that each vibration bites into the surface to be sculpted.

Figures 3-1-3 through 3-1-5 illustrate a clinical application of the above principle. This is a typical contour of a groove or bowl which is about two thirds completed. Note that areas A and B readily lend themselves to further sculpting given the favorable angle of attack. However, area C presents the same unfavorable tip to surface configuration as Figure 3-1-1. Area C can be readily sculpted if the nucleus is rotated 180° so that C is in the area formerly occupied by A; this contra-incisional position presents an optimum angle of attack and allows for completion of the groove, which is in turn a prerequisite for efficient nuclear cracking, which is in turn required for many nuclear subdivision methods.

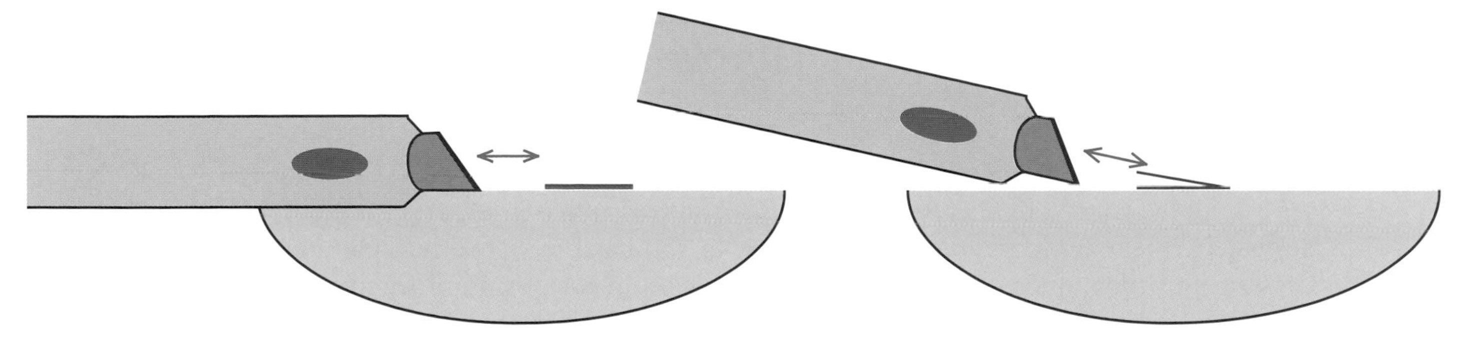

Figure 3-1-1 **Figure 3-1-2**

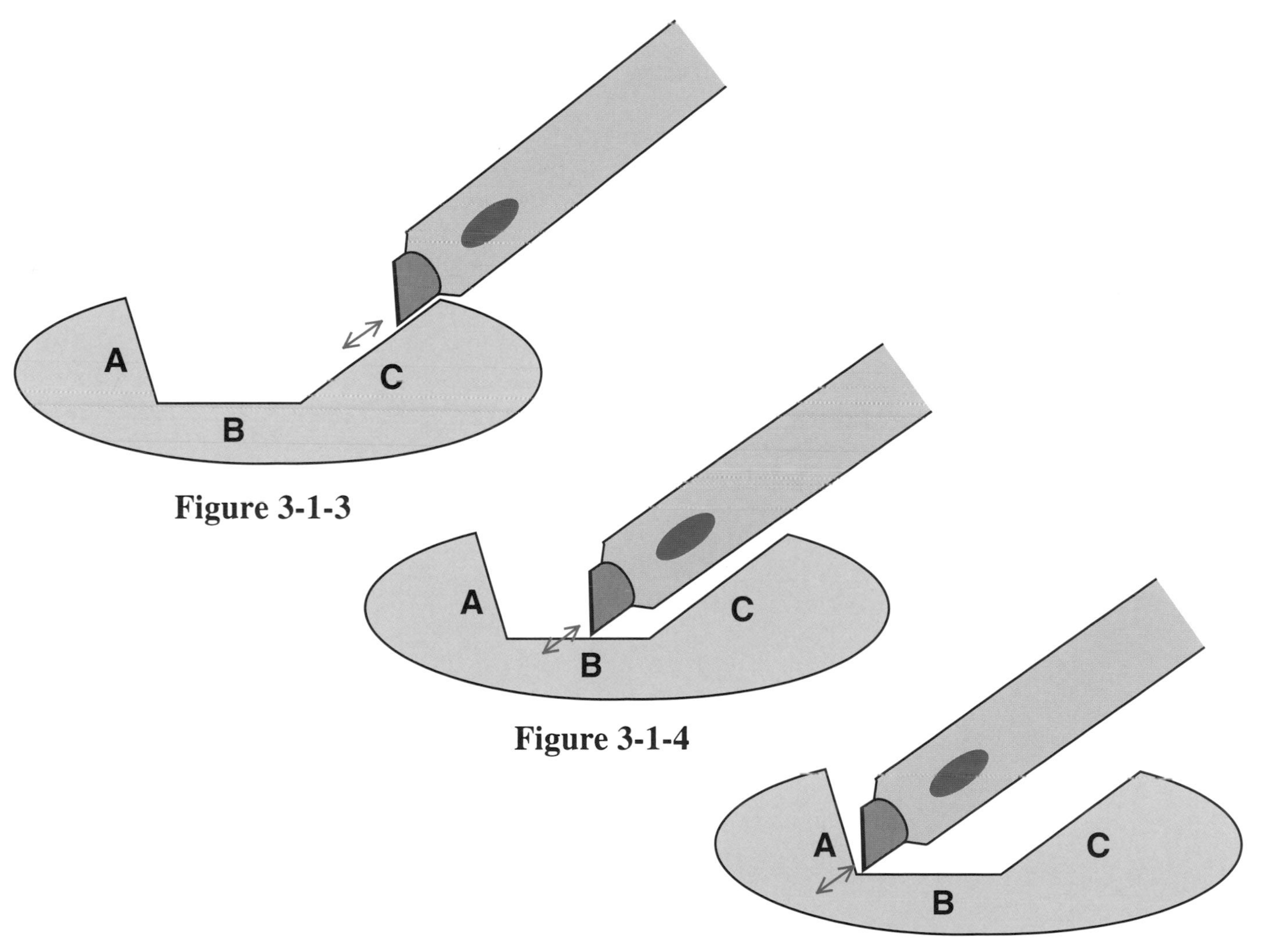

Figure 3-1-3

Figure 3-1-4

Figure 3-1-5

Figure 3-1

Minimum Groove Width

A rough rule of thumb for most phaco methods is that harder nuclei can potentially be sculpted more completely (ie, debulked) in early phases of the procedure. The rationale for leaving more nucleus initially with soft cataracts is to provide more of a handle with which to manipulate the nucleus in subsequent steps. For example, if a very wide groove is sculpted in a soft nucleus, the second instrument may simply cheese-wire through the little remaining nucleus without encountering enough resistance to induce nuclear rotation.

The reasoning behind minimum groove width involves potential impediments to sculpting, especially with harder nuclei. Simply glancing at Figure 3-2-1 would not indicate any reason why deeper sculpting could not occur. However, Figure 3-2-2 reveals that the phaco needle's silicone sleeve will not fit into the narrow groove. Always be aware of this potential obstruction. Otherwise, you may try to compensate by using unnecessarily high ultrasound power or pushing the handpiece harder and stressing zonules. Neither of these solutions will overcome the problem; you simply have to widen the groove before proceeding deeper as depicted in Figure 3-2-3. This maneuver readily exposes the nucleus to further sculpting by the emulsifying action of the tip without obstruction from the non-emulsifying silicone sleeve.

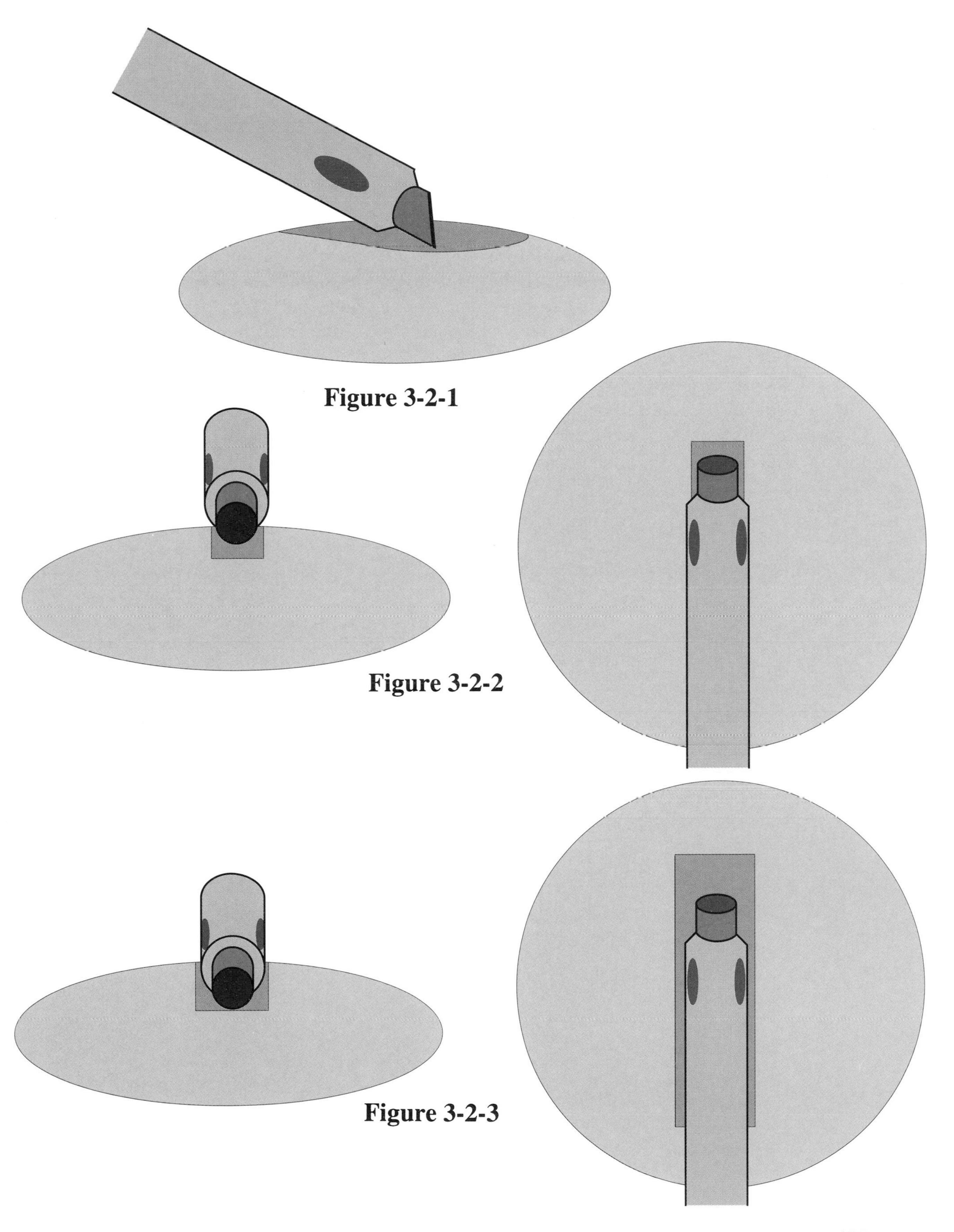
Figure 3-2-1

Figure 3-2-2

Figure 3-2-3

Figure 3-2

Posterior Groove

Although the groove may be wide enough for the complete phaco tip and sleeve (Figure 3-3-1), the posterior contour may be such that it obstructs the silicone sleeve and prevents further posterior sculpting (Figure 3-3-2). This is simply an extension of the concept of maintaining an adequate minimum groove width, but it can be more misleading when more than half of the groove depth is sculpted because it appears that the groove width is adequate from your anterior microscope's perspective since the sleeve seems to be fitting down into the groove. Only by careful attention to the posterior contour can this potential pitfall be noticed and rectified as in Figures 3-3-3 and 3-3-4. The techniques utilized to correct the posterior contour are essentially the same as those used to widen the peripheral groove contour in Figure 3-8.

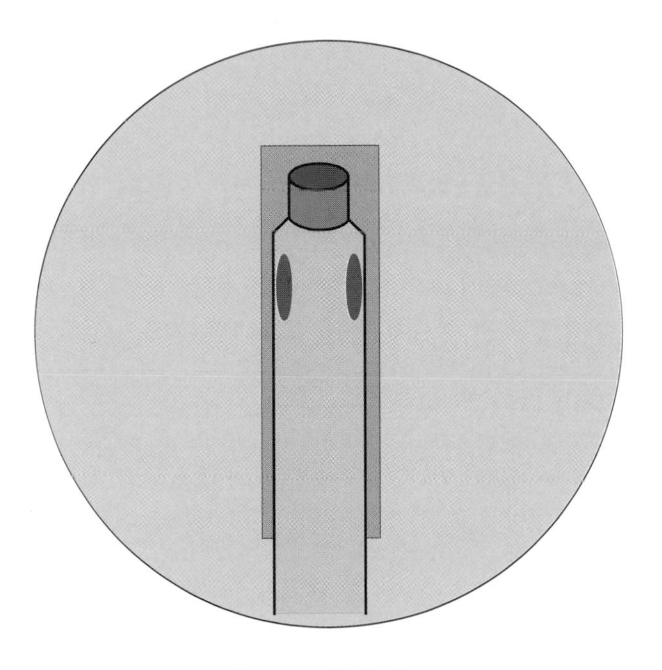

Figure 3-3-1

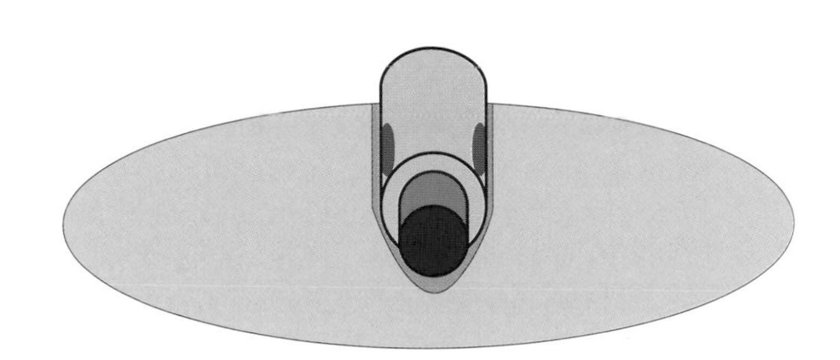

Figure 3-3-2

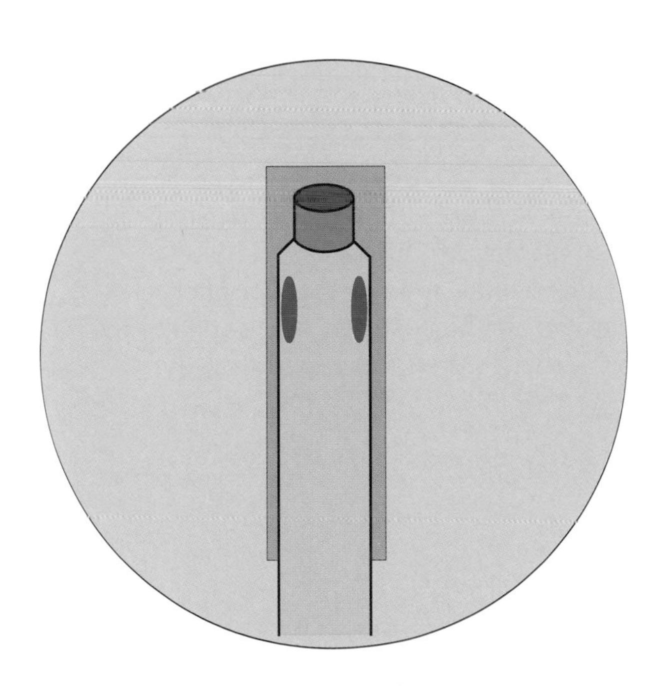

Figure 3-3-3

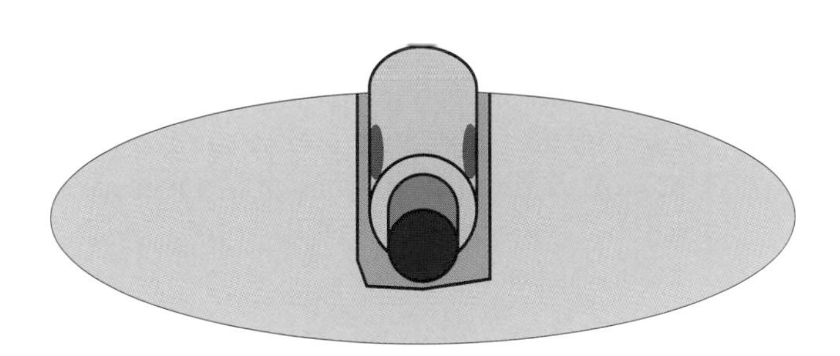

Figure 3-3-4

Figure 3-3

Judging Groove Depth

One of the most prominent fears of the beginning phaco surgeon is sculpting too deeply and inadvertently rupturing capsule. The tendency is to think one may have sculpted a Grand Canyon, when in reality the nucleus receives little more than an abrasion. Just as when using insufficient phaco power, sculpting inadequately gives only a false sense of security and in fact makes all subsequent steps more difficult; both nuclear cracking and rim removal are most efficiently accomplished after deep sculpting.

There are several ways for you to judge groove (or nuclear bowl sculpting) depth. Good stereopsis is facilitated by using lower rather than higher microscope magnifications so that the depth of field is maximized. The red reflex typically gets brighter where sculpting has reduced the thickness of nucleus which the microscope light must traverse. This technique is especially effective when the cataract has significant nuclear sclerosis; the change in brightness with progressive sculpting is not as evident with a posterior subcapsular opacity with minimal or no nuclear sclerosis. A useful technique for judging depth with posterior cortical or subcapsular opacities is utilizing parallax; gently manipulate the nucleus from side to side and observe the movement of the posterior opacities relative to the base of your groove. With decreasing nuclear thickness separating the groove base and the opacities, the opacities will move less relative to the groove base with induced parallax (Figures 3-4-1 and 3-4-2).

The groove depth can be directly measured using the phaco needle as the unit of measurement. Recall that a standard phaco needle is approximately 1mm in outer diameter (make sure you know the measurement for any needle that you are using). Since the average adult anterior-posterior lens diameter is about 4mm, the phaco needle can be used to estimate the groove depth as shown in Figure 3-4-3. A measure that accounts for possibly thick epinucleus and provides a good safety margin for most cases is two to three needle widths centrally and one to two needle widths toward the periphery. Remember that the contour of your groove must approximate the posterior convexity of the lens; your groove will therefore by definition be deeper centrally than peripherally.

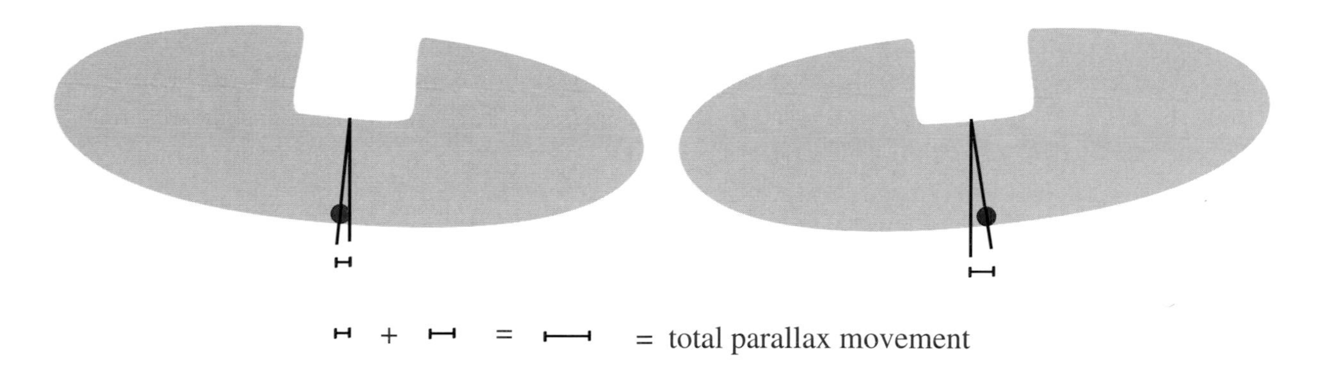

Figure 3-4-1

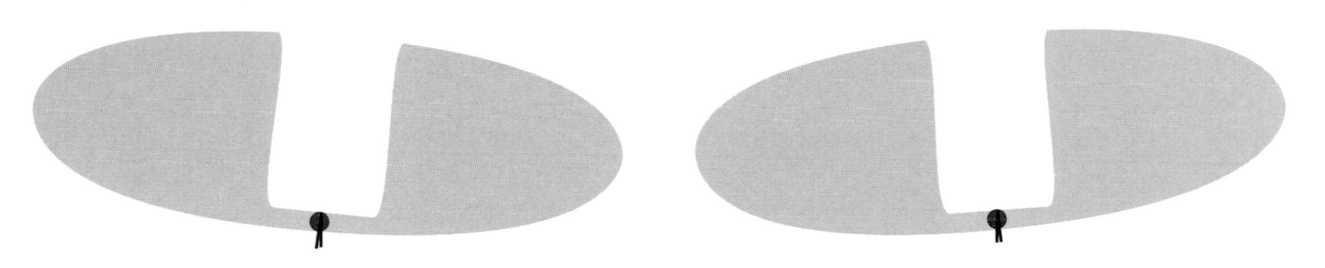

total parallax movement is negligible with deep sculpting

Figure 3-4-2

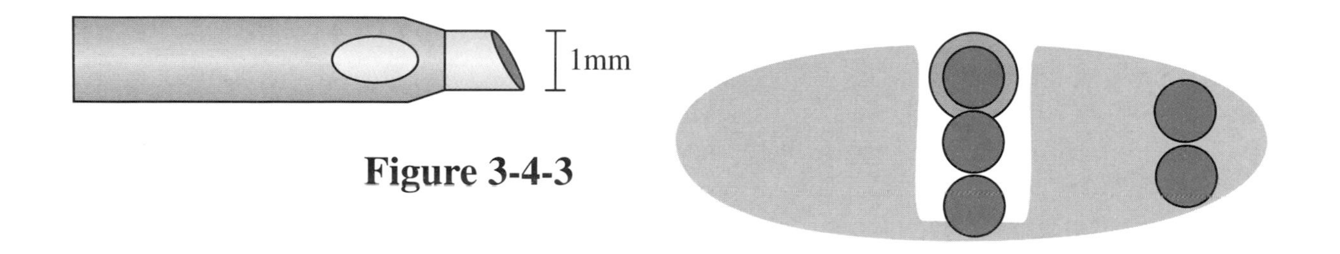

Figure 3-4-3

Figure 3-4

Peripheral Groove

Figure 3-5-1 depicts a physical impediment to further peripheral sculpting because of the silicone sleeve being obstructed by too narrow a peripheral groove; please note that this identical configuration could be present if you simply buried the needle into the face of a nuclear half in preparation for making a quadranting groove. The problem is readily fixed by widening the groove to allow further peripheral extension (Figure 3-5-2). How far do you extend it? The circular "golden reflex" of the hydrodemarcation provides a useful guide; it separates the harder inner nucleus from the soft epinucleus. Because the epinucleus is usually removed relatively easily as a pliable bowl at the end of phacoemulsification, it is unnecessary to sculpt into it beforehand; moreover, the epinucleus serves to keep the capsule protected and formed, and should therefore be left intact and undisturbed for as much of the operation as possible. The object of initial sculpting in any method is to prepare the inner nucleus for fracturing or rim removal. Therefore, the hydrodemarcation reflex marks a functional limit for peripheral extension (of the groove in a cracking method or of central sculpting in a Kratz method or one-handed method).

In Figure 3-5-3, the above objectives have been accomplished. Although the silicone sleeve would obstruct further peripheral sculpting, there is no need to widen the peripheral groove because there is no need for further peripheral groove extension. There are several potential outcomes if you ignore this fact and attempt to overcome the sleeve obstruction simply by maintaining or increasing ultrasound power and/or pushing the handpiece harder. The best possible outcome in this case would be for nothing to happen. More probable outcomes include zonular stress and tears, extension of pre-existing capsular tears (especially with can-opener capsulotomies), and creation of new capsular tears. Finally, because the phaco aspiration port is against the soft epinucleus, increasing power will easily emulsify and aspirate it, thus exposing the peripheral capsule to aspiration and rupture (Figure 3-5-4). The message to take home is that Figure 3-5-3 is a good endpoint for peripheral extension of a groove (either half or quadrant). Notwithstanding the foregoing, some cataracts may crack sufficiently with the groove just short of the hydrodemarcation line, as in Figure 3-5-1. If cracking does not occur at this point, the groove can be extended to the line as described, but not beyond it. Move on from this point to subsequent steps in your procedure, such as completing the groove 180° away or proceeding with fracturing.

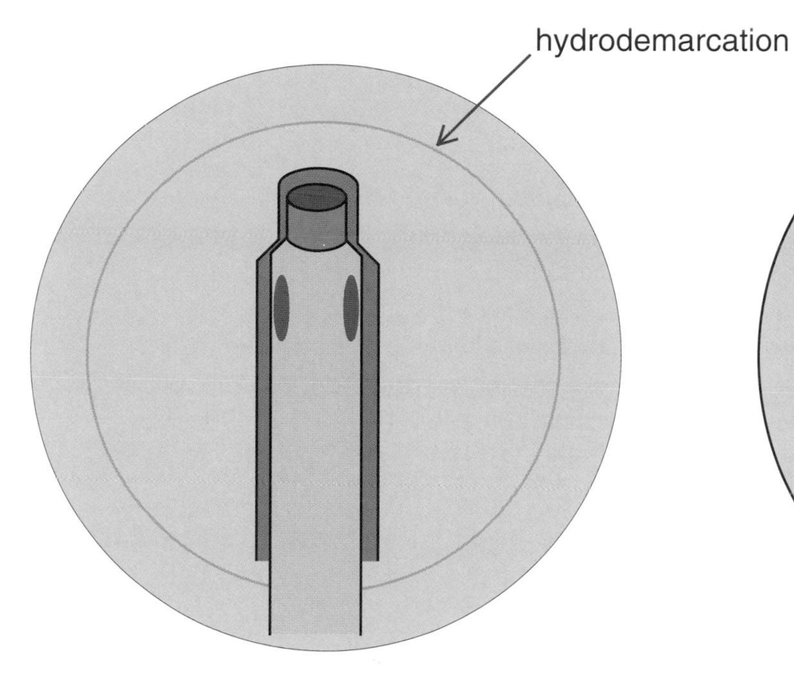

Figure 3-5-1

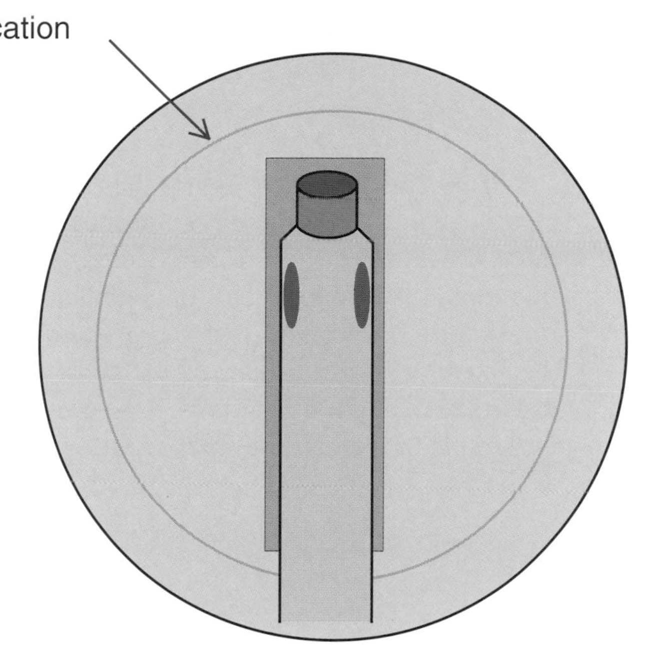

Figure 3-5-2

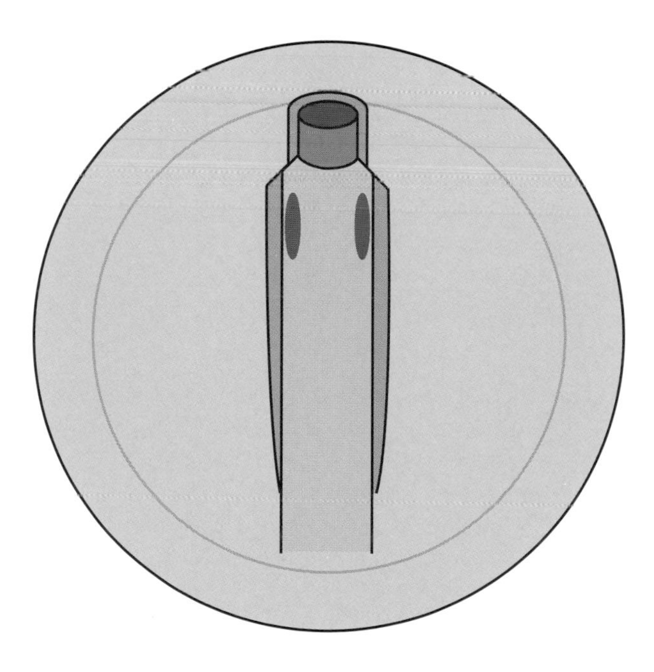

Figure 3-5-3

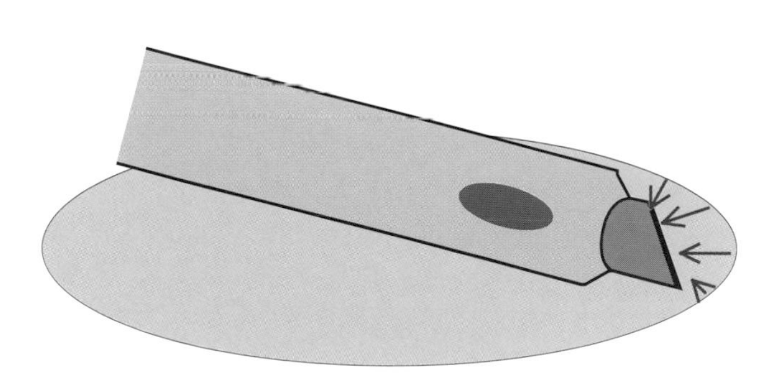

Figure 3-5-4

Figure 3-5

Physical Obstructions to Sculpting

The silicone sleeve is not the only physical impediment to free movement of the phaco needle. A decentered or misshapen lid speculum can catch on the hub of the phaco tip as illustrated in Figure 3-6. Similarly, the hub or handpiece can run into a fold of the lid drape. Insufficient slack in the handpiece tubing can also limit your mobility.

If phaco sculpting is not proceeding smoothly, there is always a reason. Look for the above possibilities as well as the factors concerning adequate groove dimensions as discussed in previous sections. Assess the phaco power variables (see Figure 2-8). Phaco is a gentle procedure; never force it!

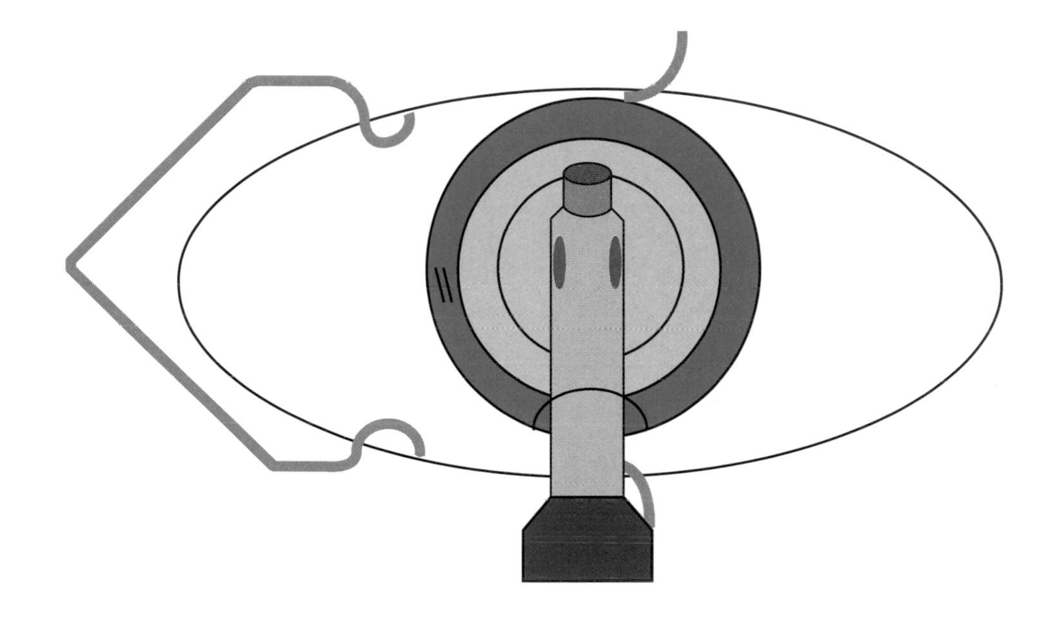

Figure 3-6

Use Low Scope Magnification

Most beginning phaco surgeons err on the side of overmagnification; the rationale behind this false sense of security is that it focuses the surgeon's concentration. It is precisely this concentrated focus which leads to problems by limiting awareness of other aspects of the procedure. Note how the limited field of view with high magnification in Figure 3-7-1 does not readily reveal the cause of an obstruction in the tip's mobility. Figure 3-7-2 (lower magnification with wider field of view) shows that the problem is the speculum as described previously. A wide field of view allows you to detect nuclear movement when sculpting so that you can adjust power, amount of tip engaged, or linear sculpting velocity as necessary. Capsular star folds from inadvertent aspiration and corneal stress lines from excessive wound distortion are both more evident with a wider field of view. Low magnification has an added advantage of providing increased depth of field. This will facilitate judging the depth and contour of grooves; it will also reduce surgeon fatigue by decreasing the amount of focus adjustments required.

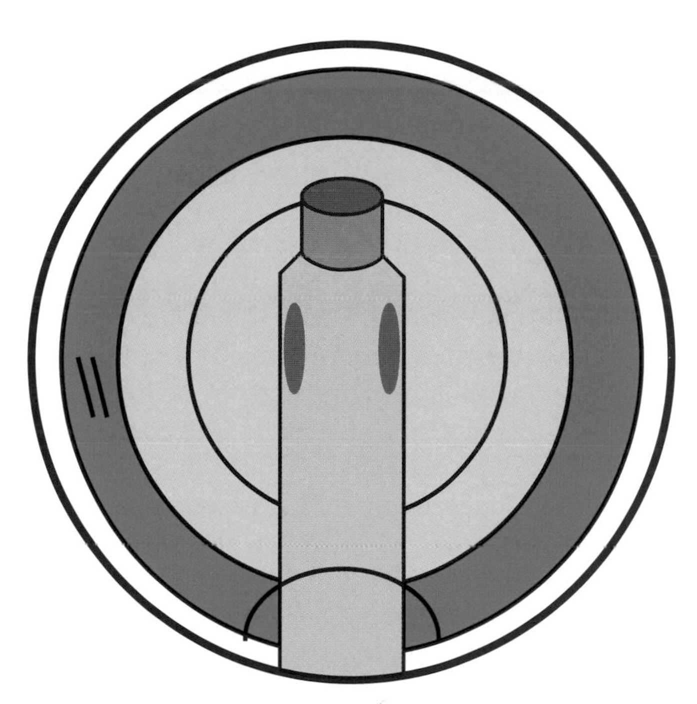

Figure 3-7-1

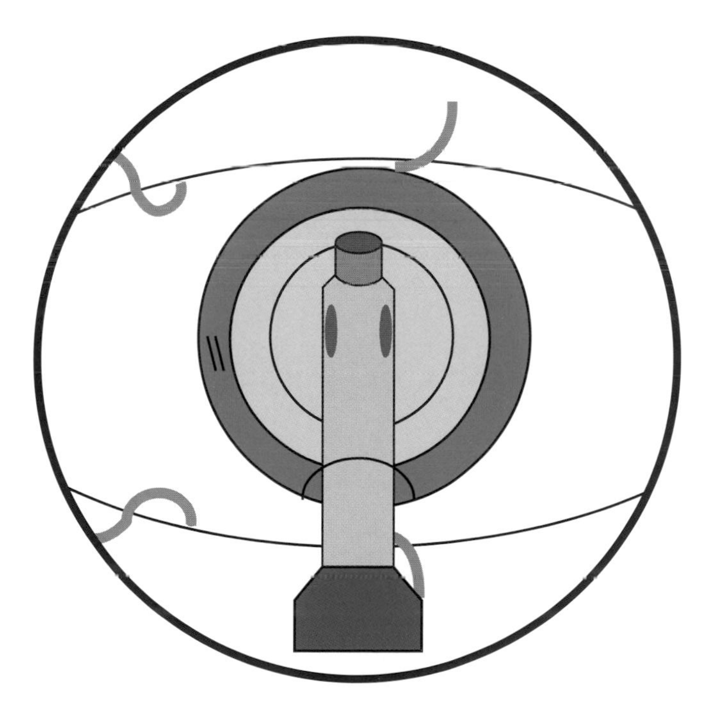

Figure 3-7-2

Figure 3-7

Tip Manipulations for Sculpting Groove

These figures address the logistics of maintaining adequate groove width. Figure 3-8-1 shows the phaco tip at one side of the groove in an attempt to sculpt more at the corner on that side. Note the distance from the end of the phaco tip to the desired end-point of groove width (red line). Figure 3-8-2 closes the distance slightly by pivoting the tip within the groove. The handpiece has been rotated 45° counterclockwise and placed against the side of the groove in Figure 3-8-3. Finally, the combination of tip rotation and pivoting in Figure 3-8-4 achieves the closest approach to the desired width of the groove. Although you will often sculpt intuitively, it is sometimes helpful to remember these fundamental techniques when having difficulty reaching a particular portion of your groove. Note that a beveled needle is used for these illustrations; a 0° tip would not require any rotation as the red line (indicating the most distal extension of the tip) would be drawn to the outer edge of the 0° tip, as opposed to the middle of the beveled tip.

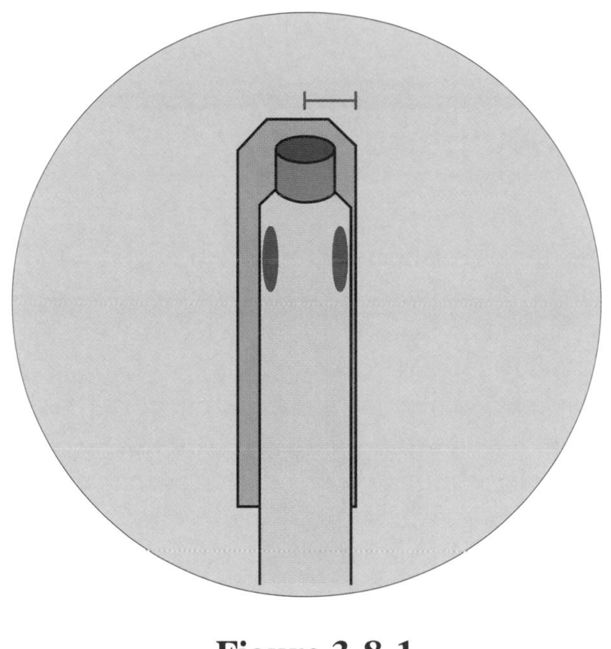

Figure 3-8-1

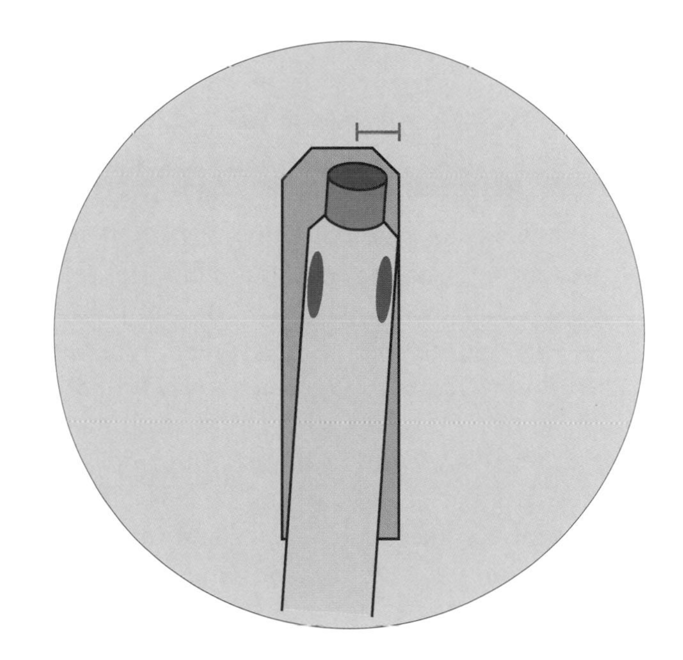

Figure 3-8-2

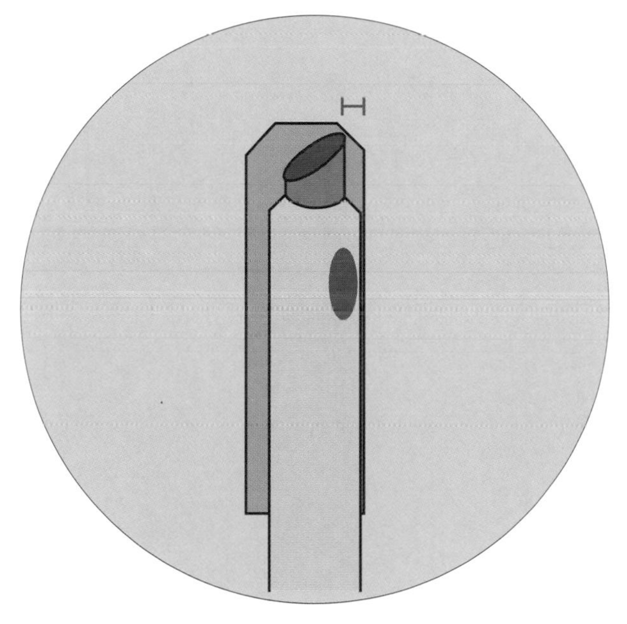

Figure 3-8-3

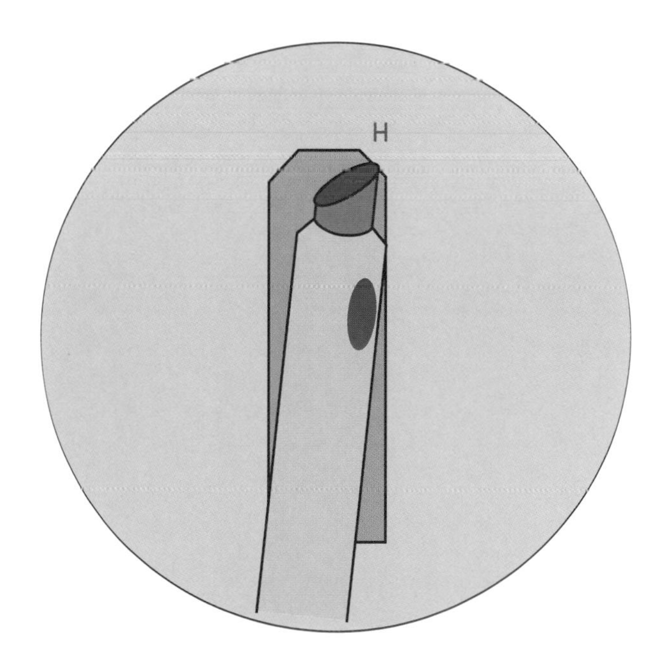

Figure 3-8-4

Figure 3-8

Avoiding Iris During Sculpting

Atrophic iris around the incision was once a hallmark of many early phaco cases utilizing older machines and techniques. This complication more typically shows up contra-incisionally with current techniques. These patients will return to haunt you at regular postop intervals; the magnified slit-lamp view of tattered edges of atrophic iris will bring back unpleasant memories of how they sought out your aspiration port throughout the surgery after the initial aspiration made that whole portion of the iris floppy. Fortunately, this complication can be practically eliminated by the following technique. Figure 3-9-1 shows the initial sculpting stopping well short of the iris (and capsulorhexis edge). This peripheral limit is respected as sculpting progresses deeper in Figure 3-9-2. Only in Figure 3-9-3 does sculpting progress peripherally; note the protective layer of anterior epinucleus which serves as a buffer between the tip and iris. Remember, it is unnecessary and often disadvantageous to remove the soft epinucleus during initial sculpting and emulsification of the inner nucleus. The epinucleus serves as a safety buffer not only for the iris but also for the capsule. This concept of iris protection is extended even further with the fault-line phaco technique (see Figures 3-21 and 3-22).

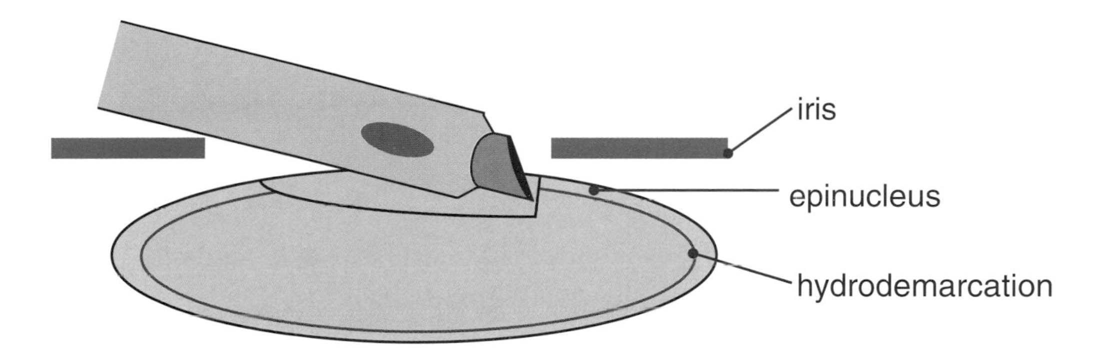

Figure 3-9-1

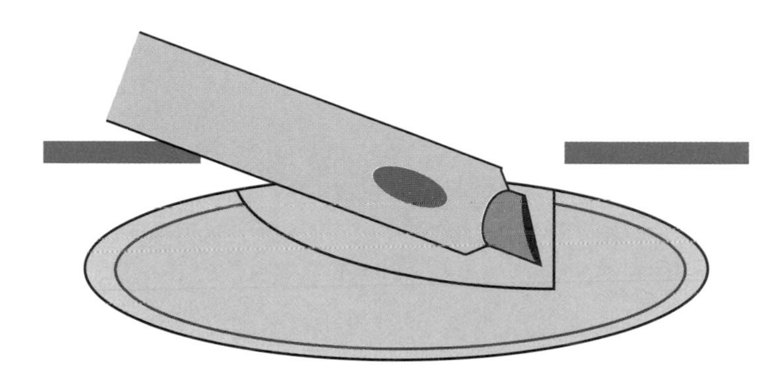

Figure 3-9-2

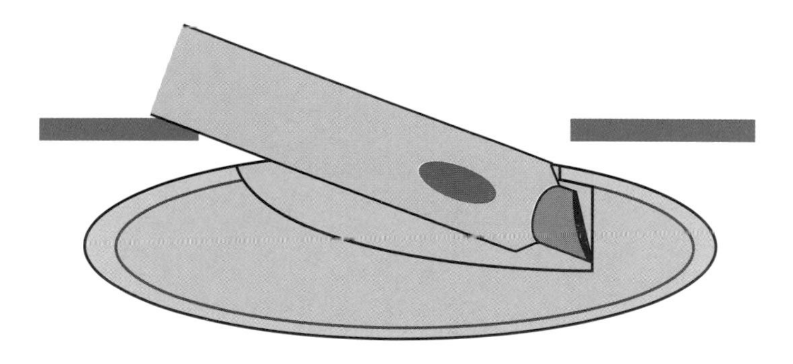

Figure 3-9-3

Figure 3-9

Layers of the Lens

Figure 3-10 shows a typical "lens within a lens" configuration with a distinct harder inner nucleus surrounded by a softer epinucleus; this appearance is typically evident on preoperative slit-lamp examination. An irrigation cannula is optimally introduced at the junction between the two to perform **hydrodemarcation** (also known as **hydrodelineation**), which facilitates free inner nuclear rotation. Hydrodemarcation also delineates the epinucleus, which helps to protect the capsule during inner nuclear manipulation and emulsification. Even relatively homogeneous nuclei are denser in the center, and hydrodemarcation can create an artifactual plane to achieve the same benefits of free inner nuclear rotation and epinuclear formation. The exception to this would be a brunescent cataract which often has very little epinucleus or cortex—Hydrosonics® may be effective in these cases. Note that the proper cannula placement for **hydrodissection** is just inside of the capsule; this will facilitate cortical and epinuclear removal as well as nuclear rotation. To the extent that the cortex is first hydrodynamically dissected, less effort is required when using the IA tip for cortical removal. Indeed, the cortex is sometimes readily removed during the aspiration of the epinucleus. Dr. I. Howard Fine coined the phrase "cortical cleaving hydrodissection" to describe this methodology.

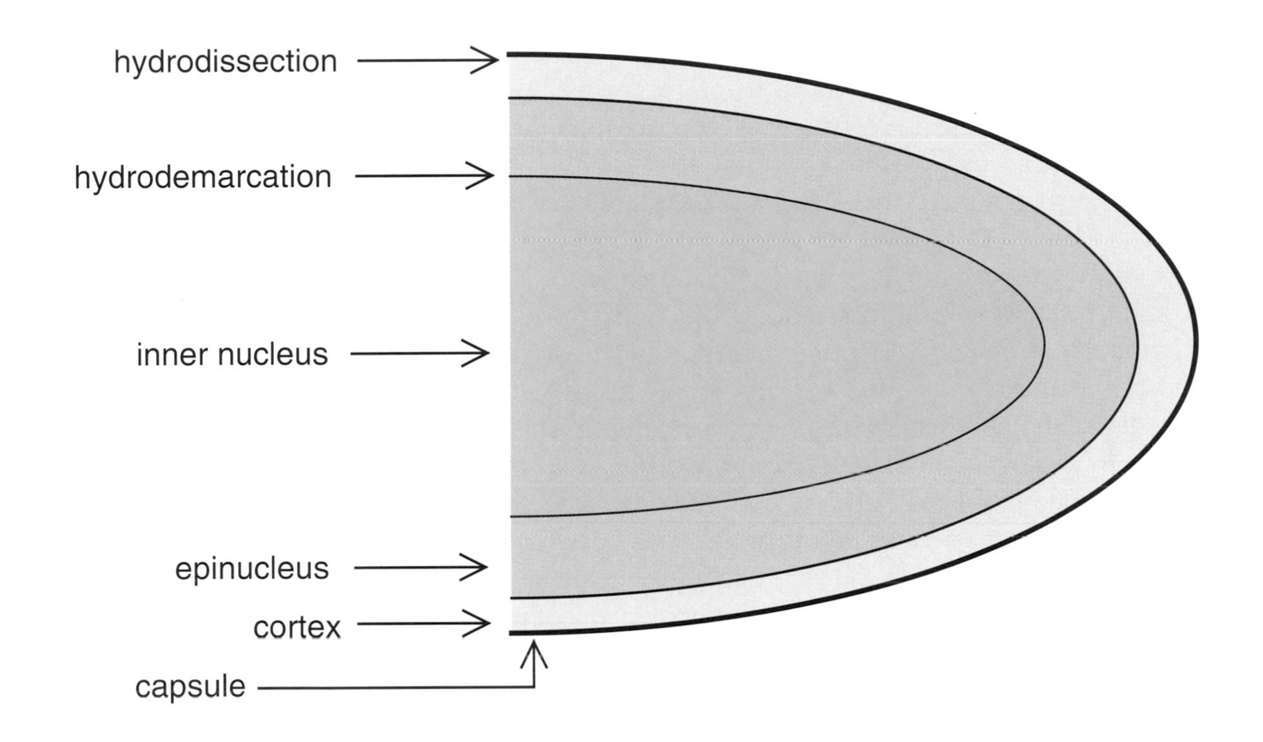
hydrodissection
hydrodemarcation
inner nucleus
epinucleus
cortex
capsule

Figure 3-10

Hydrodissection Fluid Dynamics

This technique utilizes a pressurized fluid wave (usually from an irrigating syringe and a 27-gauge cannula) to disrupt the adhesions between the capsule and cortex as illustrated in Figure 3-10. Once the initial adhesion is overcome and a dissection plane is established, hydrodissection requires less pressure on the syringe because of the inertia of the advancing fluid wave; therefore, try to complete the procedure in one step with steady pressure on the syringe as opposed to intermittent pulses which will require increased starting pressure each time to reestablish fluid wave inertia. Use just enough pressure to maintain this inertia. Less pressure would not accomplish the goal of a steady convex fluid wave passing across the posterior surface of the lens (Figure 3-11-1). More pressure might compromise the posterior capsule or abruptly eject the nucleus into the anterior chamber. Although this latter result might have seemed advantageous in the days of anterior chamber phaco, it now would require an additional step of using viscoelastic to replace the lens in the bag to facilitate the safer in-the-bag or even iris plane techniques. This principle of maintaining fluid wave inertia applies just as readily to hydrodemarcation as it does to hydrodissection.

Although it is possible to perform hydrodissection with a can-opener capsulotomy, it is far more efficient with a capsulorhexis because the intact capsular edge provides a good seal against backflow of fluid. However, even with this advantage, cannula placement is important. Note the three potential cannula positions in Figure 3-11-1; each one represents good placement in that the tip is well under the capsulorhexis and oriented perpendicular to its edge. Now look at Figure 3-11-2; each represents suboptimal placement which allows the fluid to follow a path of least resistance by refluxing into the anterior chamber instead of proceeding posteriorly with hydrodissection (see curved blue arrows). Cannula A is not placed far enough under the lip of the capsulorhexis. Cannula B is almost tangent to the capsulorhexis edge rather than perpendicular. Cannula C combines both bad aspects of cannulas A and B. Furthermore, the off-axis cannula positioning in Figure 3-11-2 (B and C) is more likely to allow the nucleus to inadvertently pivot anteriorly around them, as opposed to the central positioning of the cannulas in Figure 3-11-1, which tends to hold the nucleus in place during hydrodissection or hydrodelineation. Although these principles of fluid dynamics and optimal cannula placement are described above for hydrodissection, they will also facilitate efficient hydrodemarcation.

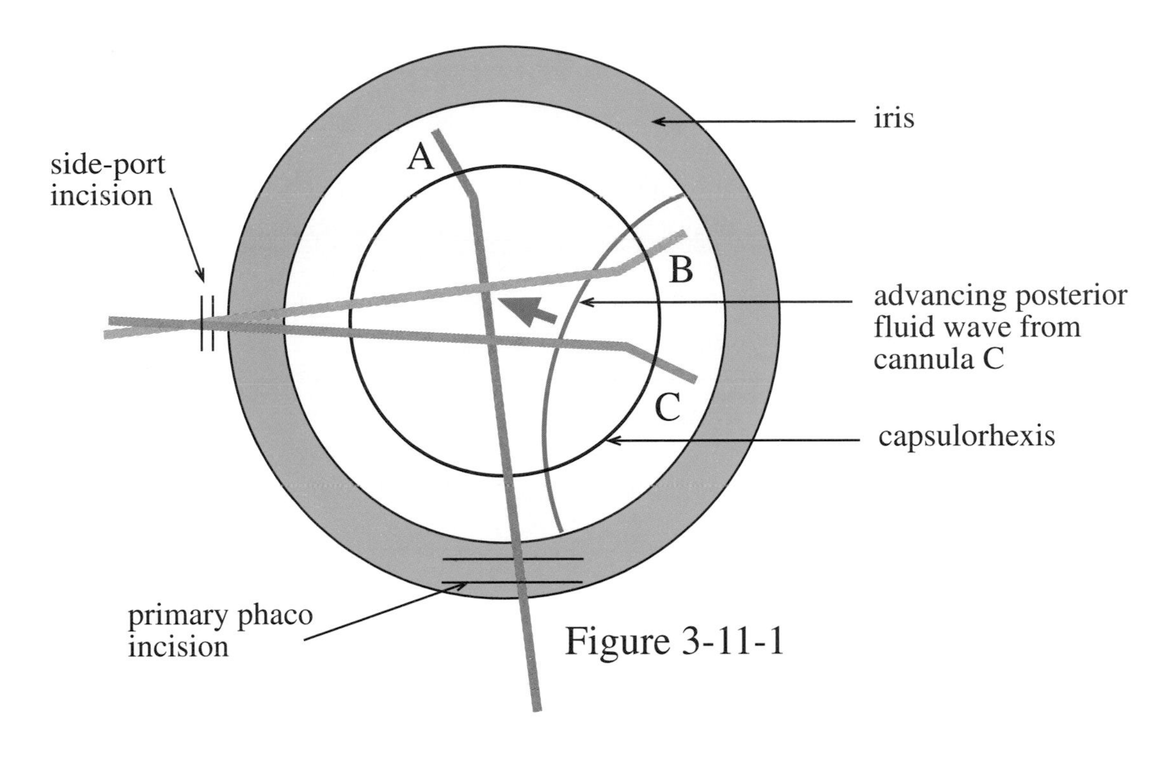

Figure 3-11-1

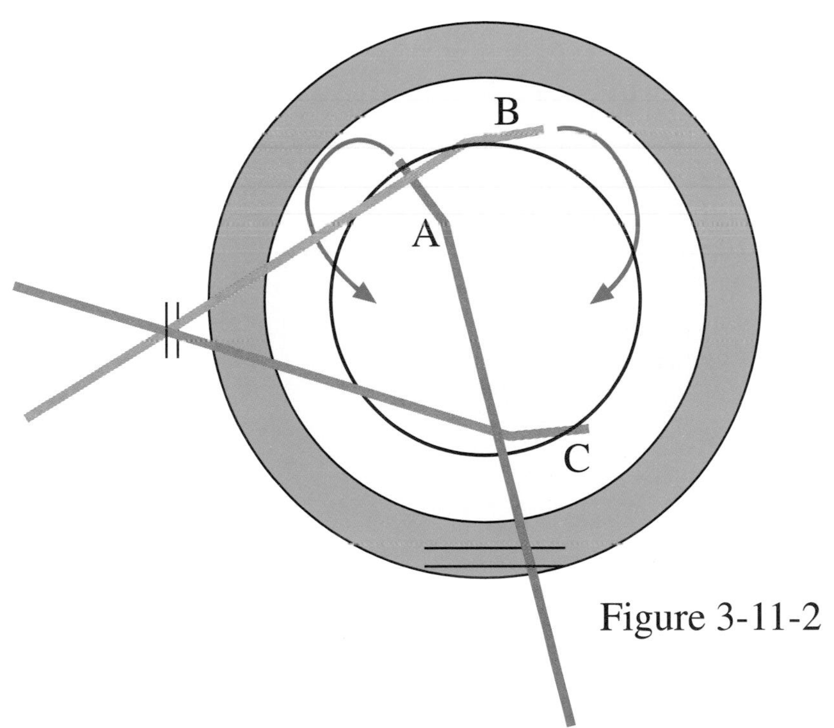

Figure 3-11-2

Figure 3-11

Nuclear Rotation: Torque Principles

I know you thought you had seen the last of physics when you finished the MCAT, but applying a few basic principles of torque and vector force analysis will greatly augment your understanding of many fundamental surgical techniques. Figure 3-12 depicts a nucleus with a groove carved from 6 to 12 o'clock; in order to most efficiently rotate it, we have to review the definition of torque:

torque = force • lever arm

where the lever arm is the distance from the axis of rotation to the point at which turning force is applied.

A force applied at point A, as indicated by the red vector arrow, does not produce any torque because its distance from the axis of rotation is 0.

torque = force • lever arm = force • 0 = 0

A force applied at point B or C produces twice as much torque it would were it applied at point D.

torque (B or C) = force • 2y = 2(force • y)
torque (D) = force • 1y = 1(force • y)

Similarly, twice as much force would be needed at point D in order to produce the same torque as a given force at point B or C.

Clinical corollary: When a certain amount of torque is necessary to rotate a nucleus, it is safest and most efficient to achieve this torque with the longest possible lever arm and correspondingly least applied intraocular force.

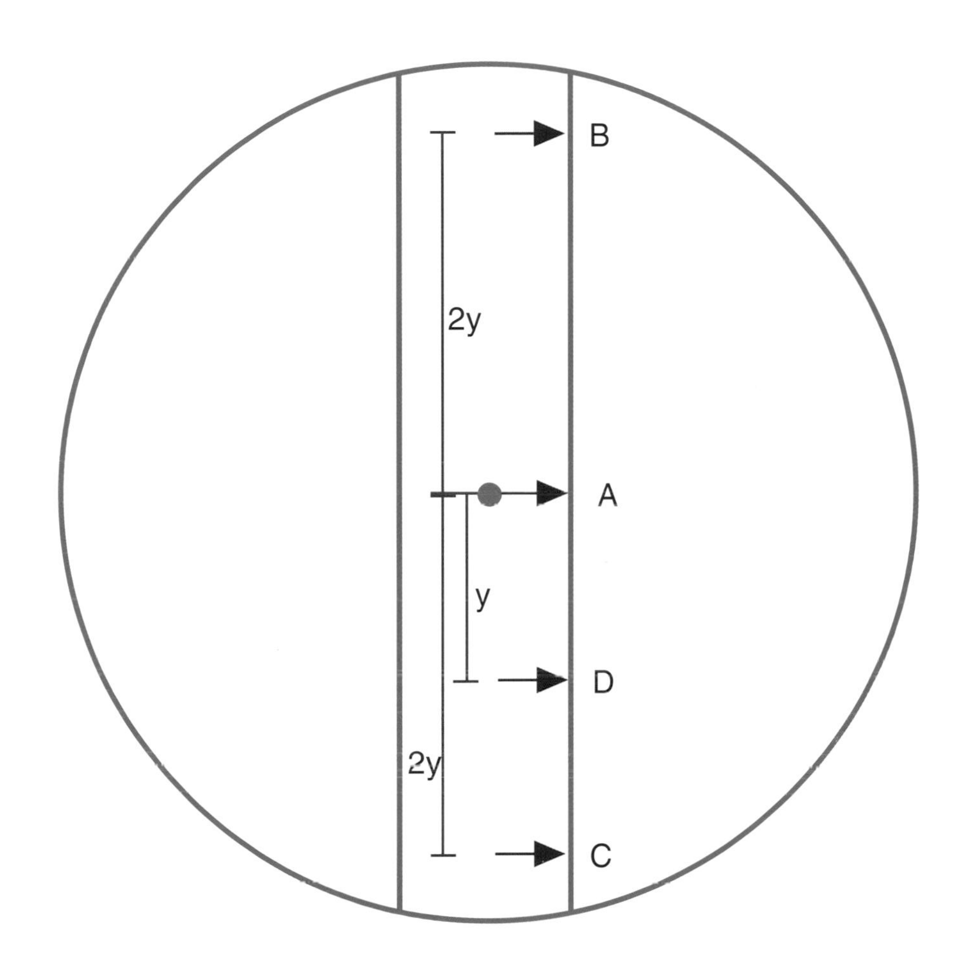

Figure 3-12

Nuclear Rotation: Clinical Application of Torque

There are several reasons why the initial groove in a quadrant/divide procedure is longer (more peripheral) at the contra-incisional position than at the sub-incisional position. One reason concerns the phaco needle angle of attack as discussed earlier in this section (see Figure 3-1). Another reason is illustrated in Figures 3-13-1 and 3-13-2; note that even with the grossly exaggerated phaco handpiece positioning shown in Figure 3-13-2, it is still impossible to sculpt as peripherally sub-incisionally relative to contra-incisionally. The nucleus may need to be rotated 180° in order to complete this groove prior to making the first nuclear crack. Figure 3-13-3 shows a nucleus manipulation instrument inserted through a side-port incision. The nucleus can be rotated either clockwise if the instrument is pushed against point A, or counterclockwise with the spatula pushing against point B. By applying the torque schematic in Figure 3-12, it can be seen that a given force will produce twice as much torque at point A relative to point B; therefore the best mechanical advantage can be achieved in this situation with clockwise rotation as illustrated in Figure 3-13-4. Note the pivoting of the spatula around the side-port incision so as to avoid wound distortion (see Figures 3-35 and 3-36).

Soft to medium density nuclei especially benefit from the above concept for two reasons. First, the cortex is more adhesive in these cases and consequently tends to resist initial nuclear rotation sometimes even after hydrodissection. Second, an instrument can push against a soft to medium density nucleus only up to a certain amount of force, past which the instrument will start to penetrate the nucleus without applying any further pushing force (see Figure 3-16). Multiplying this maximum possible force by the longest possible lever arm produces the maximum potential torque, whereas trying to obtain this same torque with a shorter lever arm would result in the instrument penetrating the nucleus, and possibly the capsule!

Each particular nucleus requires a certain amount of torque for rotation. Use the above principles to most efficiently apply this torque with the least possible intraocular force; using more force or torque than necessary decreases your safety margin.

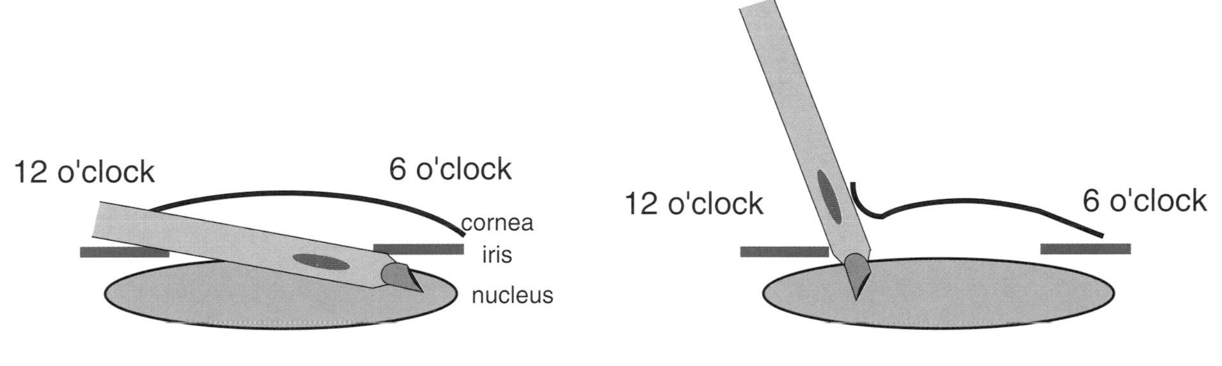

Figure 3-13-1

Figure 3-13-2

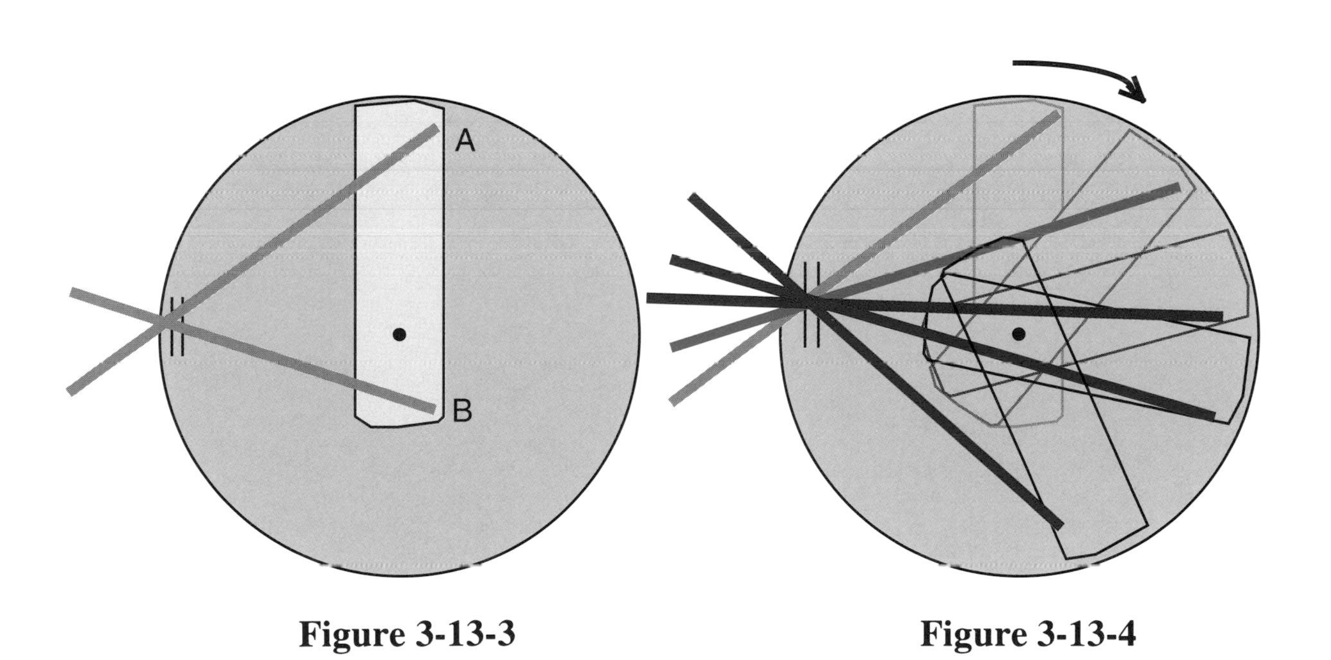

Figure 3-13-3

Figure 3-13-4

Figure 3-13

Rotating Nucleus: Pulling with Phaco Tip

As discussed several times in Section One, the phaco tip's aspiration port must first be completely occluded in order to obtain a vacuum seal before the occluding material can be manipulated (ie, rotated). An important consideration with this technique is the angle of the phaco needle bevel relative to the surface to be occluded (see Figures 1-47a and 1-47b). Figure 3-14 shows a nuclear bowl (ie, after central sculpting as in a one-handed method) which needs to be rotated, although these principles apply equally well to manipulating nuclear halves and quadrants as well as a thick epinuclear bowl. Tip A is incompletely embedded into the inner wall of the nuclear rim. Because the aspiration port is exposed to the anterior chamber where indicated by arrow x, vacuum cannot build adequately (see Figures 1-10, 1-24, and 1-25); pulling the tip would simply pull the tip out of the rim rather than rotating or pulling the nuclear rim. Maintaining the same tip orientation, but placed slightly to the left of tip A's position, tip B completely embeds the aspiration port within the nuclear rim. With this occlusion, vacuum can build and the phaco tip can be used as a handle to manipulate the attached nuclear bowl. Note that tip C is also completely embedded into the nuclear rim; however, the tip of the phaco needle is dangerously close to the nuclear periphery and capsule (see arrow z); furthermore, the vacuum seal is marginal because of the proximity of the aspiration port to the anterior chamber fluid at arrow y (see A-1 and A-2 in Figure 3-28). By rotating the tip 180° so that the bevel would be parallel to the surface of the inner rim at this position, a more efficient and safer complete occlusion like tip B could have been accomplished; this principle is essentially the same as that which was discussed with Figures 1-47a and 1-47b.

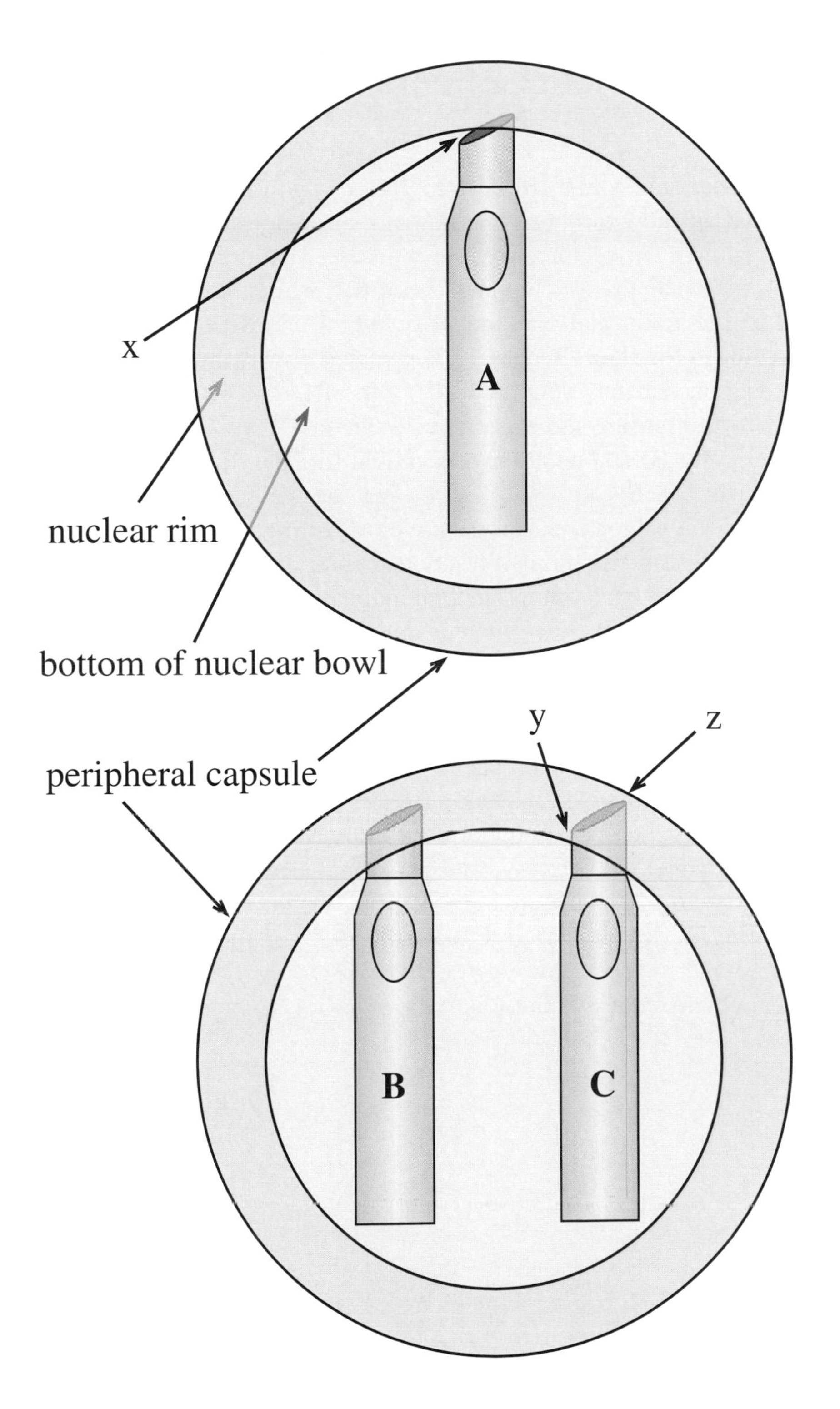
x
A
nuclear rim
bottom of nuclear bowl
peripheral capsule
y
z
B
C

Figure 3-14

Rotating Nucleus: Effects of Friction

Figure 3-15-1 demonstrates why it is easier to pull a wagon rather than to push it. Vector force A is applied as shown to push the wagon over a floor. Recall that vectors are comprised of their component vector forces. In this case, vector A is directed downward at a 45° angle and is made up of component vector B, which is in the direction of pushing and parallel to the floor, and component C, which is directed straight down against and perpendicular to the floor. Because C is directed downward, it increases the friction between the wagon and the floor as well as the friction of the axles on the wheels. Compare this to the pulling force exerted by vector D, which has component vectors E (identical to vector B) and component F (equal in magnitude but opposite in direction relative to vector C). Because F is decreasing the weight of the wagon and thereby reducing friction, the wagon is easier to move by pulling.

These principles can be directly applied to nuclear rotation as shown in Figure 3-15-2. In this case we are using a quadranting method and have already removed the first two quadrants. We now want to rotate the nucleus counterclockwise within the epinuclear bowl so that its flat surface will face the surgeon to allow sculpting of the last quadranting groove. If phaco needle Y is used to push the nucleus around with vector force D, component force F will increase the friction between the nucleus and epinucleus. However, by pulling the nucleus with vector force A, component vector C serves to decrease friction and facilitate rotation. Taking friction into account is especially important with softer nuclei which have stickier adhesions between nucleus, epinucleus, and cortex; this can be true even after hydrodissection and hydrodemarcation. Note that rotating component vectors E and B are equivalent. Also note that when the phaco needle is used for pushing, it does not need to be embedded completely as is the case for pulling (see Figure 3-14); indeed, pushing should be performed in pedal position 1 as opposed to pulling which requires pump activity to produce vacuum and holding force (position 2).

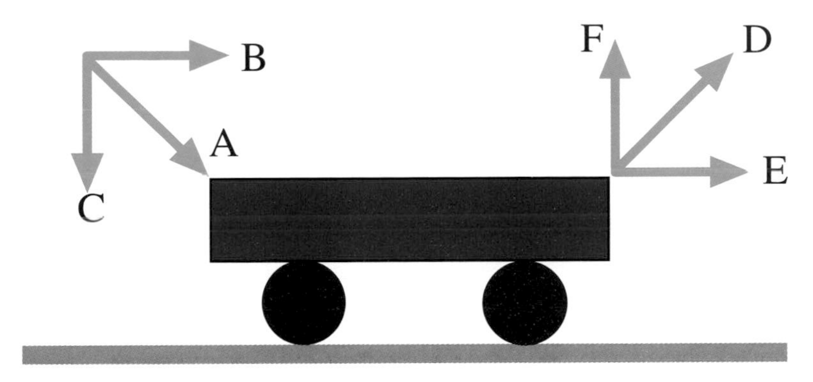

Figure 3-15-1

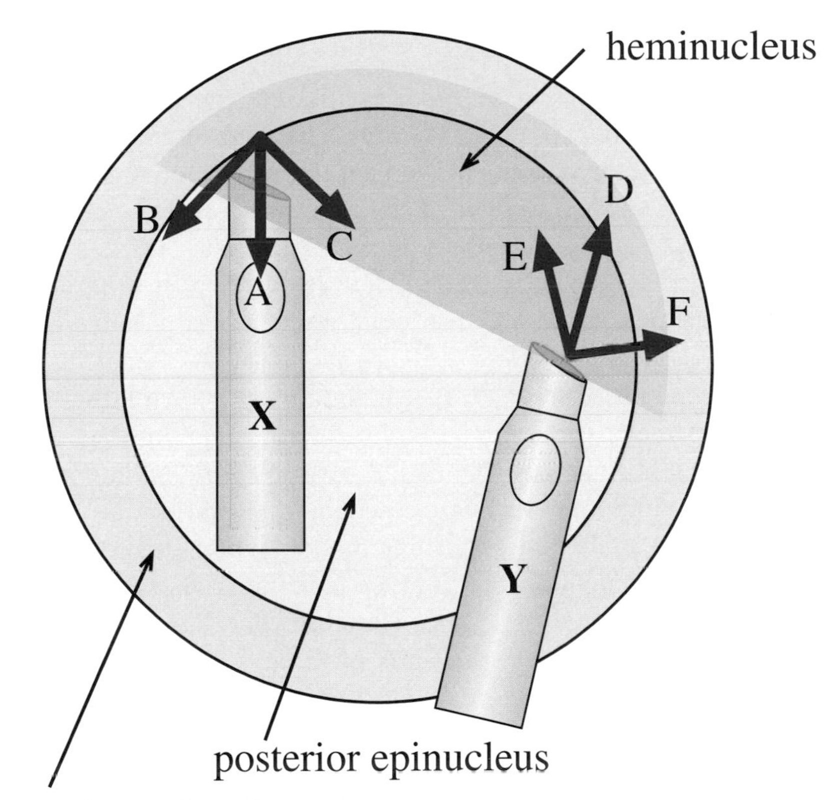

Figure 3-15-2

Figure 3-15

Optimal Instrument Placement for Nuclear Manipulation

When attempting to manipulate the nucleus (ie, rotation, cracking, etc), both shape and the placement of the manipulating instrument are important. In Figure 3-16, each instrument is pushed against the nucleus with the same amount of force (large green vector arrow). It can be seen that the effectiveness with which this force is transferred to the nucleus varies. For example, the cyclodialysis spatula has a small frontal surface area (essentially the same as the cross-sectional surface area of the instrument shaft). The force of the instrument applied over this small surface area produces a relatively high pressure (force per area) which tends to penetrate the nucleus rather than transferring the instrument's pushing force; note the significant nuclear penetration and small transmitted force vector of cyclodialysis spatula A. Cyclodialysis spatula B has less penetration and more transmitted force because of its placement in the central densest nucleus as opposed to the less dense epinuclear placement of instrument A.

The Seibel Nucleus Chopper was developed with these phacodynamic principles in mind to serve not only as a chopper but also as a universal nuclear manipulator. The distal curve allows optimal placement of the instrument tip into a groove for contact against the central densest nucleus. Furthermore, the distal tip is a polished olive shape which has a much larger surface area than the cyclodialysis spatula; note the greater area of contact indicated by more blue arrows in the magnified view of the chopper relative to the spatula. This expanded surface area allows the instrument force vector to be spread out over a larger area of the nucleus, resulting in less pressure at each point of contact and therefore more effective transmission of force with less penetration; note the minimally diminished transmitted nuclear force vector (green arrow) in the bottom diagram.

The above reasoning is sometimes confused with the logic behind a smaller aspiration port having less holding force than a port with a larger surface area (see Figure 1-48). However, the instrument shape logic states that a smaller surface area of contact produces a higher pressure (which is more likely to penetrate rather than push the nucleus). The difference between the two rationales is that the phaco machine's pump is producing a negative **pressure**, which has the units of force (numerator) per surface area (denominator); therefore, more surface area yields more force (pressure is multiplied by aspiration port surface area, the unit of which cancels the pressure's denominator surface area unit, leaving only a unit of force). In the instrument diagrams, the instrument has an applied **force**, not a pressure. Therefore, when this force is applied over a larger surface area (ie, larger denominator), it produces a lower pressure with units of force over surface area, with the pressure per unit surface area decreasing as the total applied surface area (denominator) increases.

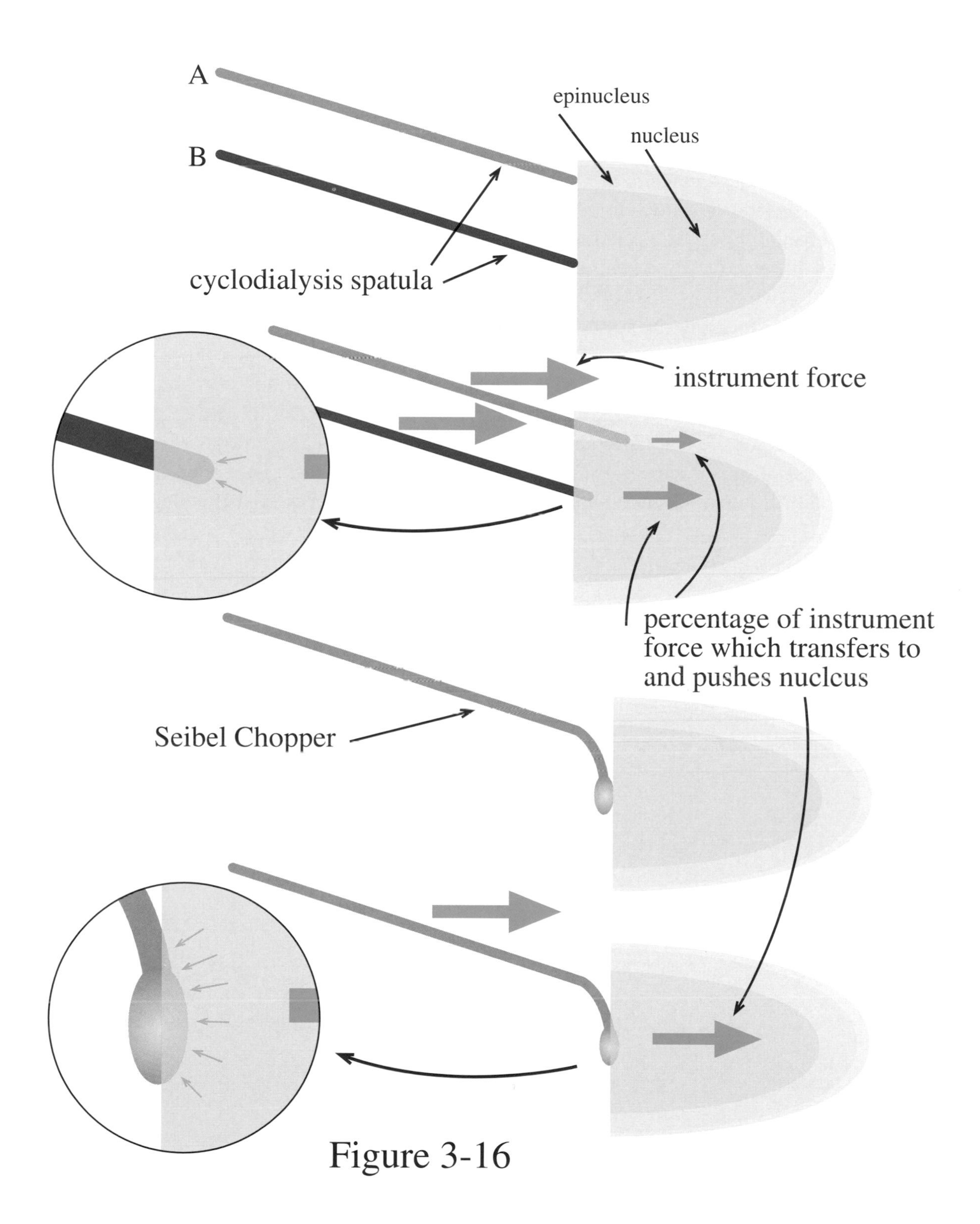
A
B
epinucleus
nucleus
cyclodialysis spatula
instrument force
percentage of instrument force which transfers to and pushes nucleus
Seibel Chopper

Figure 3-16

Nuclear Segmentation 1

As discussed in Figure 3-16, instrument placement is important with regard to effective transmission of force from the instrument to the cataract. There is additional logic behind instrument placement when performing cracking maneuvers. Figure 3-17 shows a cross-section of a nucleus with a well-prepared, deep groove as an initial step in either a stop and chop or a quadranting maneuver. The nucleus is still connected at the bottom of the groove by a bridge of posterior nuclear material; our goal is to split the nucleus into two halves (the following principles apply to quadrants as well). In theory, the ideal place to apply the splitting force would be in the middle of the bridge (area A). In practice, the same effect can be approximated by applying force at the bottom of the groove (area B). If force is applied as shown at area C, a torque is created with a lever arm from A to C. To the extent that the force is converted into torque, it is not effectively applied at the bridge to split it apart. Instead, it will create a pivoting effect around the most posterior aspect of area A without pulling it apart. The lever arm from A to B is so short that any induced torque from force application at area B is negligible.

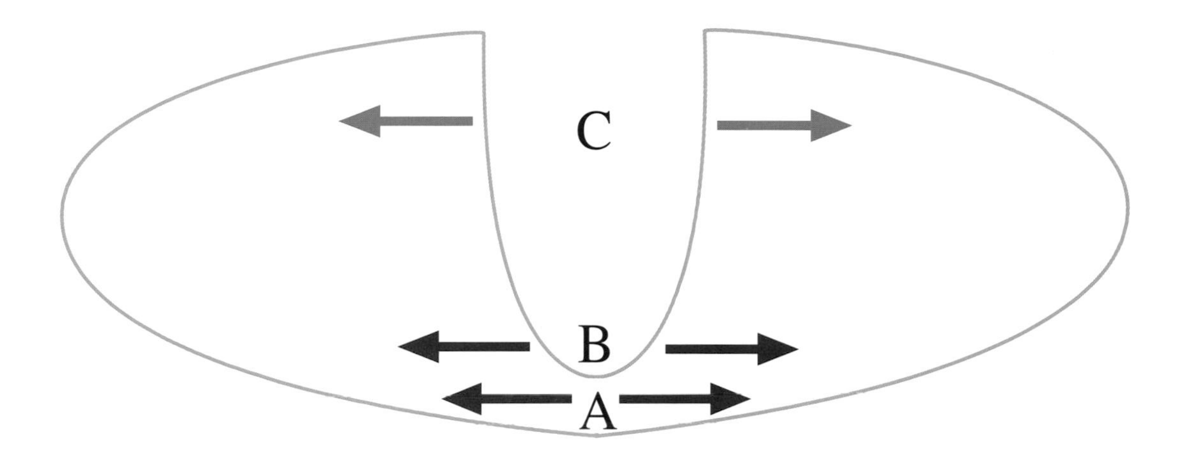

Figure 3-17

Nuclear Segmentation 2

Figure 3-18-1 shows instruments well placed at the bottom of the groove. The phaco needle can easily be positioned posteriorly in the groove because it is oriented parallel to the groove. Because the second instrument is perpendicular to the groove, it is useful for it to have a curve such that the distal tip can also be placed down in the groove as shown by the Seibel Chopper illustrated here. The nucleus is bisected with a minimum of instrument and nuclear movement. Note also that the force has been effectively applied at the bridging tissue such that the split faces are parallel (ie, they were split directly apart).

Figure 3-18-2 has instruments placed in a poor position anteriorly in the groove. The nucleus is pushed apart much further than in Figure 3-18-1, yet the top portion of the bridge is only split apart the same amount. Moreover, the bottom of the bridge is not split at all because the anterior placement of the instruments has created a torque in this area rather than a splitting force.

If posteriorly placed instruments penetrate the nucleus instead of pushing it apart, try moving them slightly anteriorly toward the central densest part of the nucleus (ie, still in the posterior half of the nuclear face; see Figures 3-10 and 3-16).

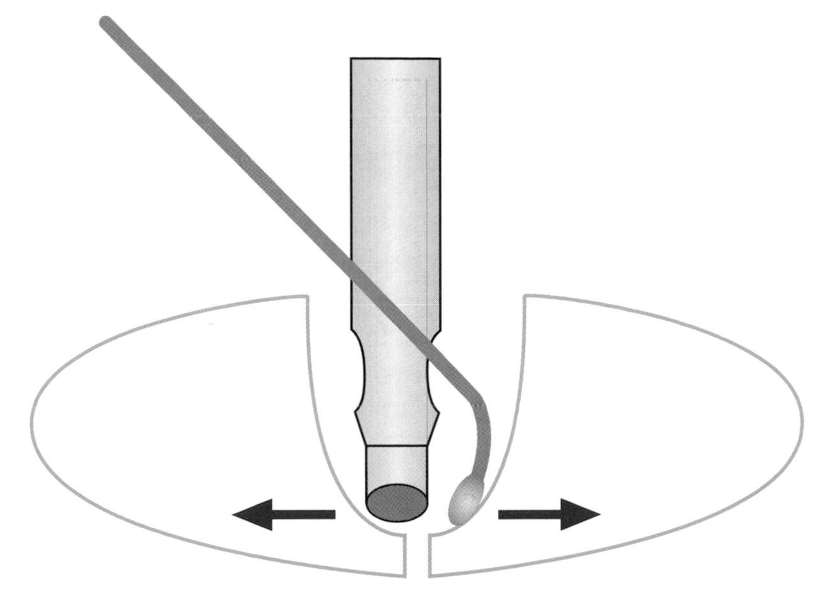

Figure 3-18-1

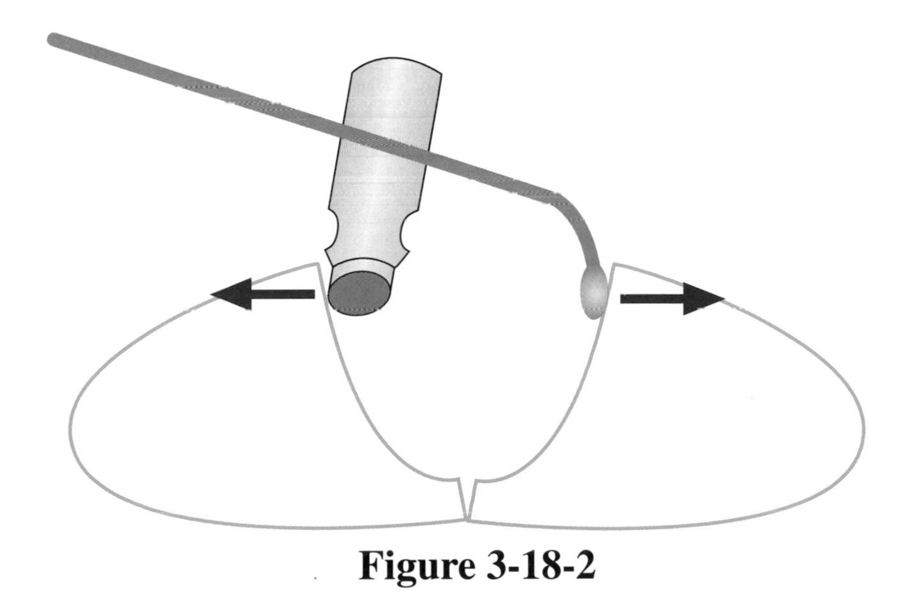

Figure 3-18-2

Figure 3-18

Nuclear Segmentation 3

Figure 3-19 superimposes the effects of anterior instrument placement (green) and posterior instrument placement (red). The separation distance necessary to break apart the bridge of connecting nucleus at the base of the groove is represented by x. Note that each nuclear half moves only half this amount with posterior instrument placement, thus imparting minimal stress to the surrounding intraocular tissues. Compare this to the anterior instrument placement schematic, in which the nuclear halves are displaced almost 10 times as much (distance y). For all of this unnecessary strain on the capsule and zonules, only the top of the bridge is split adequately, with the bottom remaining intact and acting as a pivot point (see Figure 3-18-2).

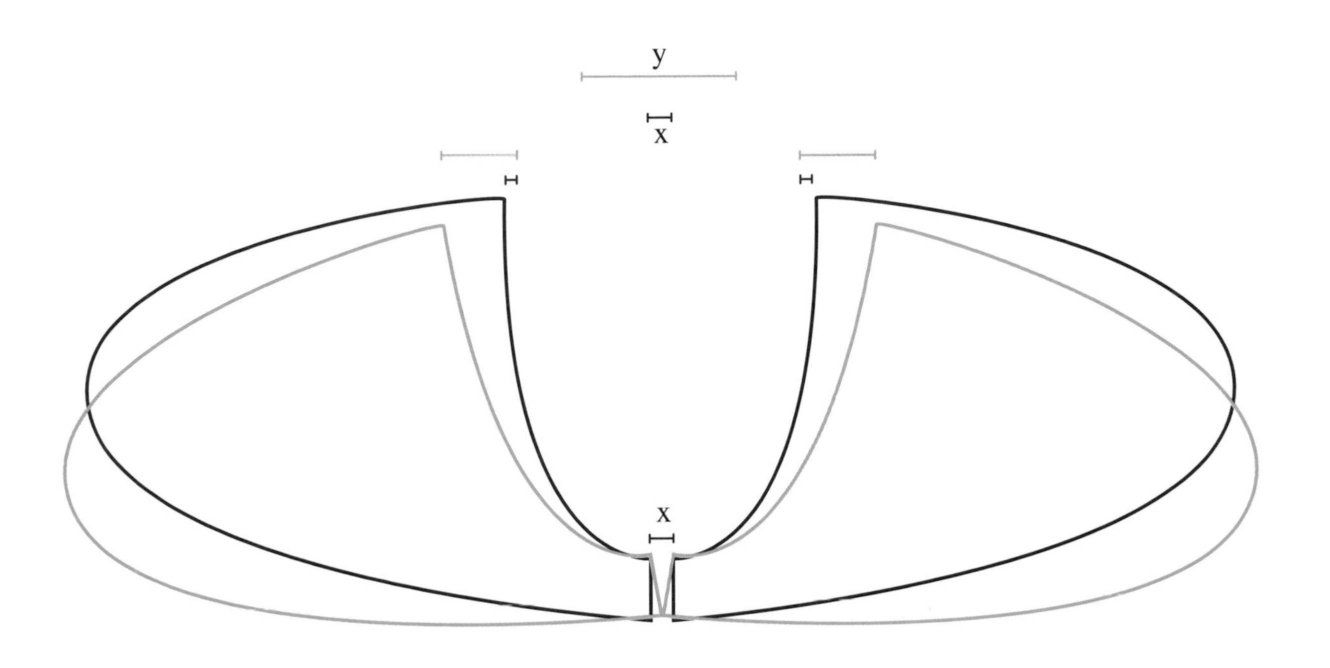

Figure 3-19

Nuclear Segmentation 4

In Figure 3-20, the remaining nuclear half has been grooved and almost completely quadranted by using the splitting methods previously discussed. However, a small bridge of tissue (A) remains. Options include repeating the previous methods, using viscoelastic with the Salz Nucleus Splitter, or using the instruments as illustrated in Figure 3-20. In this case, the phaco needle is occluded and exerting a pulling force with the foot pedal in position 2. At the same time the Seibel Chopper is inserted through the side-port incision and is used to exert a pushing force. The combination of these forces produces a shearing force across the bridge A, effectively separating the half into quadrants. Since one quadrant is already engaged on the phaco needle, it can readily be mobilized into the center of the posterior chamber or iris plane and emulsified.

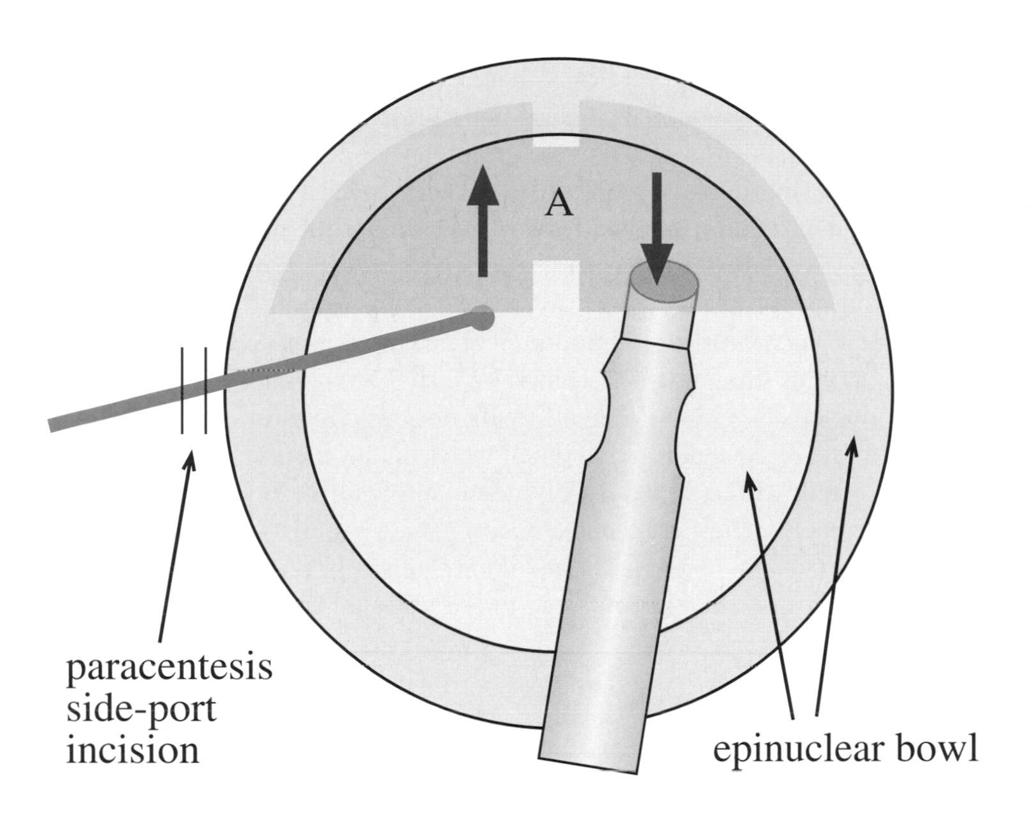

Figure 3-20

Fault-Line Phaco

I developed this segmentation technique as an exercise in the application of phacodynamic principles to both instrument design and surgical methodology. The development began with a mechanical analysis of the human crystalline lens, which is an oblate spheroid of increasing density from the periphery toward the center. Grooving methods of nuclear segmentation use considerable sculpting as they progress from anterior to posterior; the grooves must also be wide enough to prevent the silicone irrigation sleeve from obstructing progress. However, all that is really required for cracking is a central channel in the densest portion of the nucleus. Figures 3-21-1 and 3-21-2 show that the height and length of this fault-line channel are such that a significant amount of the central densest nucleus is emulsified, allowing for propogation of cracking (red arrows) when force is directed against the inner walls of the channel (green arrows). Toward this end, the width of the channel only needs to be sufficient for the phaco tip and the cracking instrument. The Flat-Head Phaco tip (see Figure 1-50) was designed specifically to create this channel such that considerably less ultrasound power and time are required in preparation for cracking relative to a traditional grooving method.

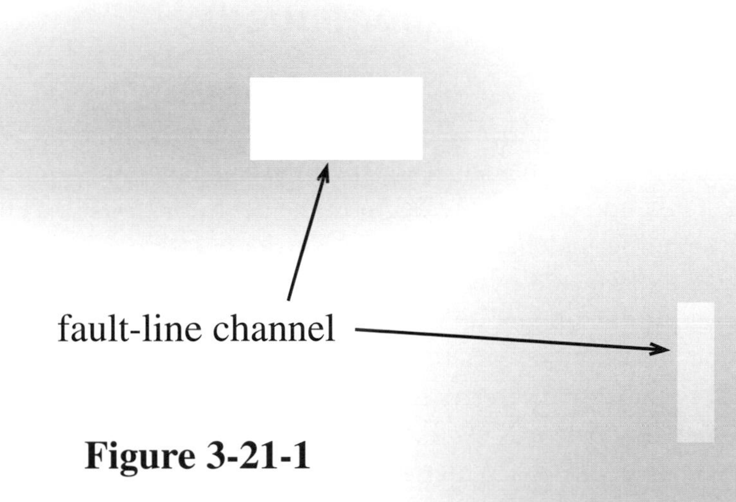

Figure 3-21-1

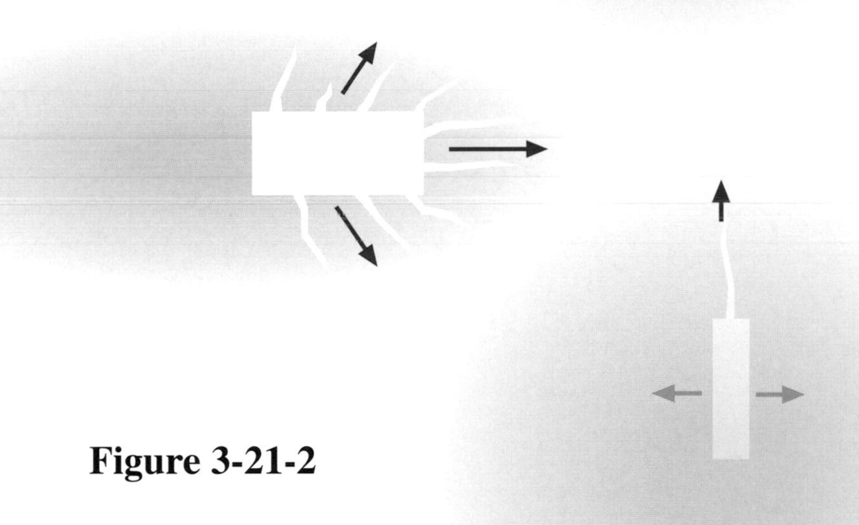

Figure 3-21-2

Figure 3-21

Fault-Line Phaco (continued)

The only sculpting in this technique occurs as the initial step when the Flat-Head Phaco tip is oriented horizontally to create a small square bowl as shown in Figure 3-22-1. This bowl will allow the fault-line channels to begin in the central densest part of the cataract. In preparation for creating the channels, the tip is oriented vertically as shown in Figure 3-22-2. Typically, only two side-by-side passes are required to provide enough room for the tip and the cracking instrument (a Seibel Chopper in this case); these passes are made with efficient occlusion mode phaco. Note the green bars in the side cross-section of Figure 3-22-2; these indicate the safety margin afforded by the central intranuclear location of the fault-line channel with respect to the posterior and peripheral capsule as well as the anterior capsule and iris. With the instruments positioned as shown in the top view of Figure 3-22-2, separating them will produce a crack as shown in Figure 3-21-2. Once this crack is created, the nucleus is rotated to facilitate more fault-line channels and cracks, creating quadrants or smaller fragments as desired.

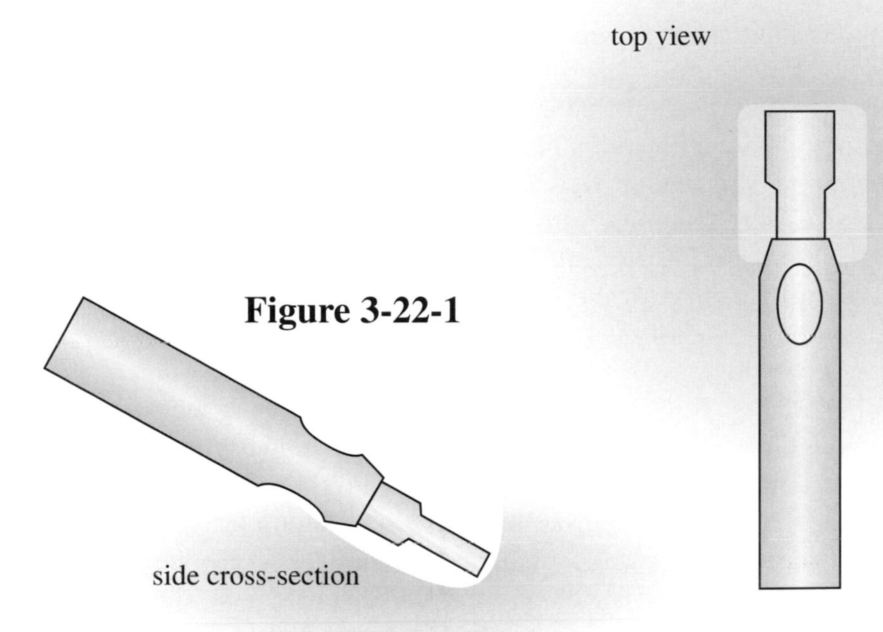

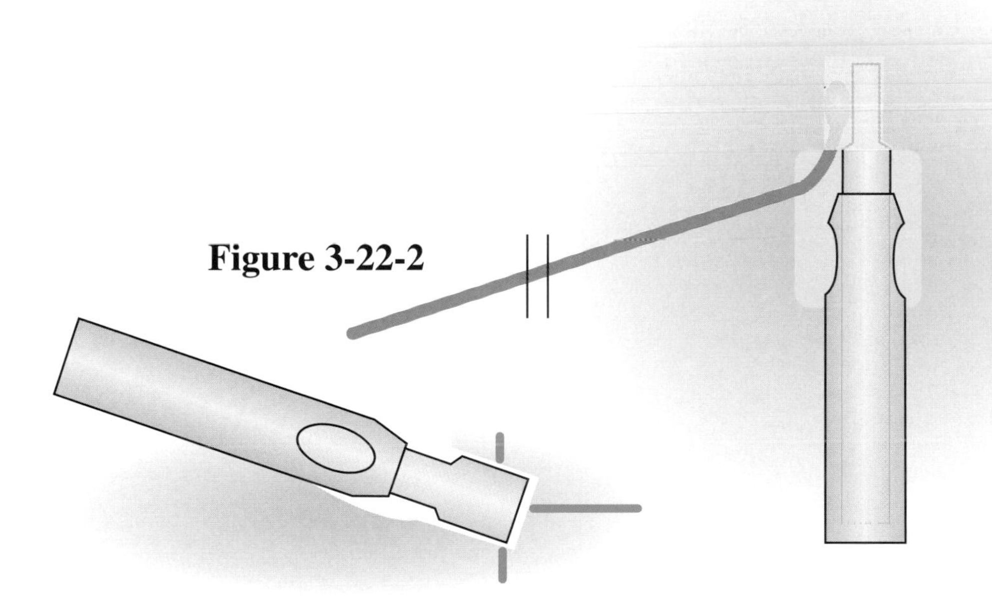

Figure 3-22

Chopping Techniques 1

Although chopping methods have been previously discussed in Figures 2-13, 2-14a, and 2-14b with regard to machine settings, the following discussions will focus on optimization of surgical technique for these maneuvers. Figure 3-23 shows multiple cross-sections of a stop and chop maneuver in which the heminucleus is impaled by the phaco tip in preparation for chopping (for the top view perspective of the stop and chop maneuver, see Figures 2-14a and 2-14b). Diagram A illustrates the importance of avoiding the anterior capsule with the chopping instrument. Diagram B illustrates the proper initial placement of the chopper just central to the capsulorhexis edge; note that the epinucleus has been removed up to the level of the capsulorhexis edge. At this point, the surgeon could attempt to press posteriorly with the chopper in order to penetrate and engage the nucleus for chopping. However, even though most current chopping instruments have a small surface area at their distal tip, this maneuver can push denser nuclei posteriorly with concomitant capsular and zonular stress; furthermore, this posterior force causes a torque and shear force on the nucleus at the phaco aspiration port which can break the vacuum seal and compromise control. Although a few choppers have been designed with sharp tips to facilitate penetration with less nuclear displacement, these instruments compromise capsular integrity in case of inadvertent contact. I feel that a better option is to bluntly dissect between the epinucleus and inner heminucleus with the chopper; note in diagram C how this maneuver has been facilitated by initially rotating the chopper so that the plane of its distal 90° bend is more parallel rather than perpendicular to the iris plane. It is returned to its original perpendicular position once it has engaged the nuclear periphery as in diagram D, where it is now able to begin chopping toward the phaco tip.

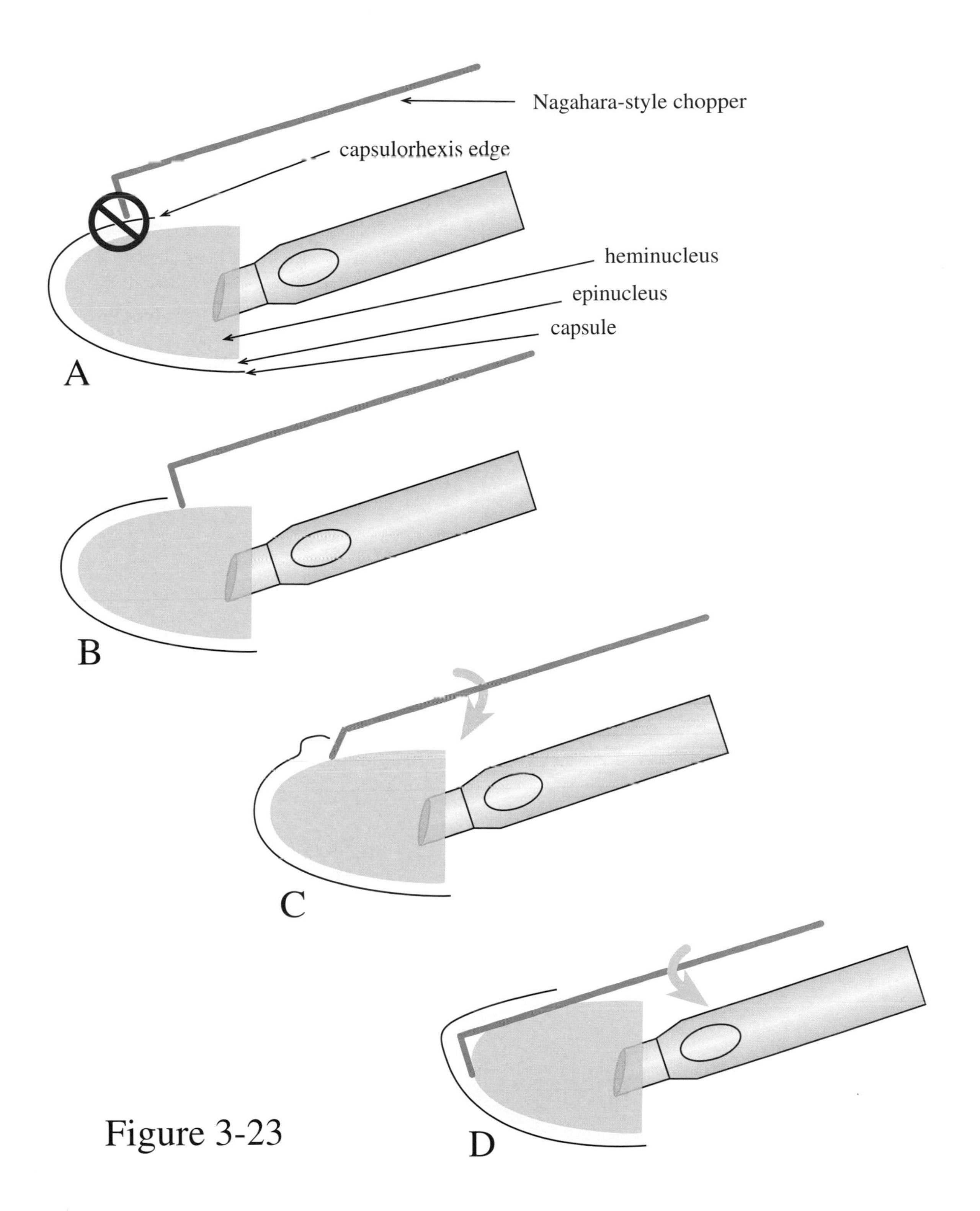
Nagahara-style chopper
capsulorhexis edge
heminucleus
epinucleus
capsule
A
B
C
D

Figure 3-23

Chopping Techniques 2

A potential liability of the method that was illustrated in Figure 3-23 is the danger of engaging the capsule with the chopper during the dissection between B and C, as well as during the chop itself which starts from position D (note the close proximity of the chopper tip to the epinucleus and capsule at these stages). The tip of most choppers is the same diameter as the rest of the distal instrument shaft; this small surface area can produce a high focal pressure which can penetrate the capsule (see discussion with Figure 3-16), leading to potential vitreous loss. In order to minimize the potential for the chopper tip to engage the capsule, Figure 3-24 illustrates the use of vacuum (holding force) used by the occluded phaco tip (pedal position 2) to draw the heminucleus centrally during the dissection with the chopper, thereby increasing the distance between the capsule and the chopper tip. **When pulling a fragment impaled by the phaco needle, recall the importance of discontinuing ultrasound; a vibrating needle will typically pull out of the fragment rather than pull the fragment with it.** The space for this central displacement was created by the initial groove formation performed with Dr. Paul Koch's stop and chop maneuver (also known as Dr. Ronald Stasiuk's mini-chop).

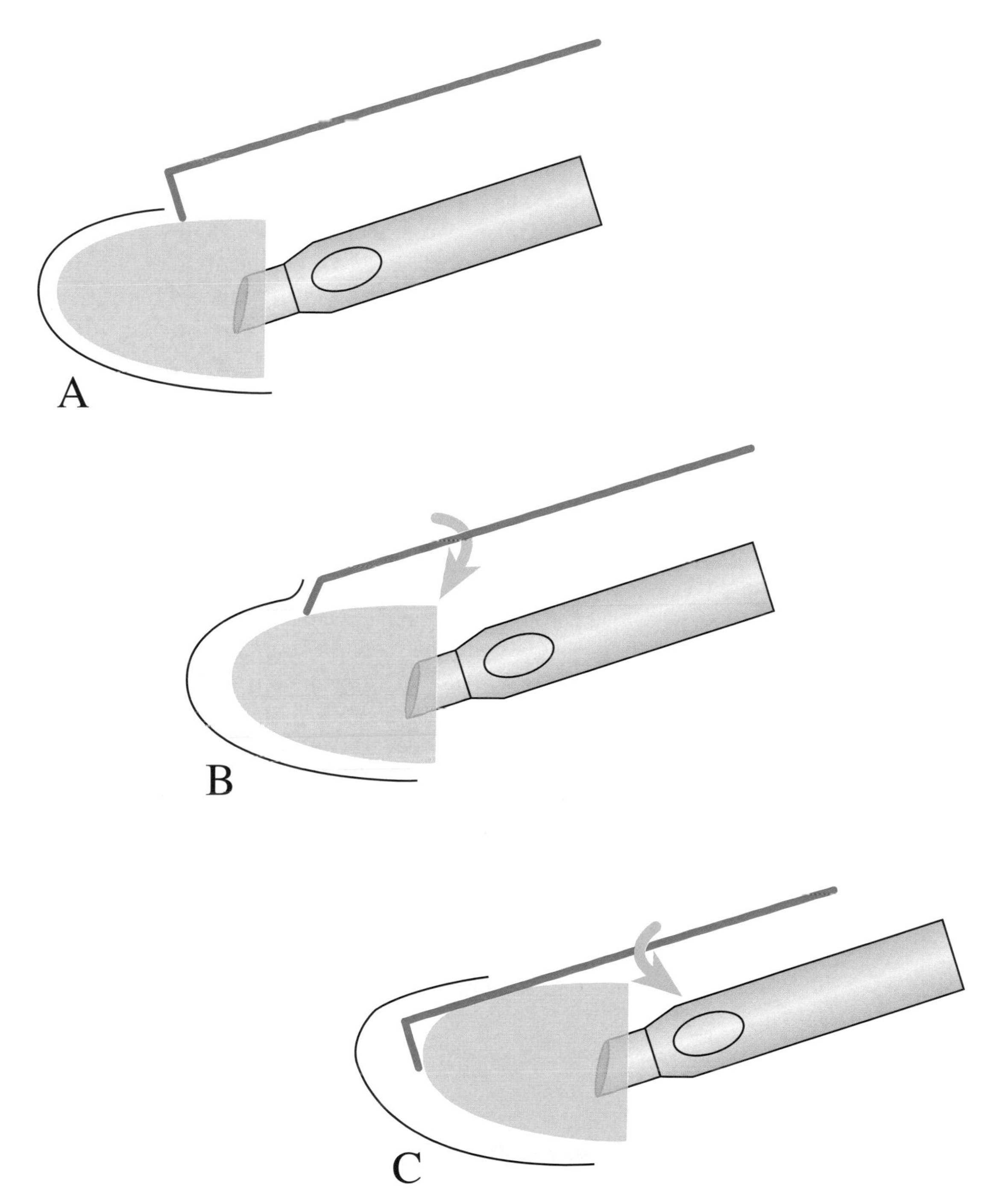

Figure 3-24

Chopping Techniques 3: Seibel Chopper

The safety and efficacy of the procedure illustrated in Figure 3-24 are further enhanced by the use of the Seibel Chopper as shown in Figure 3-25. The polished distal olive-shaped tip has a much larger surface area than the tips of standard choppers; therefore, the olive tip is much less likely to damage or penetrate the lens capsule (anterior, peripheral, or posterior) in case of inadvertent contact (see Figure 3-16). The olive tip's shape and larger surface area further facilitate the blunt dissection between the nucleus and epinucleus; nevertheless, the technique is still optimized by initially rotating the instrument so that the plane of the distal bend is closer to the plane of the anterior surface of the nucleus and the anterior capsule (see curved green arrows in diagrams B in Figures 3-24 and 3-25 as well as diagram C in Figure 3-23). The junction of the olive tip and the curved shaft creates an angle that positively engages the nuclear periphery (red arrow in diagram C, Figure 3-25); this angle maintains engagement during the actual chop. Note also how the curved shaft more anatomically approximates the nuclear periphery (blue arrows in diagram C, Figure 3-25) relative to the abrupt 90° bend of standard choppers (eg, diagram C of Figure 3-24); the gently radiused 75° curve also better facilitates entry and exit through the side-port paracentesis incision relative to standard choppers' abrupt 90° bend. The chopping edge of the curved shaft is offset 45° to facilitate use as shown in the top (surgeon's) view illustrated in Figures 2-14a and 2-14b; note the 45° angle between the straight instrument shaft and the direction of the chop (top diagrams in Figure 3-25). Note that the curved shaft tapers to a very small radius of curvature at the chopping edge in order to concentrate the instrument's force into a pressure (see Figure 3-16) that will cleave virtually any cataract; however, it is intentionally not sharpened to a knife edge so that the instrument has a good safety margin when using the inner curved segment to manipulate the intraocular lens, iris, etc.

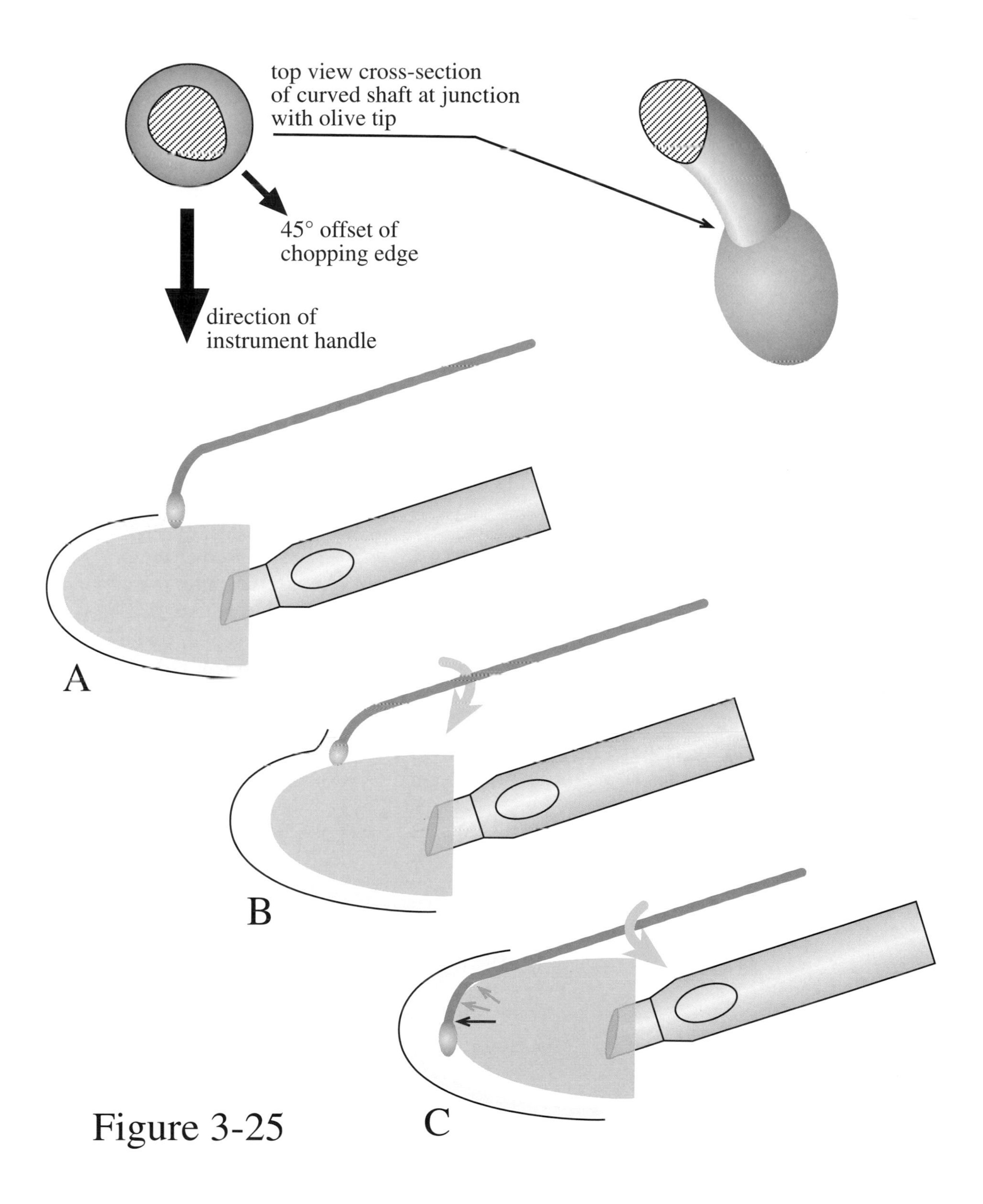
top view cross-section
of curved shaft at junction
with olive tip
45° offset of
chopping edge
direction of
instrument handle
A
B
C

Figure 3-25

Chopping Techniques 4: Flat-Head Phaco Tip

The Flat-Head tip, seen in Figures 1-50 and 3-22, is also useful for chopping in two ways. First, the fault-line channel created when the tip impales the heminucleus provides a cleavage plane which the chopper can meet halfway; this would be the case if the chopper had been placed at point y in diagram A (Figure 3-26) and than drawn toward the tip as indicated by the red arrow. Recall the shape of the fault-line channel (see Figure 3-22-2) which is taller in anterior-posterior dimension than a standard round phaco needle; it therefore eliminates more of this densest portion of the nucleus in the chopping plane and better facilitates a complete chop.

The second way in which the Flat-Head tip may be used is directly illustrated in Figure 3-26. This method is particularly useful with dense fibrous nuclei which may not chop completely such that a posterior bridge of connecting material remains, such as point z in diagram A. For this method, the chopper engages the heminucleus at point x such that the chop will extend just to the side of the phaco tip and leave it embedded in the fragment to be chopped as shown. Because the Flat-Head tip is a rectangular shape which is surrounded by the rectangular shape which it created by boring into the nucleus, it can effectively be used like a flat-head screwdriver to transmit torque to the impaled fragment in order to complete the segmentation by splitting the remaining posterior adhesion. This can be performed by a counterclockwise rotation (diagram B) which produces a splitting force right at the connecting bridge (see Figures 3-17 and 3-18-1); alternatively, a clockwise rotation can be employed (diagram C) which will produce an anterior shearing force at the connecting bridge (see Figure 3-20). Both ways are effective, and neither technique can be effectively used with a standard round needle, which would tend to rotate within the cylindrical hole which it bored rather than transmitting torque to the impaled fragment.

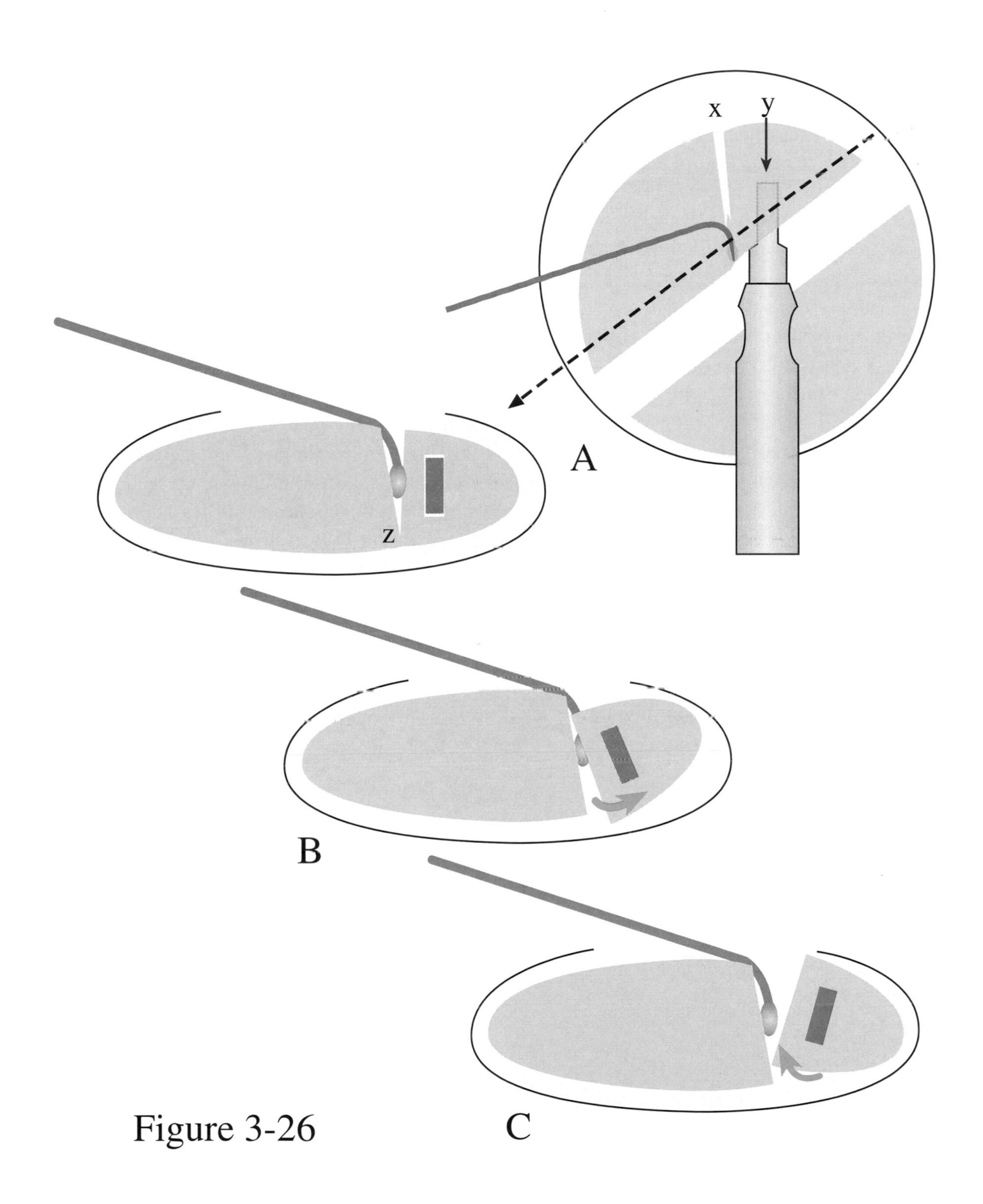

Figure 3-26

Vacuum Seal

Whenever the phaco needle is used to pull the cataract (or segment thereof), the aspiration port must be completely occluded in order to effectively transfer the pump's vacuum as a gripping force (see Figures 1-10, 1-22, and 1-25). In order to optimally occlude the aspiration port, a good vacuum seal must be achieved (Figure 3-27, diagram A). Note that the tip is embedded 1 to 1.5mm into the nuclear fragment. Note also the tip's central location in the fragment's anterior-posterior dimension; this is the most homogeneously densest part of the cataract and will provide the best vacuum seal.

Diagram B shows the phaco tip engaging the cataract so anteriorly that the aspiration port is exposed to the anterior chamber fluid (red arrow); this incomplete occlusion will preclude optimum gripping of the nuclear fragment. When pulled, the phaco tip will most likely pull out of the fragment rather than pull the fragment with it. Diagram C has the aspiration port completely occluded, but it is still too anteriorly positioned. Recall that the anterior (as well as posterior and peripheral) nucleus is often not as dense as the central nucleus, and higher vacuum levels might preferentially aspirate the less dense material, compromising the vacuum seal as shown in diagram D (red arrow). This situation could also have occurred if the surgeon used too high an ultrasound level to initially embed the tip.

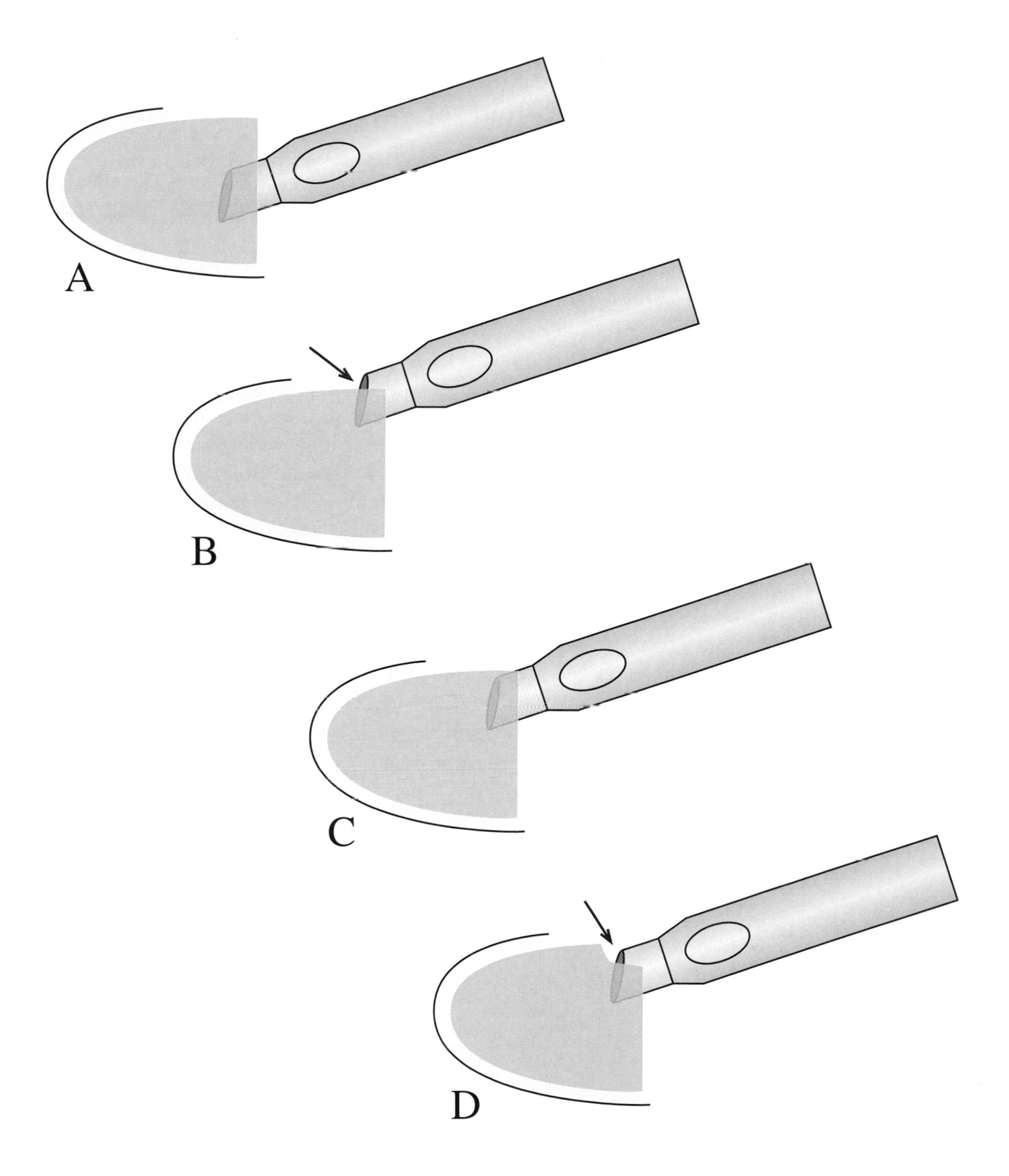

Figure 3-27

Vacuum Seal (continued)

In diagram A-1 of Figure 3-28, the aspiration port is completely occluded in the correct central face of the nuclear fragment as described on the previous page. However, the tip is not embedded to a sufficient depth. Note in Figure 3-28-A-2 how a slight manipulation of the phaco needle (blue arrow) has caused a break in the vacuum seal (red arrow). By embedding the aspiration port to an adequate depth of 1 to 1.5mm, the vacuum seal can better resist routine manipulations of the tip without breaking and causing loss of gripping control.

Diagram B of Figure 3-28 illustrates the phaco tip embedded to an adequate depth and positioned properly in the central densest nucleus, with a good potential for a vacuum seal. However, that potential has been eliminated in diagram C because too much nuclear material has been removed around the tip, thereby precluding complete occlusion of the aspiration port. Two conditions could lead to this problem. First, using too high an ultrasound power and/or maintaining it for too long a time when embedding the tip will produce this clinical picture. The tip should be embedded with mild linear controlled ultrasound with correspondingly minimal cavitation in order to achieve the tight fit shown in diagram B; furthermore, ultrasound power should be discontinued immediately once the tip is embedded to an adequate depth by disengaging pedal position 3 while maintaining pedal position 2 to maintain and build vacuum and gripping force. The second condition that could lead to diagram B is the use of too high a vacuum level for the density of nucleus which is engaged. Vacuum should ideally be titrated with linear control to an appropriate level which will grip the engaged fragment without being so high that it abruptly aspirates the material just around the aspiration port.

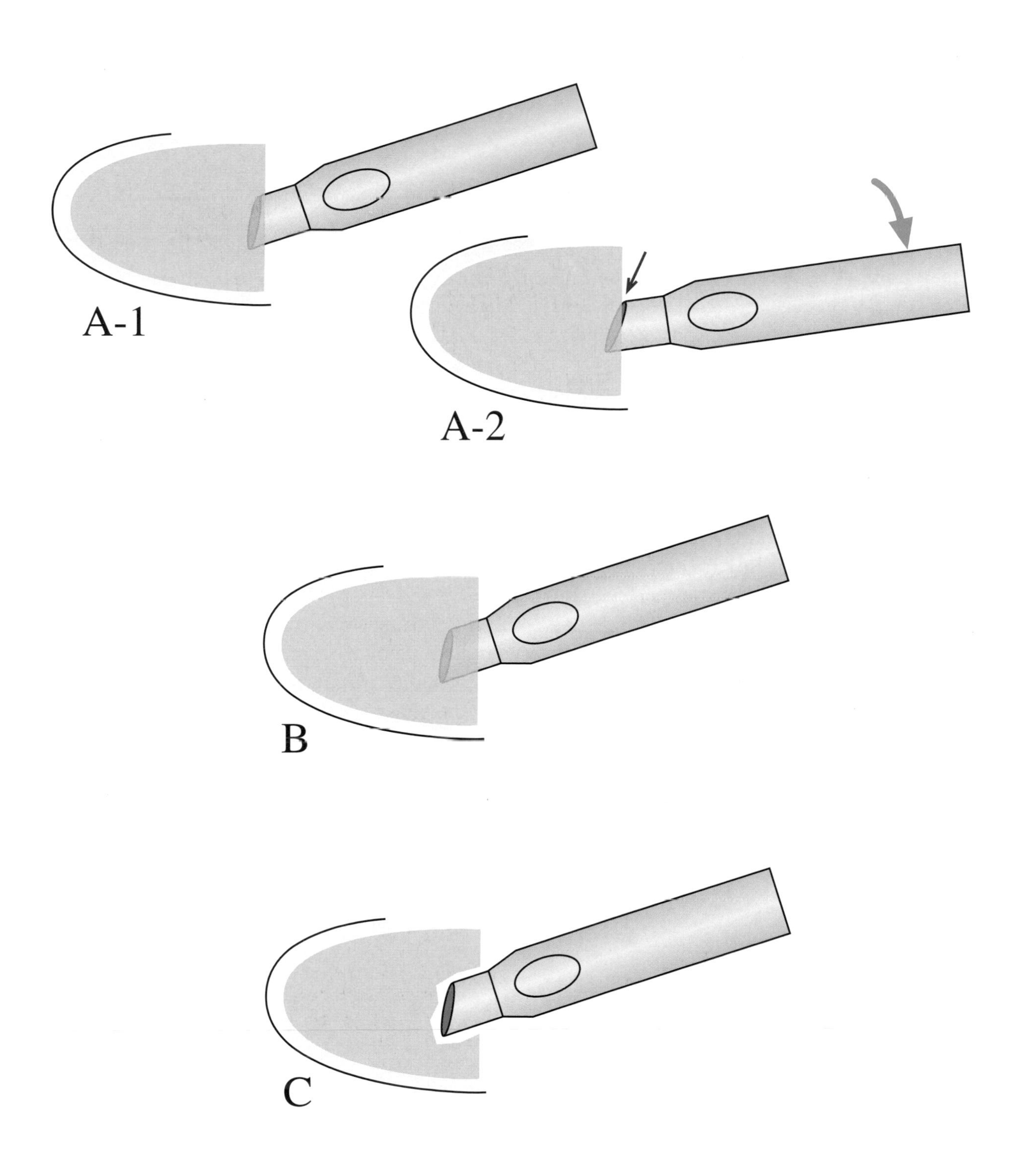

Figure 3-28

Fragment Manipulation 1

Nuclear quadrants (or smaller segments produced by phaco chopping) are ideally pulled with the phaco tip to the center of the posterior chamber or iris plane where they can then be safely emulsified as a free-floating mass which readily carousels into the phaco port. Care should be taken when initially moving the quadrant so that any sharp edges do not threaten the capsule, notwithstanding Dr. Robert Osher's grand prize-winning video on the subject from the 1997 ASCRS Film Festival. Figure 3-29-1 has the phaco tip embedded in the anterior portion of the quadrant with ultrasound engaged. Note how the softer outer portion of the nuclear fragment by the upper part of the needle bevel is more rapidly emulsified and aspirated relative to the harder inner portion engaged by the lower part of the needle bevel. This differential causes a quadrant rotation with the sharp quadrant point being rotated directly against the capsule. Figure 3-29-2 depicts a safer method of engaging the quadrant by applying ultrasound power in the center of the quadrant where the density is homogeneous (see Figure 3-27); the quadrant is drawn directly onto the phaco needle without rotation. With it safely engaged in this fashion, it can then be moved centrally and anteriorly for complete phacoemulsification and aspiration. The variable nuclear density which was a disadvantage in Figure 3-29-1 can theoretically be used to your advantage as seen in Figure 3-29-3. Note how the same principles are applied in reverse to induce rotation of the sharp point away from the posterior capsule by initially placing the phaco needle posteriorly instead of anteriorly; however, this maneuver places the aspiration port in potentially dangerous proximity to the posterior capsule.

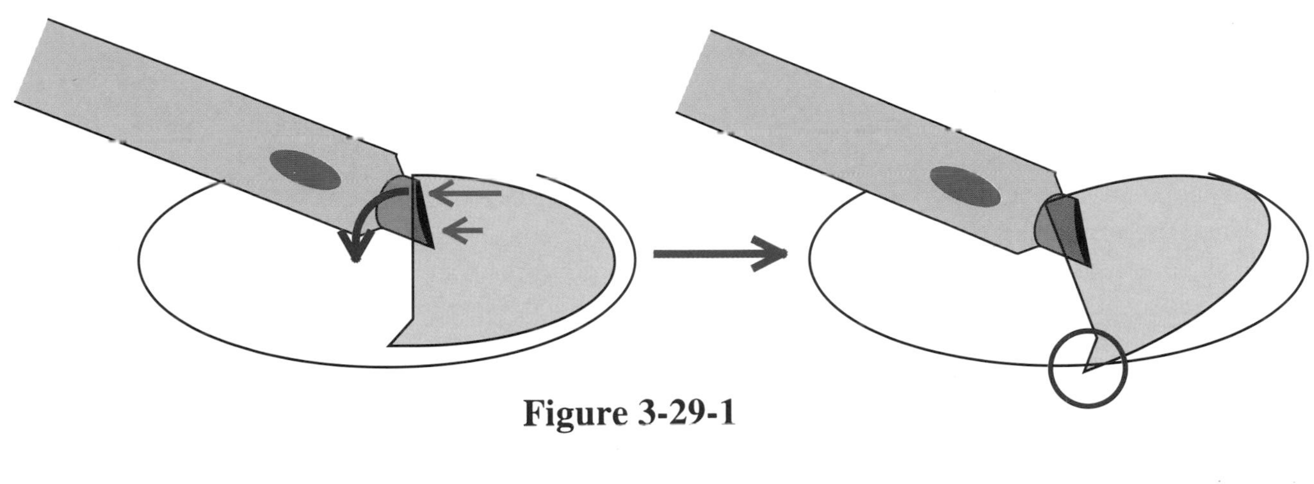

Figure 3-29-1

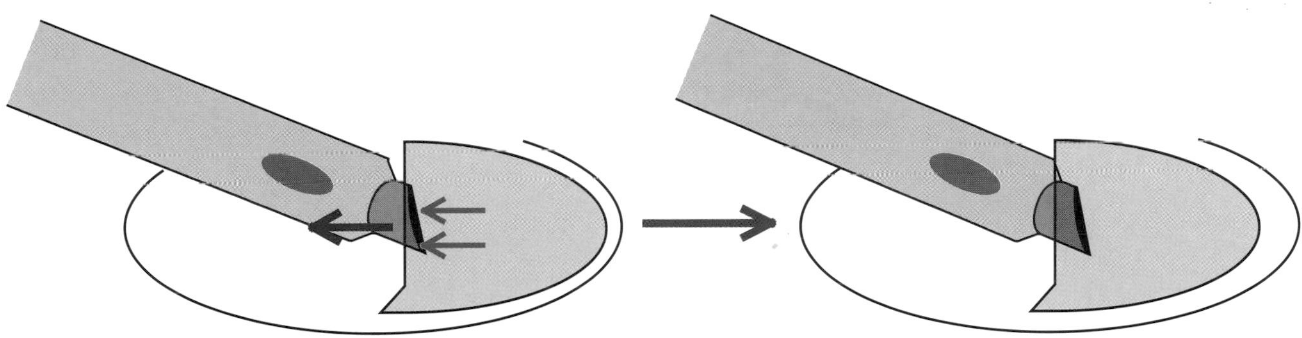

Figure 3-29-2

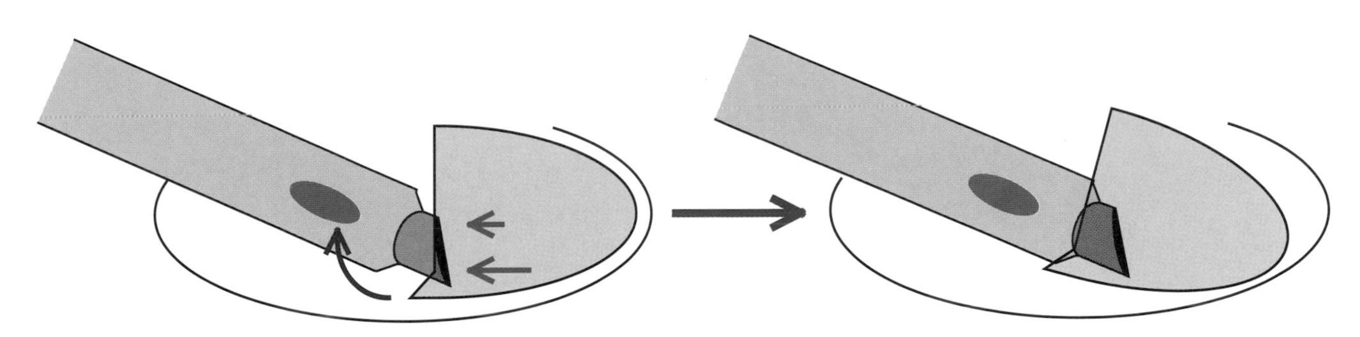

Figure 3-29-3

Figure 3-29

Fragment Manipulation 2

Another method of handling the sharp point of the quadrant is by engaging it within the lumen of the phaco needle. This maneuver can be accomplished by first moving to pedal position 0 on the foot pedal, thereby decreasing the IOP (see Figures 1-6 and 1-22). The vitreous pressure will then make the center of the posterior capsule protrude anteriorly; this along with gentle manipulation by the second instrument tips the sharp point anteriorly (Figure 3-30-1), where it can be engaged by the phaco needle (Figure 3-30-2). The foot pedal is then depressed into position 1 to repressurize the anterior chamber (Figure 3-30-3). Once positive control of the sharp point by the phaco needle is established, you can then move into position 3 to embed the tip and then position 2 to mobilize the fragment to a safer central location in preparation for carouseling emulsification. Alternatively, one could maintain position 3; because the phaco needle is engaging the posterior nucleus, activating ultrasound power will continue to rotate the point safely up as in Figure 3-29-3. As with Figure 3-29-3, caution must be exercised because of the proximity of the phaco tip to the posterior capsule.

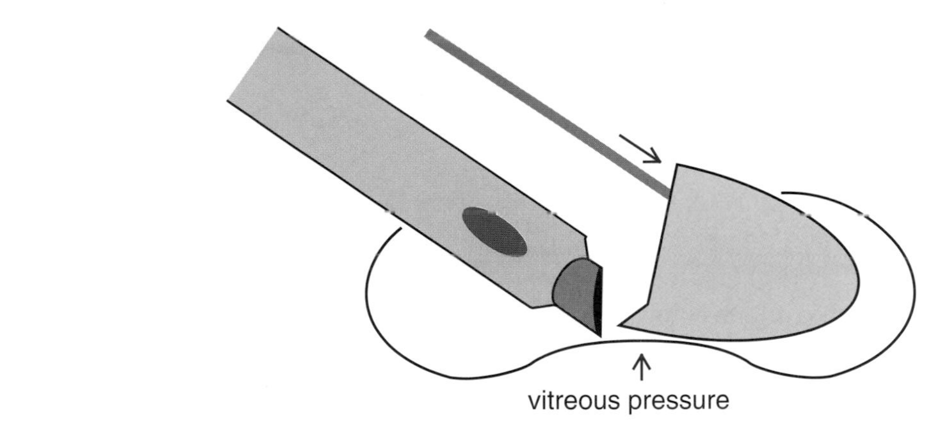

Figure 3-30-1

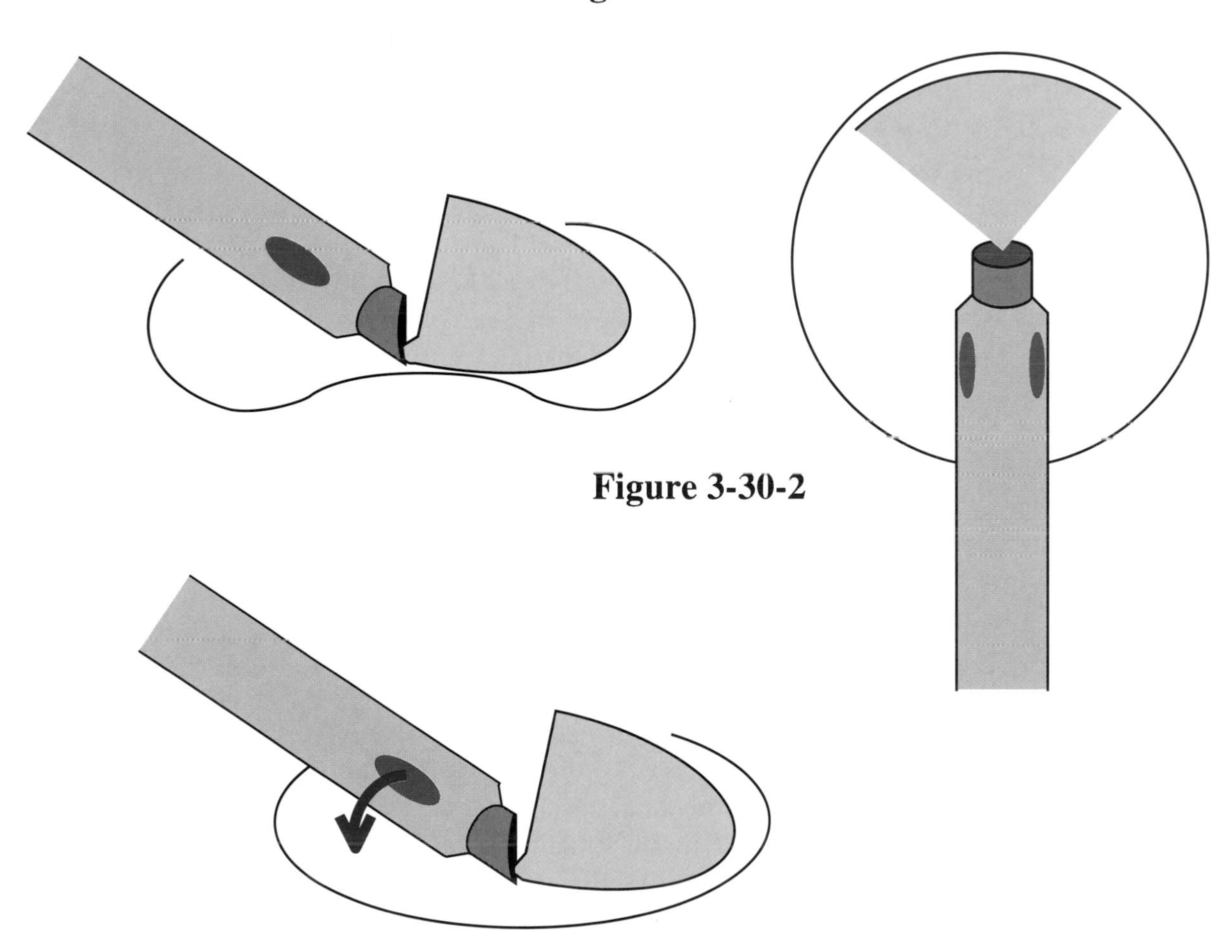

Figure 3-30-2

Figure 3-30-3

Figure 3-30

Fragment Manipulation 3

The phaco tip in Figure 3-31-A has impaled a nuclear fragment, boring almost completely through it. Maintaining pedal position 3 in this case invites disaster because of the aspiration flow (red arrow) tending to draw unwanted material like iris or capsule into the port. Furthermore, without complete occlusion of the aspiration port, vacuum cannot aid in aspirating the fragment; similarly, the flow does not help to aspirate the fragment because fluid is drawn into the tip prior to affecting the fragment. Recall that because of the axial orientation of ultrasound needle vibration, continuation of position 3 will not accomplish any further emulsification of the fragment; the needle will simply vibrate back and forth along the axis of the hole it has bored. Lastly, the phaco needle cannot progress any further through the fragment because of the physical obstruction from the silicone irrigation sleeve (see Figures 3-2 and 3-3). The correct move in this case is to back off to position 1 to maintain the anterior chamber; then use a second instrument through the side-port incision to push the fragment off of the phaco tip and then reengage to emulsify in a carousel fashion, manipulating and feeding the fragment to the tip with the second instrument as necessary (Figure 3-31-C). Note how the segment's sharp tip was ultrasonically removed prior to carouseling in order to prevent it from spinning into the capsule or cornea.

Engaging fragments in a tangential fashion for carouseling enables efficient emulsification as both flow and vacuum continue to feed new material into the phaco tip as the previously engaged portion is emulsified and aspirated in an efficient occlusion mode of operation. Note the non-tangential fragment engagement shown in Figure 3-31-B in which the phaco needle has bored into a thick part of the fragment; maintaining position 3 with a dense nuclear sclerotic fragment would not produce any further emulsification because the silicone sleeve will prevent vacuum from drawing the fragment any further into the needle. Furthermore, because the aspiration port is completely occluded, maintaining position 3 will cause potentially dangerous heat buildup from incisional friction caused by the vibrating ultrasonic needle in the absence of a cooling flow current. Fragments engaged in this fashion should be removed by refluxing or with a second instrument so that they can be reengaged for emulsification in a carousel fashion as in Figure 3-31-C. **Larger fragments generally require more manipulation by a second instrument to maintain optimum tangential positioning for carouseling; therefore, chopping methods are typically more efficient than quandranting techniques because smaller nuclear fragments are generated.**

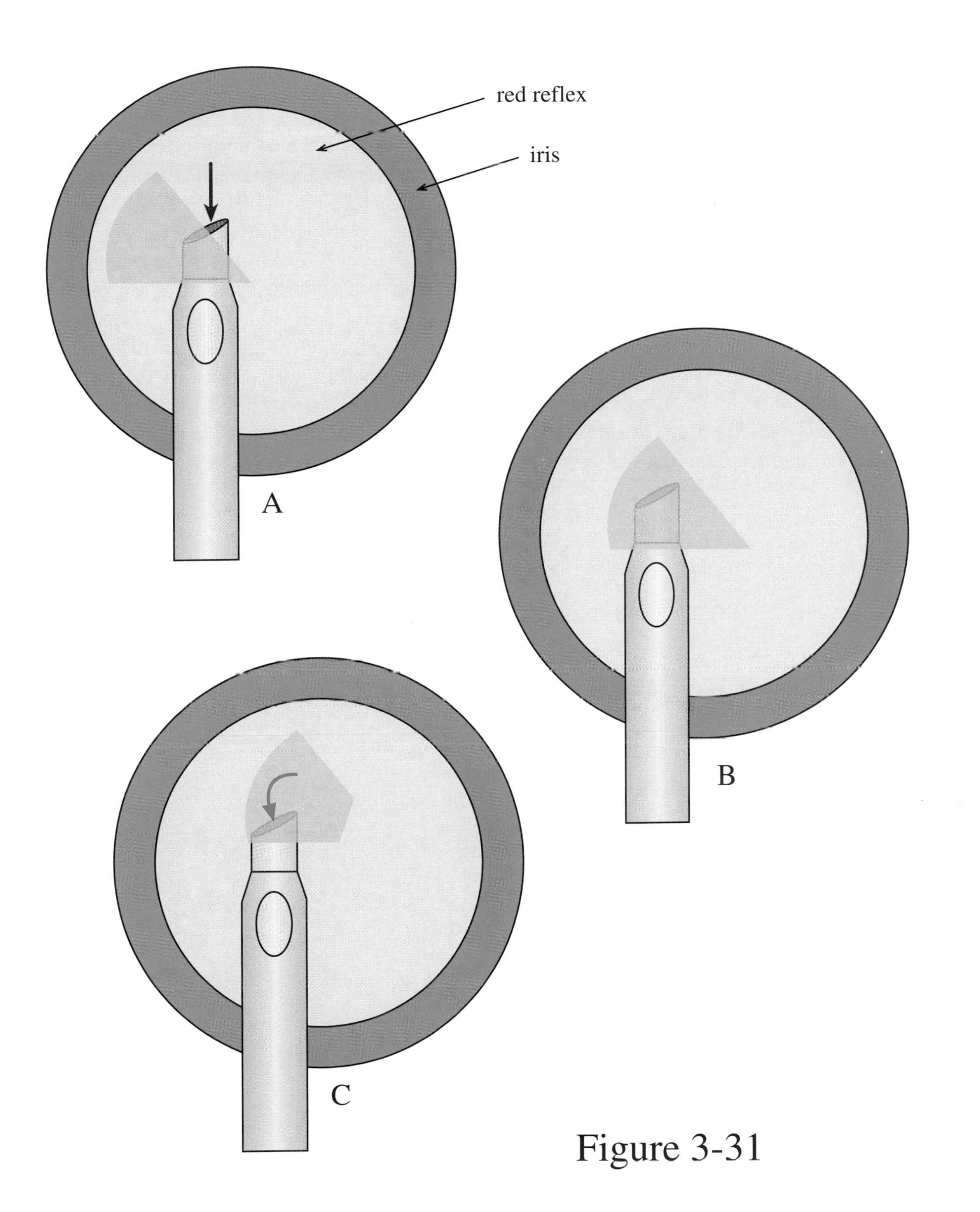

Figure 3-31

Fragment Manipulation 4: Viscodissection

Sometimes you will paint yourself into a corner and have the last remaining quadrant at the sub-incisional position. If you are unable to rotate it to the contra-incisional position with an instrument from the side-port incision, use the technique in Figure 3-32-1. The viscoelastic cannula is introduced through the side-port incision with the tip placed under the sub-incisional rim of the capsulorhexis as if to perform a hydrodissection; in this case, it will be a viscodissection. Note in Figure 3-32-2 how the fragment has been moved to a position where it can be readily engaged with the phaco tip; moreover, it is stable in this position because of support from the viscoelastic. This technique is equally successful in dealing with epinucleus at the sub-incisional position. Additionally, viscodissection is a valuable technique for **dealing with very soft nuclei** (eg, posterior subcapsular cataract in a young adult) which can be difficult to manipulate with cracking, chopping, or rotational maneuvers in order to achieve mobilization to the central anterior chamber for safe aspiration.

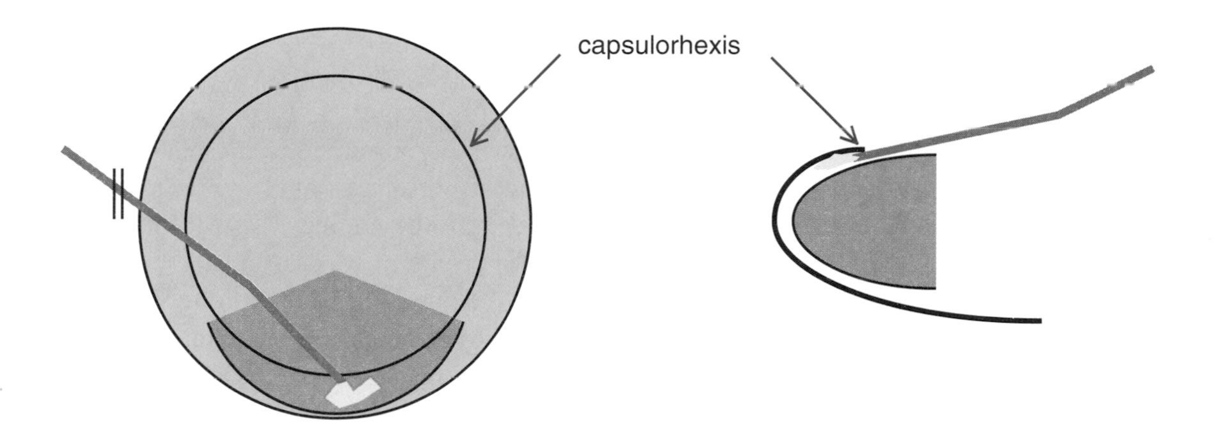

Figure 3-32-1

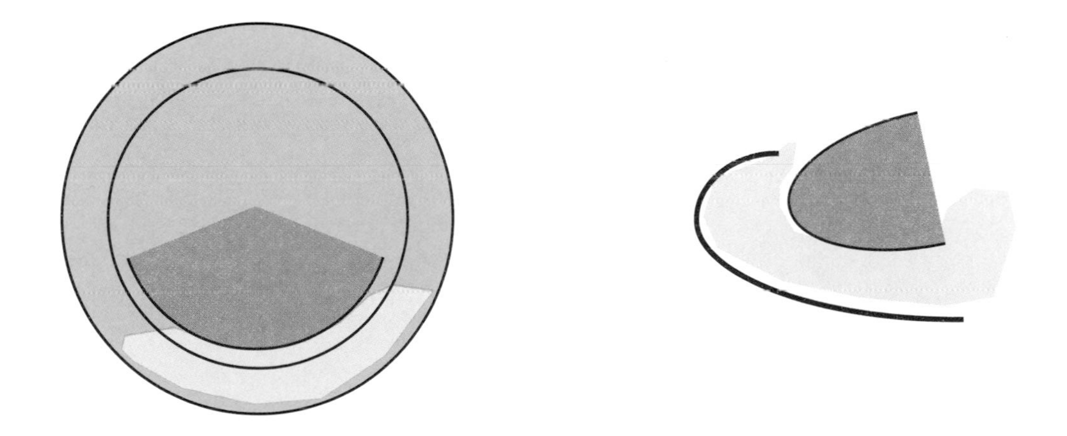

Figure 3-32-2

Figure 3-32

One-Handed Strategies 1

A fundamental goal of one-handed techniques, as well as the Kratz/Maloney two-handed technique, is to remove the bulk of the nuclear top, center, and rim so that the remaining posterior nuclear plate is small enough to be freely attracted to the phaco tip for safe carouseling/emulsification in the center of the posterior chamber or iris plane. Both techniques begin with deep central sculpting to debulk the nucleus. Dr. Maloney's original technique involved removal of the rim from peripheral to central at the area closest to the main surgical incision. As an alternative, the one-handed technique shown in Figure 3-33-1 depicts removal of the rim from central to peripheral at the contra-incisional location. Note that in this figure that removing the rim in this sculpting fashion will leave a nuclear plate with the same diameter as that of the original whole nucleus. Note the different way in which the nuclear bowl has been sculpted in Figure 3-33-2; the contour is such that a thin weak area has been created as indicated by point A. The location of this fault-line predetermines the diameter of the subsequent nuclear plate. Gentle ultrasound is used to embed the phaco tip; the foot pedal is then backed off to position 2 so that when the tip is withdrawn, it uses vacuum to carry the rim with it after breaking it free from the nuclear plate at the weakest area (point A). This technique effectively accomplishes the goal of a resultant nuclear plate with a substantially smaller diameter than that of the original nucleus.

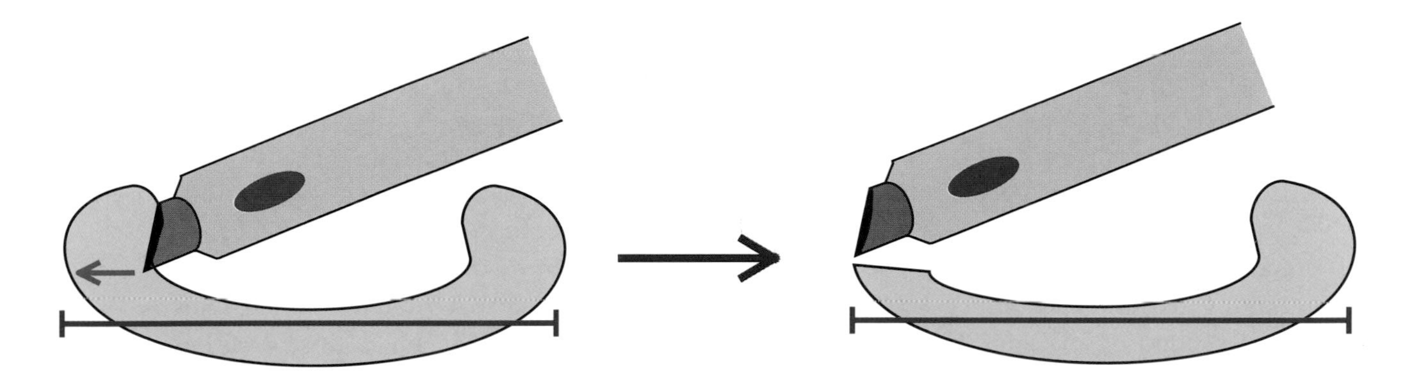

Figure 3-33-1

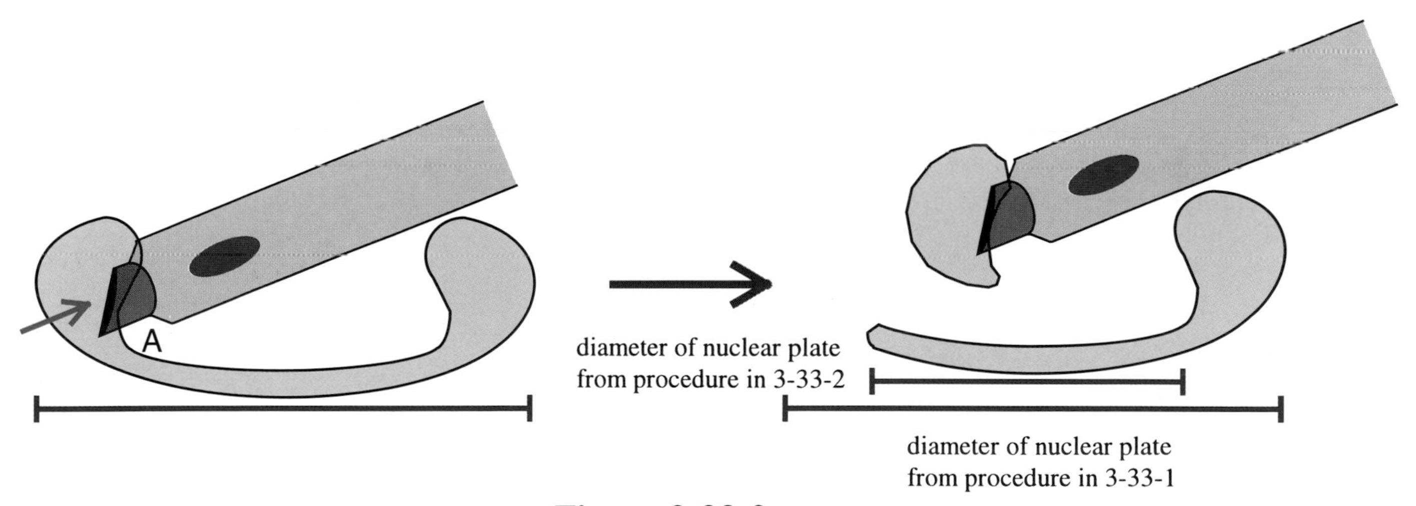

Figure 3-33-2

Figure 3-33

One-Handed Strategies 2

An important key to efficiency in phaco surgery is to be always thinking several steps ahead of your current step; by planning each step so that it will facilitate subsequent steps, you will avoid painting yourself into a corner. As an example, let's continue with the procedure begun on the previous page. Figure 3-34-1 shows the microscope's anterior view of the nuclear bowl which has been sculpted out so that a faultline has been created around the perimeter of the planned nuclear base. The phaco tip is embedded in the nuclear rim as shown using mild ultrasound power and then reverting to pedal position 2 only; the rim segment is then broken free while pulling while maintaining position 2 in Figure 3-34-2. You will sometimes have to facilitate removal of this first section by making phaco nicks in the rim on either side of it. Once this piece has been safely emulsified in the center, the tip is positioned so as to reengage the rim as illustrated in Figure 3-34-3.

At this point, the tip could be pulled to break off another section of rim, but doing so would simply remove the contra-incisional portion of the rim while leaving poor access to the remainder of the nucleus; remember by definition that a one-handed strategy does not give you access to a second instrument which could rotate the nucleus to provide more rim in the 6 o'clock position. The most effective way to rotate the nucleus with the phaco tip is by pulling (see Figure 3-16), but that will not be possible with the entire inferior section of rim removed. It is possible to rotate it by nudging the nuclear plate, but this has both a poor mechanical advantage as well as a poor safety margin. A better option that sets up subsequent steps is shown by the green arrows in Figure 3-34-3, in which the tip is used to rotate the nucleus so that the engaged portion may be removed at the same clock position as the original segment. By repeating this process, each step sets up the subsequent step until the rim is completely removed and a nuclear plate remains.

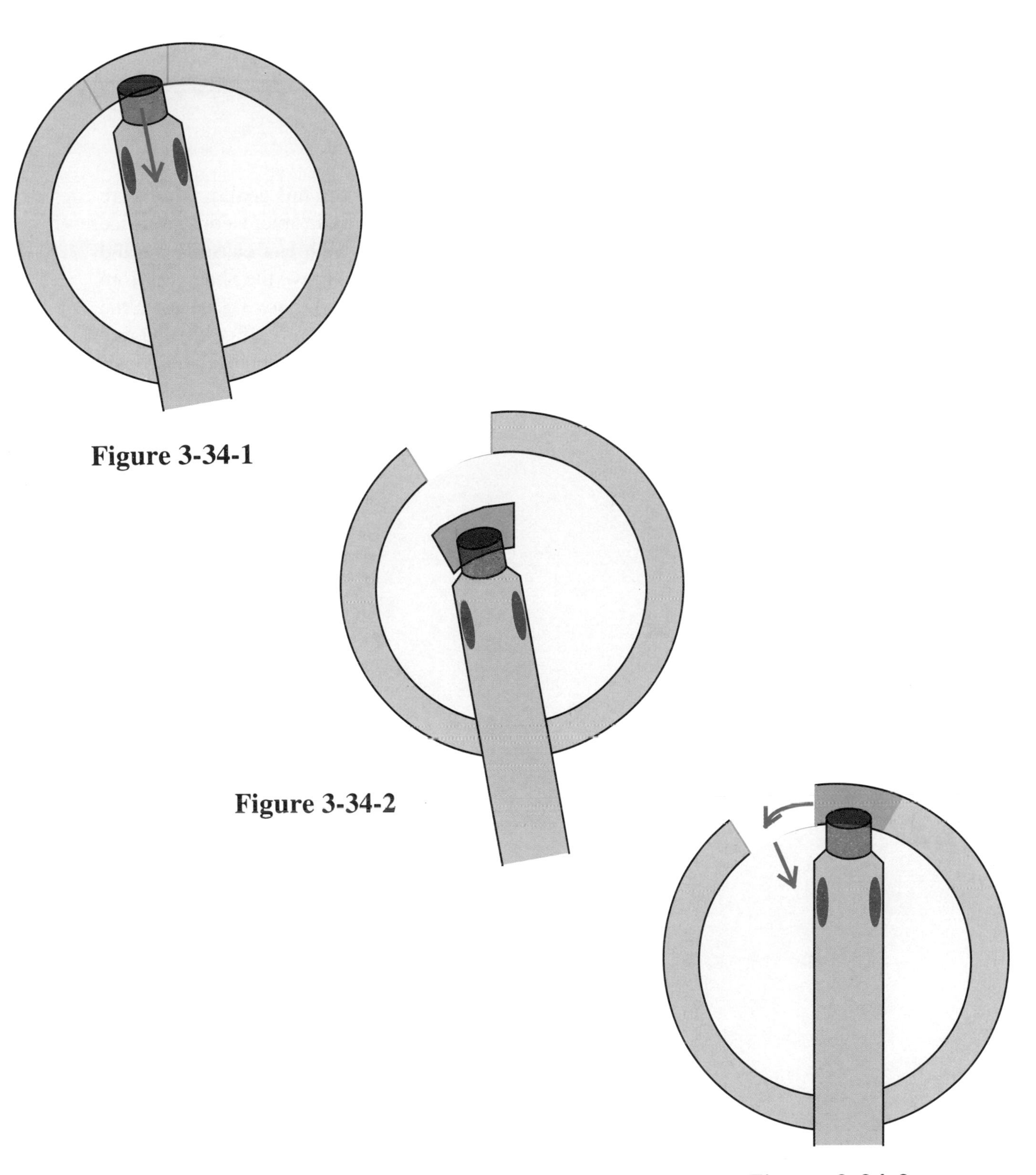
Figure 3-34-1

Figure 3-34-2

Figure 3-34-3

Figure 3-34

Pivot Around Incisions 1

All intraocular maneuvers need optimum visualization. With this goal in mind, care must be taken to pivot around side-port and tunnel incisions to avoid corneal striae which inhibit visualization and to avoid wound distortion which can cause leaks and chamber collapse (Figure 3-35-1). In Figure 3-35-2, we wish to move the phaco tip from point A to point B. The shortest, intuitive movement is shown in Figure 3-35-3; note the resultant corneal striae. By pivoting around the incision as in Figure 3-35-4, this wound distortion is avoided. Sometimes corneal striae are unavoidable, especially when dealing with an anterior corneal entry found in sutureless-style sclerocorneal and clear corneal incisions; however, careful attention to pivoting can still lessen the effect.

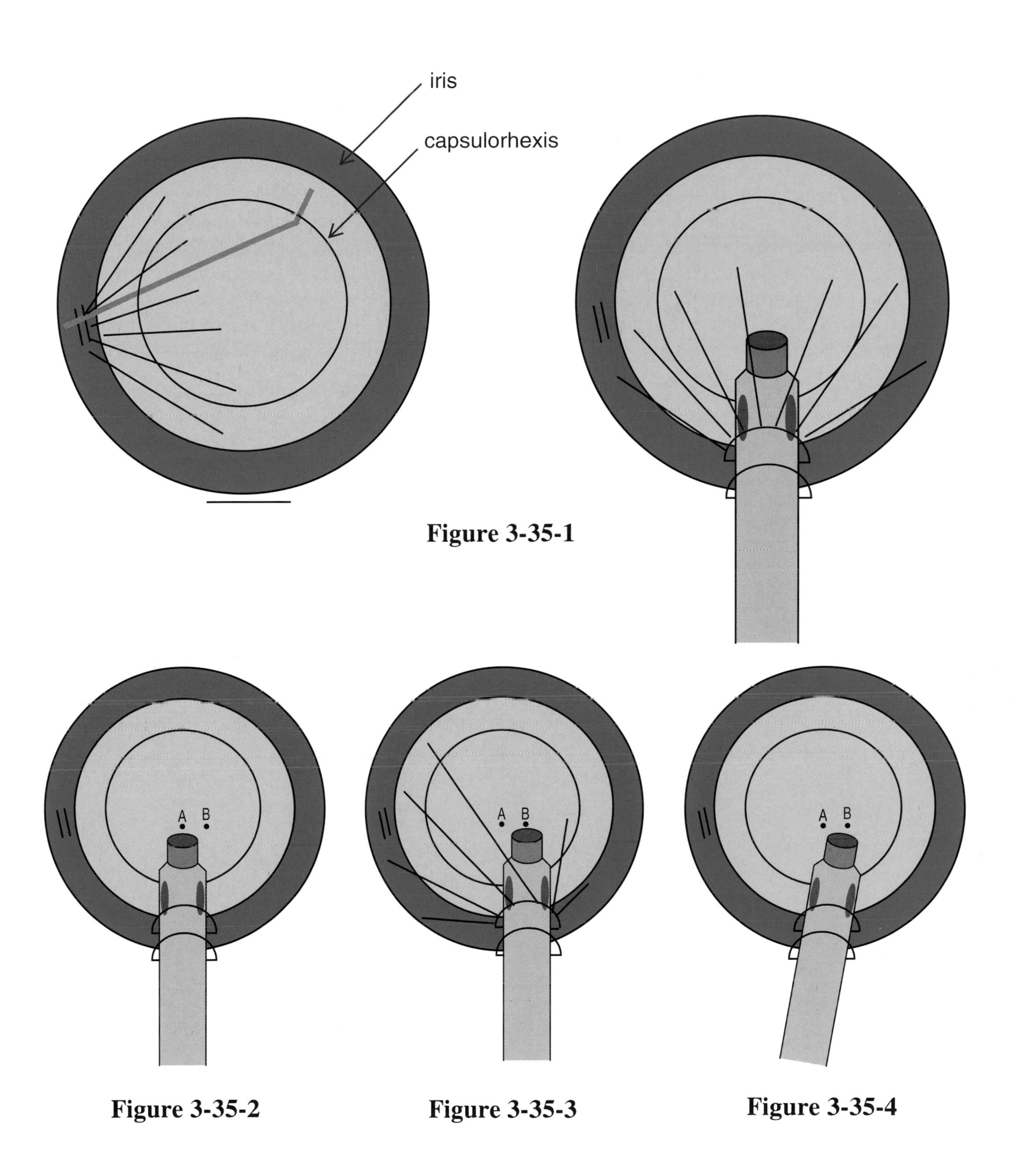

Figure 3-35-1

Figure 3-35-2

Figure 3-35-3

Figure 3-35-4

Figure 3-35

Pivot Around Incisions 2

Figure 3-36 illustrates another disadvantage of not pivoting around incisions; the eye is easily decentered, requiring frustratingly frequent X-Y scope adjustments. As a corollary, remember that you can intentionally move the eye in this fashion to, for example, enhance the red reflex. Using both the main incision and the side-port incision, you can coarsely manipulate the eye in X-Y fashion by simply moving the instruments inserted through these incisions. Once the eye is in the desired position, you can then pivot the instruments within the incisions to reach any part within the eye without affecting the eye's position.

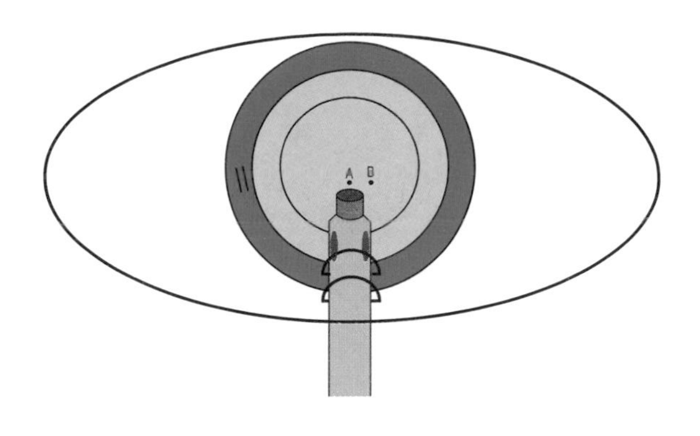

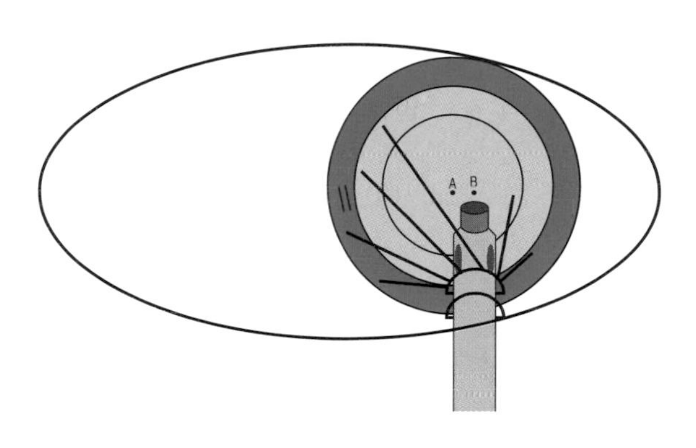

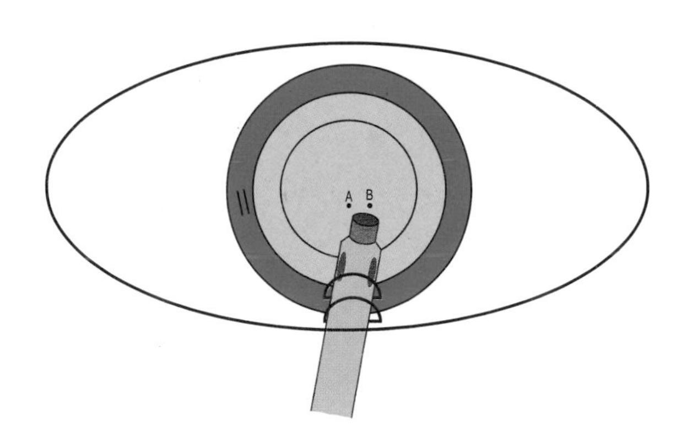

Figure 3-36

SECTION FOUR

Irrigation and Aspiration Techniques

Cortical Classification

When phacoemulsification is complete, we would all like to be left with cortex such as that engaged by tip A in Figure 4-1. This soft, thick material is readily engaged and aspirated. However, this is not the case with the thin, diaphanous strands of cortex drawn into tip B. Because these strands lack sufficient volume to completely occlude the tip, flow is often of greater importance than vacuum in optimizing machine parameters; the frictional force of a rapid flow over the cortical strands functions to pull them along with the flow current. When using a vacuum pump, flow and vacuum **autoregulate** their effect on the strands relative to the proportion of the tip that is unoccluded vs occluded, respectively; if the strands are not being effectively aspirated, the surgeon simply increases the commanded vacuum level.

The effect of flow and vacuum is perhaps better illustrated when using a flow pump. If a low flow rate is used (ie, 10cc/min), the strands at tip B might be drawn into the aspiration port, but it is unlikely that they will be effectively aspirated from the eye, even if a high vacuum preset level is set. The reasoning is two-fold. First, low flow rates will not effectively build vacuum even with an unoccluded IA tip even if a high preset vacuum limit is chosen (see Figure 1-35b). Furthermore, the slow flow exerts insufficient frictional force on the strands to draw them away from their capsular adhesions. Therefore, one should use a more effective higher flow rate when dealing with cortical strands (eg, about 30cc/min); moreover, the vacuum limit must be set high enough so that the pump does not stop when resistance to flow raises the vacuum in the aspiration line. For example, note in Figure 1-35b that a commanded flow of 30cc/min produces a vacuum inside the 0.3mm IA tip of 200mm Hg. The preset vacuum level should therefore be set higher (eg, 350mm Hg) so that flow can be maintained through a partially or non-occluded tip. If a vacuum limit of 100mm Hg were instead used, the flow would never build past 20cc/min even though the commanded flow was set to 30cc/min; the reason would be the feedback loop from the vacuum limit stopping the pump when vacuum had built to the preset of 100mm Hg from fluidic resistance through the unoccluded IA tip at 20cc/min.

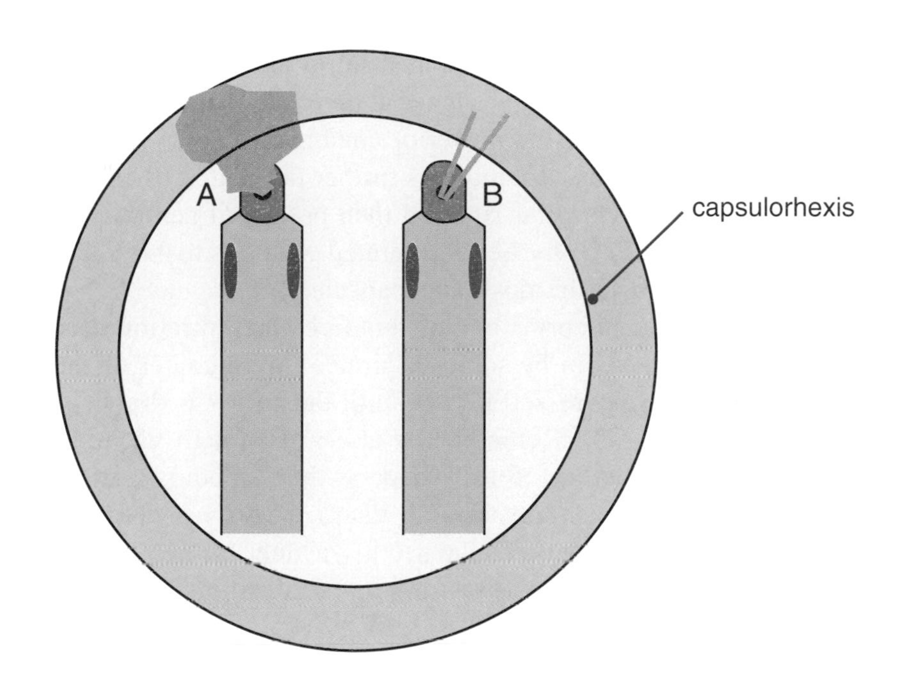

Figure 4-1

Cortical Removal: Large Pieces Instead of Small Bites

With the IA tip positioned as in Figure 4-2-1, you have a couple of options. You could fully depress the IA pedal and readily aspirate a chunk of cortex (assuming a high vacuum preset level); however, this maneuver would have some disadvantages. First, you would have to reengage and reaspirate many times to remove all of the cortex if you are taking only a small amount at a time. Secondly, aspiration of in situ cortex increases the danger of inadvertently aspirating adjacent structures such as iris and capsule. A better technique is to use linear vacuum control and to only depress the foot pedal far enough into position 2 to firmly engage the cortex without aspirating it. As the tip is moved toward the center of the posterior chamber, the cortex is gently peeled away as shown in Figure 4-2-2. This technique is further facilitated by initially engaging the cortex under the **anterior** capsular rim and then peeling it centrally; any inadvertant capsule incarceration would be far better tolerated with this technique as opposed to engaging the cortex adjacent to the **posterior** capsule.

With a large piece of cortex completely free, the aspiration port is then turned superiorly so that the cortex can be safely aspirated in the center of the posterior chamber. The foot pedal is then depressed further until the cortex is drawn as a continuous piece into the tip (Figure 4-2-3). Remember to use just enough vacuum to accomplish your goal. It might be unnecessary to fully depress the IA pedal in order to completely aspirate the cortex, and using more vacuum than necessary decreases your safety margin. When you make an incremental increase in vacuum by depressing the pedal to a new position, remember to wait for rise time before deciding whether to increase vacuum still further (see Figures 1-20 and 1-33).

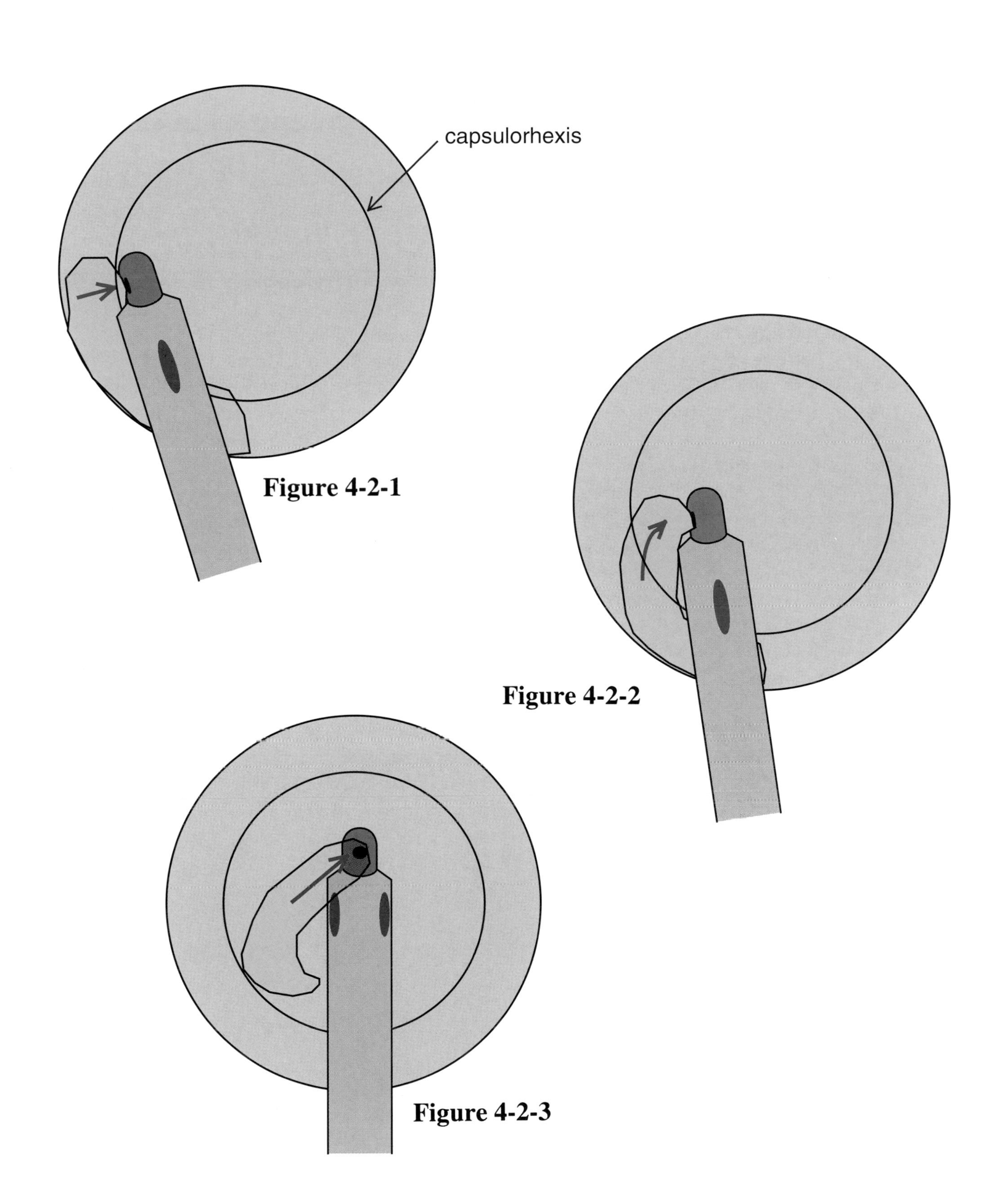

Figure 4-2-1

Figure 4-2-2

Figure 4-2-3

Figure 4-2

IA Port Turned Posteriorly

This is a technique that is often helpful for removing cortex at the sub-incisional position with the straight tip. As long as the aspiration port is occluded with cortex, the posterior capsule is safe (Figure 4-3-1). However, if this occluded cortex is suddenly aspirated instead of gently engaged and pulled as in the previous page, the posterior capsule can be directly exposed to the aspiration port's reestablished flow and potential surge (Figure 4-3-2). A characteristic star fold pattern is produced when the IA tip grabs the posterior capsule as shown in Figure 4-3-3. The probability of posterior capsule rupture in this situation depends on several factors. The most dangerous set of variables would include a vacuum pump machine with a high maximum vacuum preset and a fully depressed foot pedal. The rapid transfer of vacuum with tip occlusion (rise time), which is characteristic of vacuum pumps, would likely deform and rupture the incarcerated capsule. The safety margin could be increased in this case by using a lower maximum vacuum preset. Also, you could utilize linear IA control with the foot pedal only partly depressed into position 2 to initially engage cortex without abruptly aspirating it, as in Figure 4-2. When using a flow pump machine, safety can be maximized by using a slower commanded flow rate; the aspiration line would not have any significant vacuum preload without occlusion, and the slow rise time would allow the maximum time for you to react before dangerous levels of vacuum were obtained.

When confronted with such a capsular star fold, you can be virtually assured of tearing the capsule if you panic and suddenly jerk the tip away while the capsule is engaged. The vast majority of these inadvertent capsular aspirations can be safely dealt with as long as you **do not move the tip**. Train yourself to react to this situation not with your hands but with your foot; go immediately to position 1 for venting of built-up vacuum (see Figures 1-13 and 1-41) or even to reflux position to disengage the capsule. Then take a deep breath and let your pulse return to normal.

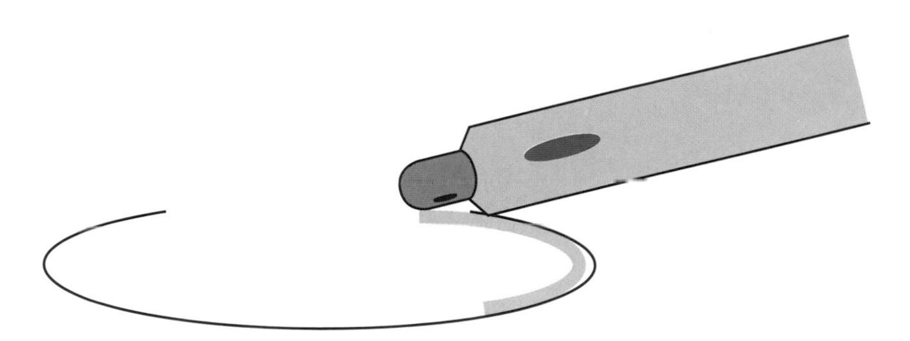

Figure 4-3-1

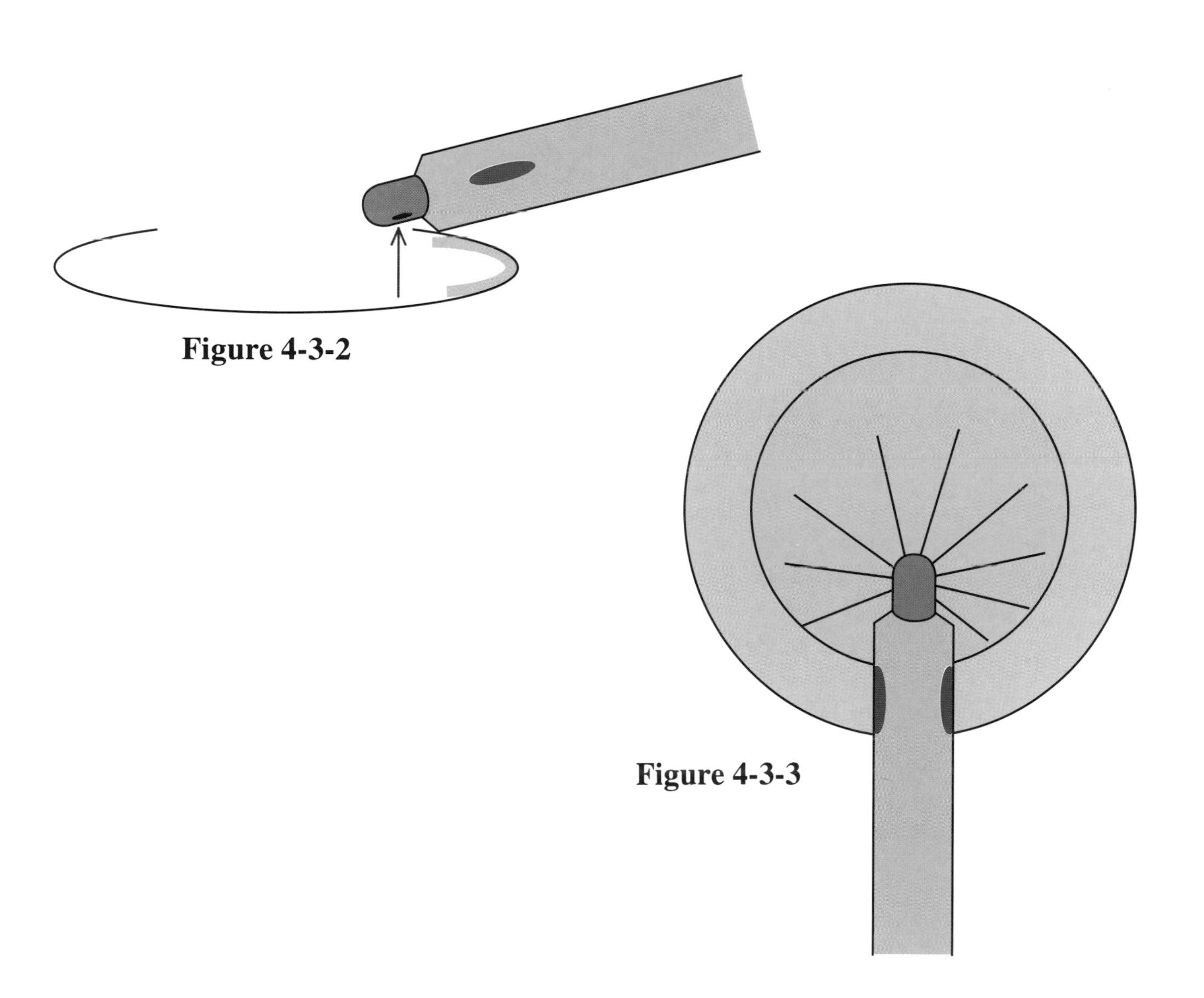

Figure 4-3-2

Figure 4-3-3

Figure 4-3

Manual Cortical Removal

A 27-gauge angled or J-shaped cannula can be used on an irrigating syringe as shown in Figure 4-4. This technique is often helpful for tenacious sub-incisional cortex. The goal is not to necessarily aspirate the cortex completely but rather to engage it and peel it away from the capsule, pulling it to the center of the iris plane. At this point you can easily remove it by replacing the cannula with the IA tip with the aspiration port safely turned superiorly; the now free-floating cortex will be readily attracted to the aspiration port even when using moderate flow rates.

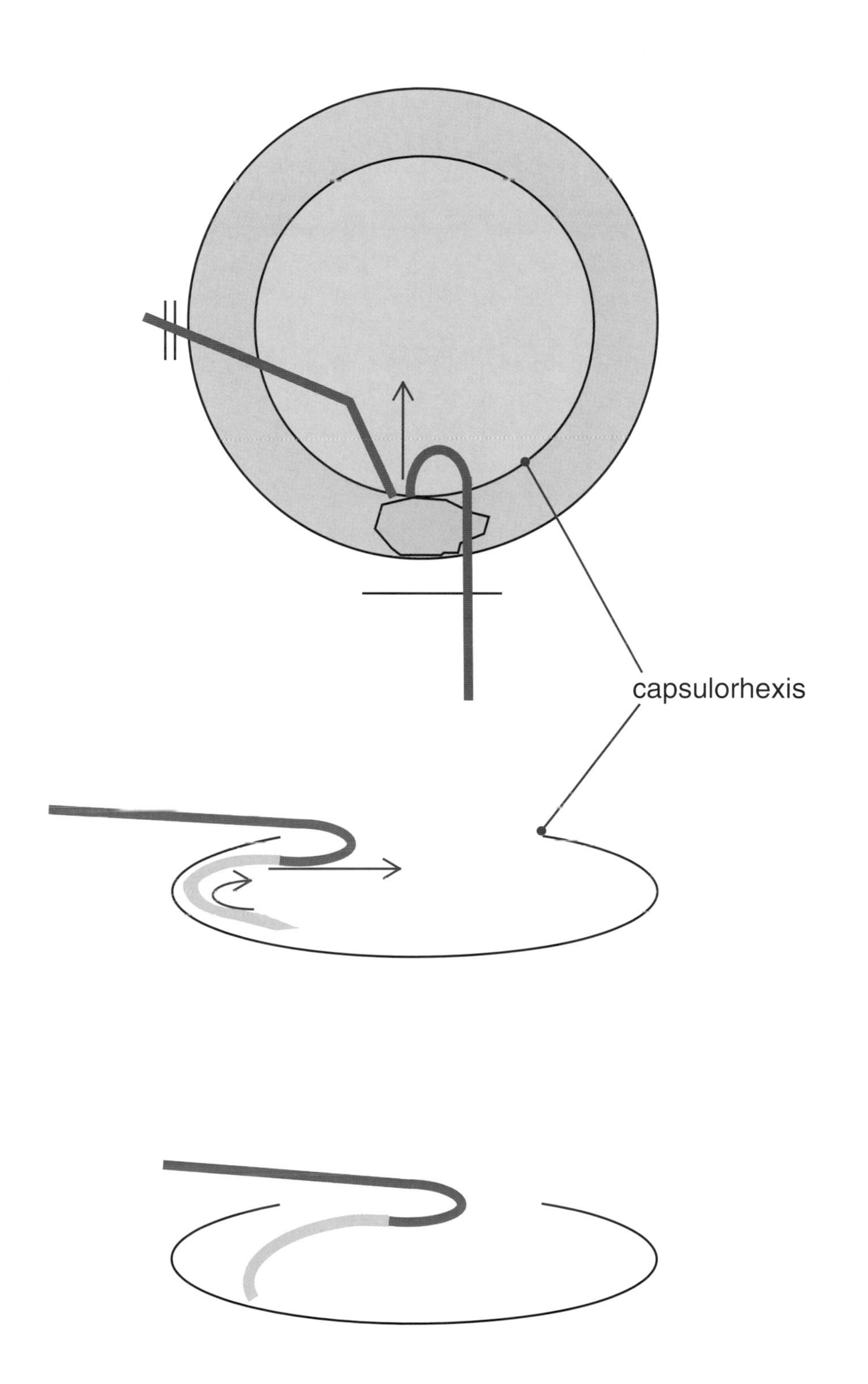

Figure 4-4

90° and 45° IA Tips

These tips provide alternatives to the standard straight tip when you encounter cortex in difficult positions, particularly at the sub-incisional location. The 90° tip has several advantages at this position. The vacuum pulls most strongly in a peripheral direction as indicated by the arrow in Figure 4-5-1. Therefore, the most likely material to be aspirated is the cortex, not the capsule. Additional capsule protection is provided by the fact that the part of the tip that contacts the capsule is 90° away from the aspiration port, thereby physically holding the posterior capsule away from the port. Contrast this configuration to the 45° tip shown in Figure 4-5-2. Note how the part of the tip contacting the capsule is only 45° away from the aspiration port; the capsule is therefore more vulnerable to inadvertent aspiration with this tip relative to the 90° tip configuration. Similarly, the vacuum pulls most strongly in a direction 45° posteriorly as indicated by the arrow; the capsule is just as likely as cortex to be aspirated in this illustration.

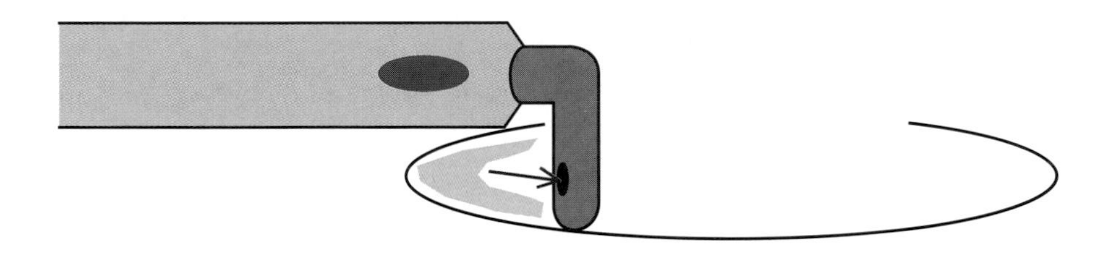

Figure 4-5-1

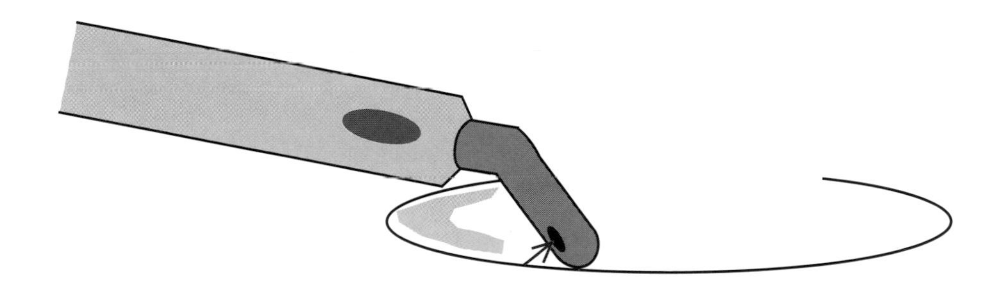

Figure 4-5-2

Figure 4-5

Using the IOL to Help Remove Cortex

The IOL, or intraocular lens, can be used to help remove residual cortex in two ways. First, rotation of the lens in the bag utilizes the haptics to help dislodge peripheral cortex so that it can be more readily attracted to the IA tip. Secondly, you can use the tip-down configuration shown in Figure 4-6. Having the aspiration port in such close approximation to the IOL surface effectively decreases the diameter of the port, much the same as pressing your thumb over the end of a garden hose creates a higher pressure system; the resultant increased vacuum preload more readily aspirates any engaged cortex. In addition, the IOL provides a physical barrier between the posterior capsule and the aspiration port.

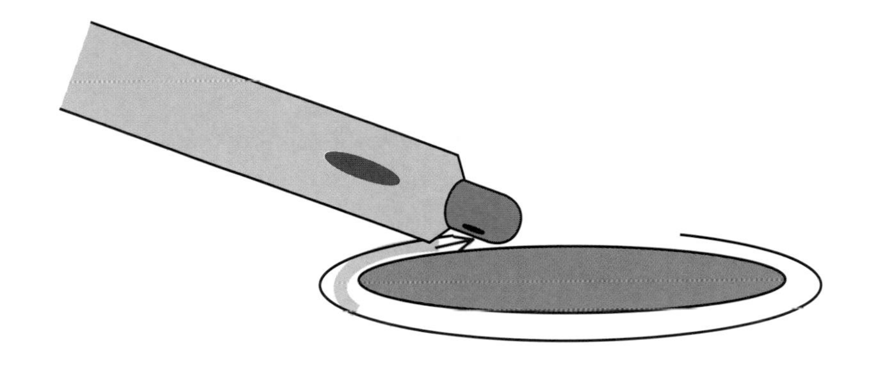

Figure 4-6

Linear Vacuum vs Linear Flow

In IA mode, some flow pumps offer the option of either linear pedal control of flow (ie, rotational speed of the pump head) or linear pedal control of vacuum. If the surgical goal is to engage cortex for peeling away from the capsule as shown in Figure 4-2, then linear vacuum control is more effective. The object in this case is to grip the cortex with just enough force (vacuum) to allow positive control (Figure 4-7-1) but not so much force that material is abruptly aspirated (Figure 4-7-2). Recall that the vacuum limit is preset on the machine's control panel and that the actual vacuum (with full aspiration port occlusion) is titrated with linear pedal movement. If the surgeon prematurely pushes the pedal slightly past the optimum gripping vacuum level (eg, material just begins to aspirate through the port), then the pedal pressure can be **slightly** reversed to reestablish an appropriate gripping level of vacuum. Contrast this scenario to that of linear flow control, under which vacuum could not be decreased after it started to cause premature aspiration of cortex (other than with a return to position 1 and venting completely back to zero vacuum relative to the IOP). Linear flow control would allow titration of the rise time, but this would still not allow diminution of vacuum once the optimum gripping level had been surpassed. The main advantage of flow control is for dealing with thin strands of diaphanous cortex as discussed in Figure 4-1. Perhaps the most effective mode of control is with a vacuum pump (or with a flow pump used in vacuum emulation); in these cases, grip could be precisely titrated to thick cortex as discussed above, and grip and flow would **autoregulate** with thin cortex as a function of applied vacuum as discussed with Figure 4-1. Alternatively, a Dual Linear foot pedal could be utilized with a flow pump so that both vacuum and flow could be simultaneously and independently adjusted as necessary.

Note that Figure 4-7-2 depicts the actual vacuum at the moment of occlusion break and aspiration of cortex; the actual vacuum will subsequently decrease with the decreased resistance through the aspiration port.

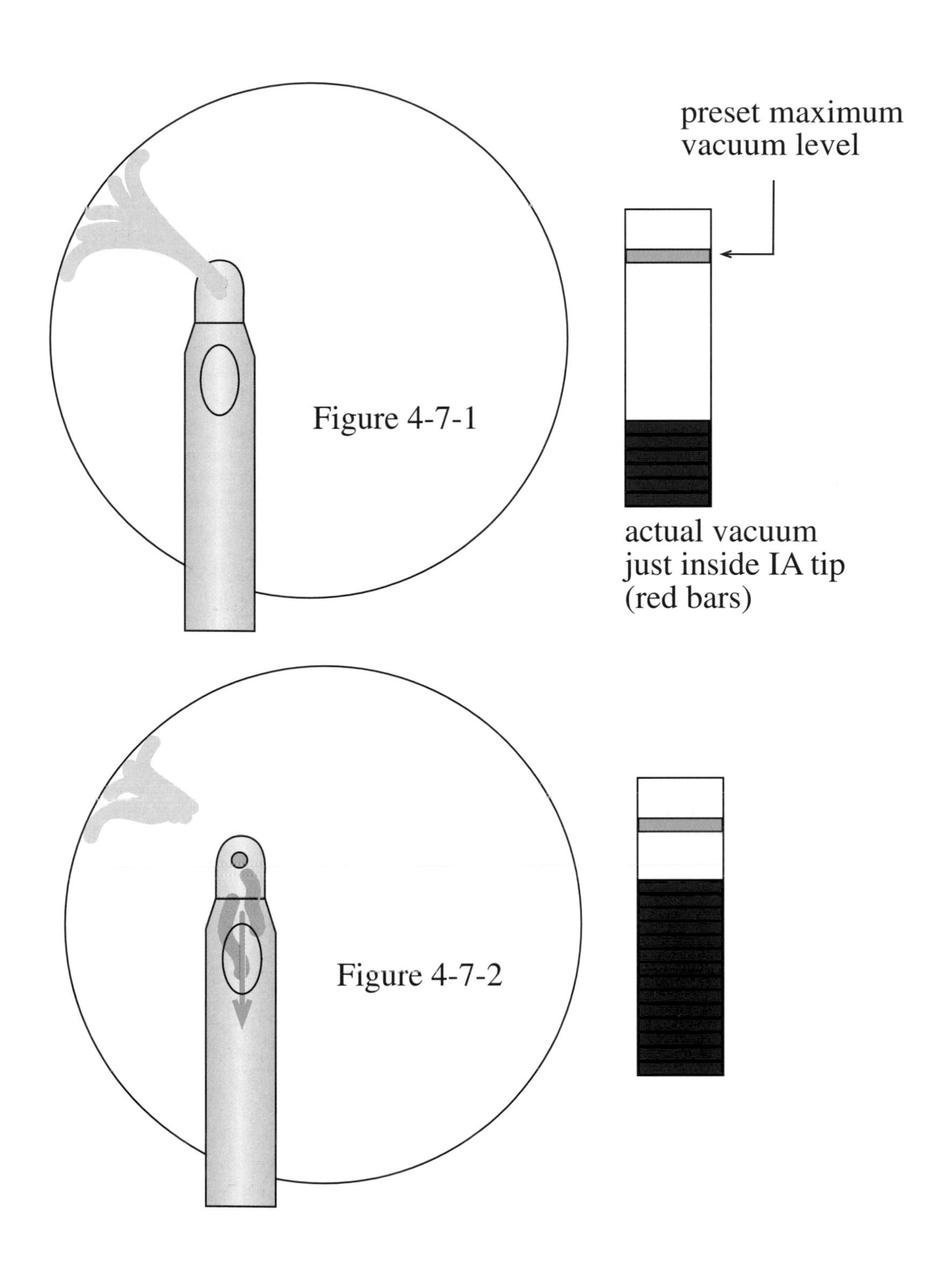
preset maximum
vacuum level
Figure 4-7-1
actual vacuum
just inside IA tip
(red bars)
Figure 4-7-2

Figure 4-7

SECTION FIVE

Physics of Capsulorhexis

Stress and Strain

The Continuous Curvilinear Capsulorhexis was independently developed by Drs. Howard Gimbel and Thomas Neuhann; it is universally acknowledged as one of the fundamental elements of modern phaco surgical techniques. An understanding of the dynamics of creating a capsulorhexis begins with an overview of material analysis. Figure 5-1-1 is a strip of material without any forces acting on it; the interdigitated central portion represents the intermolecular attractions at this location. Figure 5-1-2 depicts the material with very mild force applied as indicated by the arrows; **stress** is the force divided by the cross-sectional area where the force is being applied (the central interdigitated area in this case). In Figure 5-1-3, the stress has increased (bigger arrows) so that the material begins to deform; note the stretching at the center. **Strain** is defined as the change in length of a deformed material divided by its original length. If strain is increased just beyond a material's elastic limit, the material will be permanently deformed even after stress is discontinued. As strain increases further beyond the elastic limit, stress usually initially increases slightly but then decreases as the material's **breaking point** is approached. When this point is reached, the intermolecular bonds are broken and the material tears apart. Note the slightly smaller force arrows in Figure 5-1-4 relative to those in Figure 5-1-3; these smaller arrows represent the force required just prior to the breaking point.

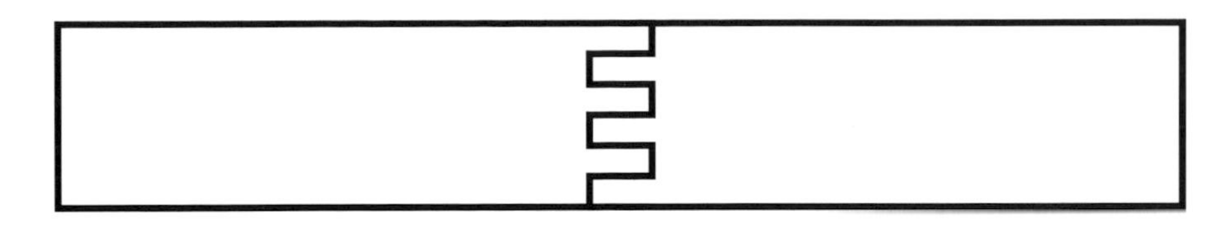

Figure 5-1-1

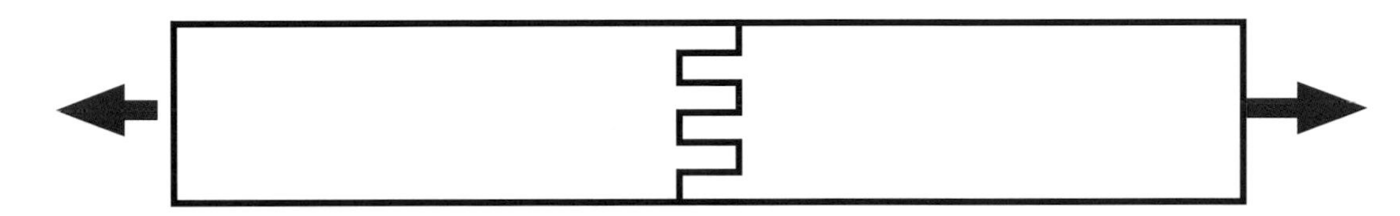

Figure 5-1-2

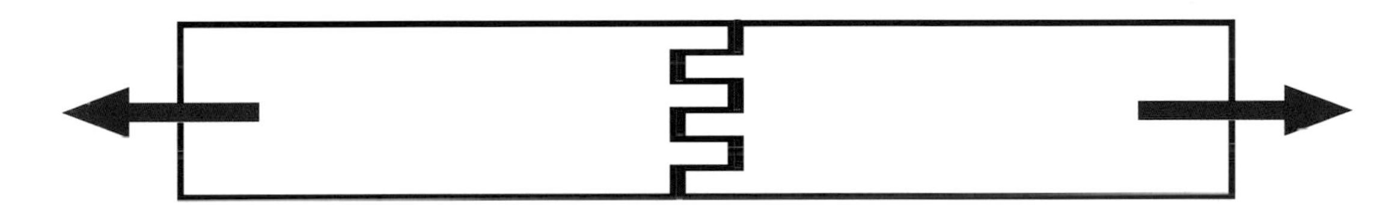

Figure 5-1-3

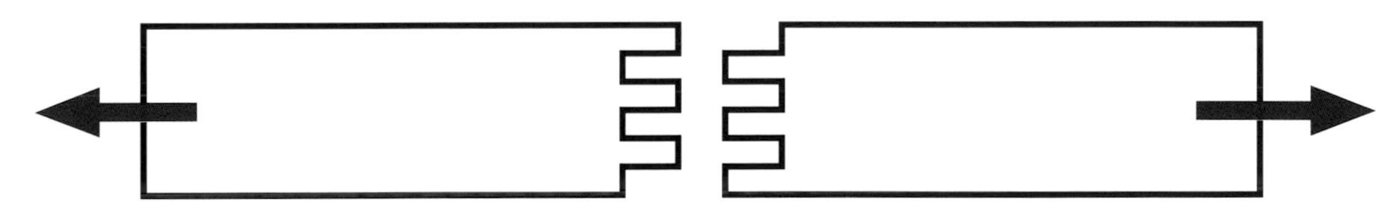

Figure 5-1-4

Figure 5-1

Shear vs Rip

Figure 5-2-1 illustrates shearing principles. Area x remains stationary while area y is pulled from point a to point b in order to tear this material from point A to point B. All of the pulling force is concentrated at the point of tearing and is in the same direction as the tear. Even though area y may still be engaged by a cystotome or forceps at point b, no further tearing will occur as long as the instrument is not moved. Contrast this with the ripping schematic shown in Figure 5-2-2, where area x is again stationary and the material is engaged with an instrument at the blue dot and pulled with vector force t (note the arrows going to the left which represent the counterforce caused by the left side of the material being stationary). Although no tearing occurs while y is pulled from a toward b, stress and strain in the material progressively increase. When point b is reached, the strain passes the material's breaking point and ripping begins in the direction noted by arrow E. Figure 5-2-2 depicts the material just as ripping begins. Point A has just ripped apart. Point B is undergoing strain. Point C has some stress without any deformation, and point D has no forces acting on it. Note the changes in the points when the rip reaches point B (Figure 5-2-3). Point C, which previously had stress without deformation, now has strain. Point D, which formerly had no forces acting on it, now has stress. The rip will tend to propagate in this fashion as long as area y is held firmly at point b, even though it is not being moved any further. Recall that the stress required at the breaking point is less than that required to reach the breaking point; the surplus force fuels the tear's propagation.

Therefore, ripping the capsule is less desirable than shearing for two reasons. First, the tear tends to uncontrollably extend when ripping even when the grasping instrument is held stationary. Second, more force is generally needed to begin a tear with ripping as opposed to shearing because the force is distributed over a larger area with ripping (ie, at points A, B, and C in 5-2-2) relative to the concentration of force just at the point of tearing with shearing (point A in Figure 5-2-1). Moreover, only a component vector (t_1) of the pulling force pulls the material apart with ripping while the residual force (t_2) serves to direct the rip in direction E; contrast this to the efficiency in shearing of all of the pulling force being utilized in the direction of the tear.

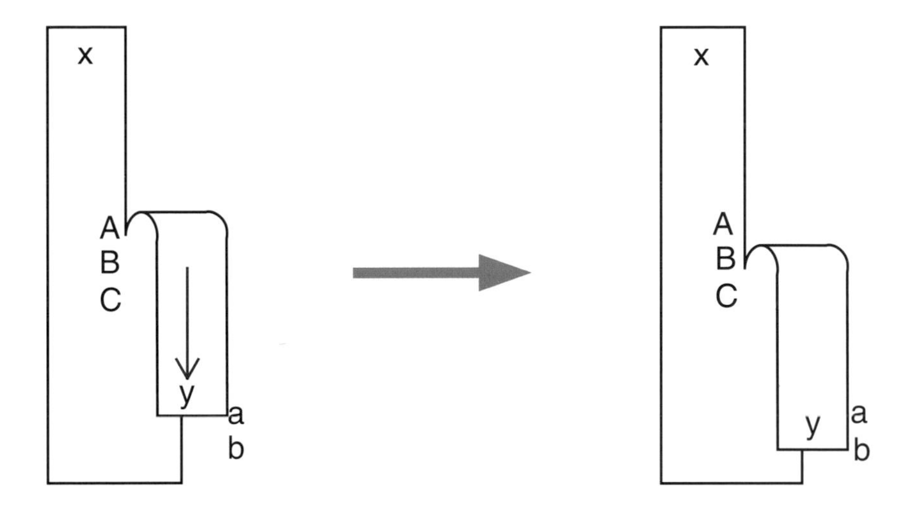

Figure 5-2-1

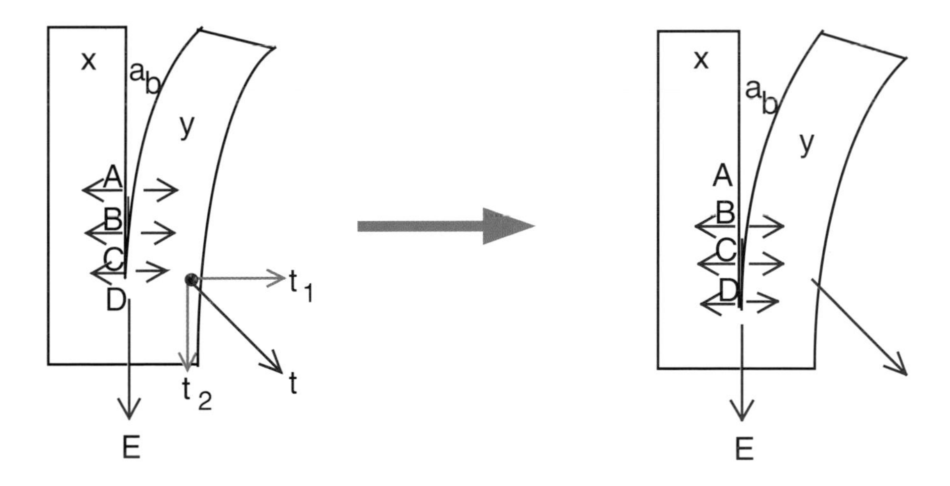

Figure 5-2-2

Figure 5-2-3

Figure 5-2

Capsulorhexis with Shearing

Capsulorhexis often begins with the formation of a flap as in Figure 5-3-1. The cystotome enters at point 1 and then proceeds to point 4 using either small, connecting can-opener bites or a side-cutting cystotome. At point 4, the cystotome is pulled in the direction of the blue arrow to create a capsular flap, which is then folded over to lay on top of intact anterior capsule as shown. The flap is engaged with a cystotome or capsular forceps at point y and pulled in the direction of the curved red arrow. When using a cystotome, press only hard enough to engage and move the flap; too much force may penetrate the flap, thus inadvertently cutting the intact capsule beneath as well as retarding progression of the flap because of resistance created by engaged cortex. Note that point y is somewhat inside of the peripheral edge of the flap in order to provide a safety margin against the cystotome slipping peripherally off of the flap and damaging intact capsule. Figure 5-3-2 shows further progress. Notice the symmetry around point a. The flap is a mirror image of the area of capsulorhexis performed thus far; furthermore, it provides a template showing where the capsulorhexis will proceed. The flap is grasped at point y and pulled in a curvilinear fashion as shown. Figure 5-3-3 shows the capsulorhexis one third completed. Notice how the point of instrument engagement (y) is adjusted to stay 2 to 3 clock hours away from the point of shearing. If the instrument were instead placed closer, such as point z, an artifactual stress line (green line) would be created which would compromise the predictability of the direction of shear propagation.

Compare the flap positions in Figures 5-3-2 and 5-3-4. Note the loss of symmetry around point a in Figure 5-3-4, which has more of a bullet-shaped configuration relative to the continuous mirror-image curve through point a in Figure 5-3-2. The reason for the difference is that the flap has not been spread out flat in Figure 5-3-4 (note the folds in the flap). If this flap is engaged at point y and pulled as shown, the capsulorhexis shear will proceed but with a smaller radius than in Figure 5-3-2. Sometimes you may elect to purposely change the size of the capsulorhexis in this manner, but be aware that only gradual changes in curvature are practical when utilizing shearing. If the flap is pulled to make an even smaller capsulorhexis than Figure 5-3-4 (ie, a more pointed bullet shape at point a), a distortion is induced at point a which converts the shear to a modified rip which often propagates peripherally. Abrupt changes in the direction of the tear are best accomplished by a planned ripping maneuver as shown in Figure 5-4.

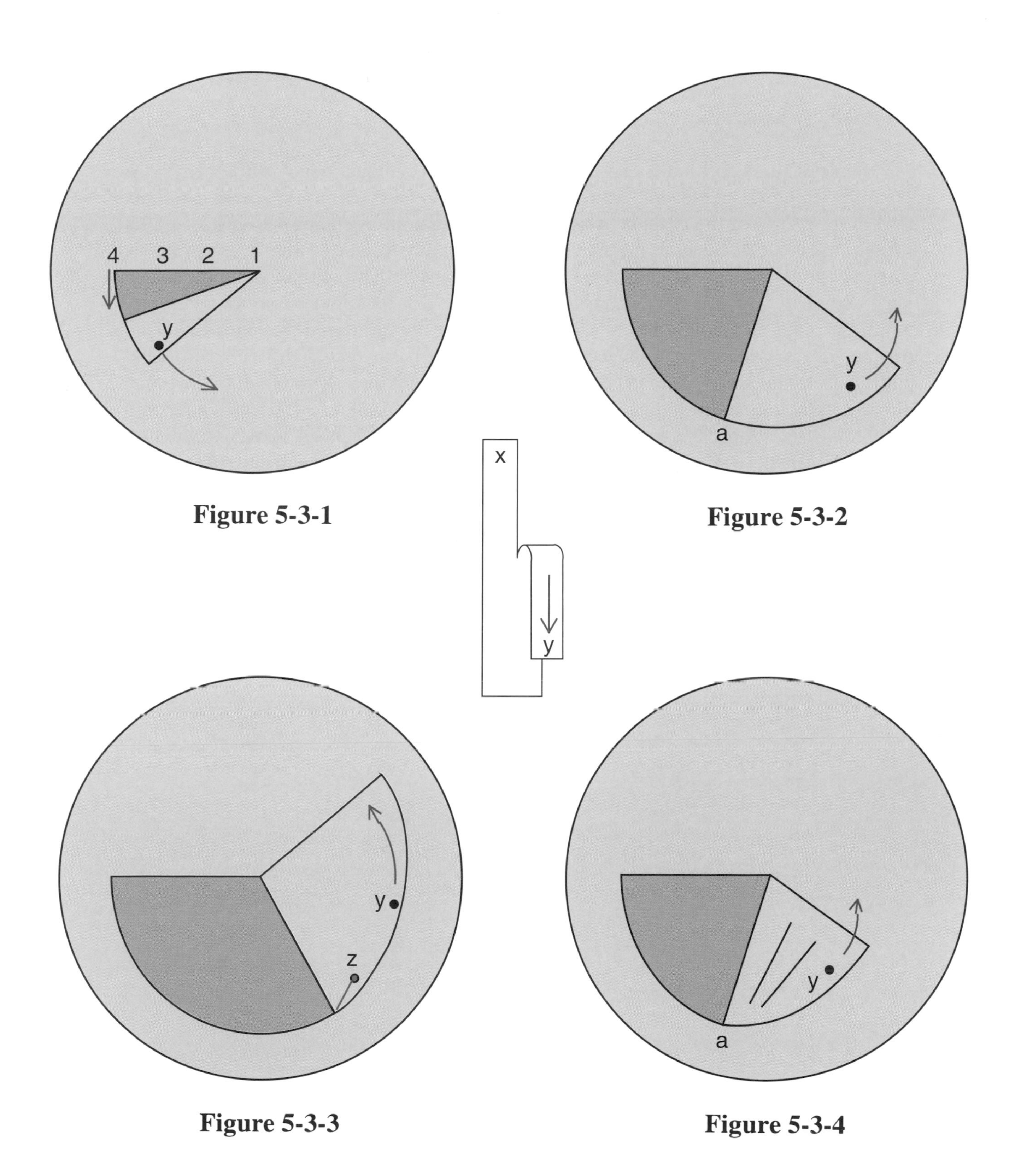

Figure 5-3-1

Figure 5-3-2

Figure 5-3-3

Figure 5-3-4

Figure 5-3

Capsulorhexis with Ripping

Figures 5-4-1 and 5-4-2 demonstrate a ripping technique, which differs from the shearing technique in several aspects. First, the direction of pulling is much more toward the center of the capsule. Also, the flap is engaged by the pulling instrument at a point that is much closer to the tear. Recall in a ripping technique how tearing force is spread over a relatively large surface area of the capsule between the grasping instrument and the tear; grabbing the capsule closer to the tear therefore improves control by minimizing any extraneous force. The reason why a ripping technique tends to extend peripherally is illustrated in Figure 5-4-4. This tendency is overcome by using sufficient pulling force in an appropriate direction (more toward the pupil center rather than directly in the direction of the desired tear) so that the capsule is distorted as shown in Figure 5-4-5, resulting in a circular propagation of the tear. Although ripping techniques are more difficult to control and are more likely to inadvertently extend peripherally relative to shearing techniques, they do have the advantage of enabling more abrupt changes in the direction of the tear.

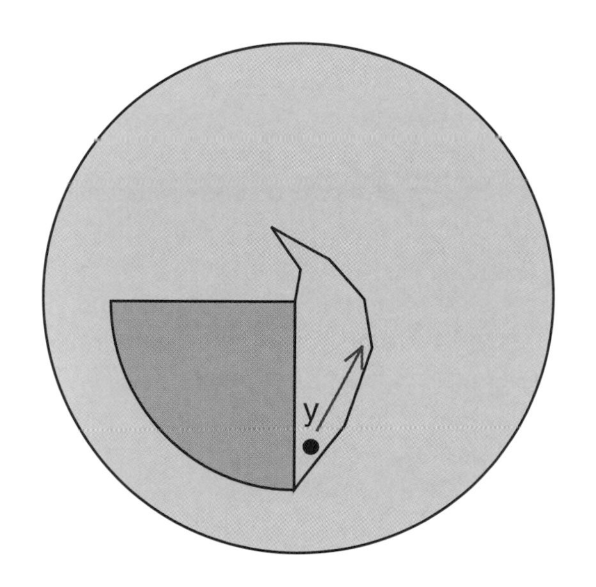

Figure 5-4-1

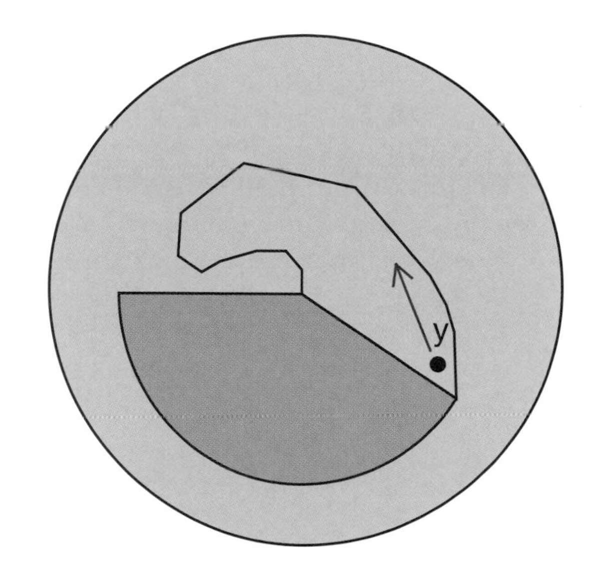

Figure 5-4-2

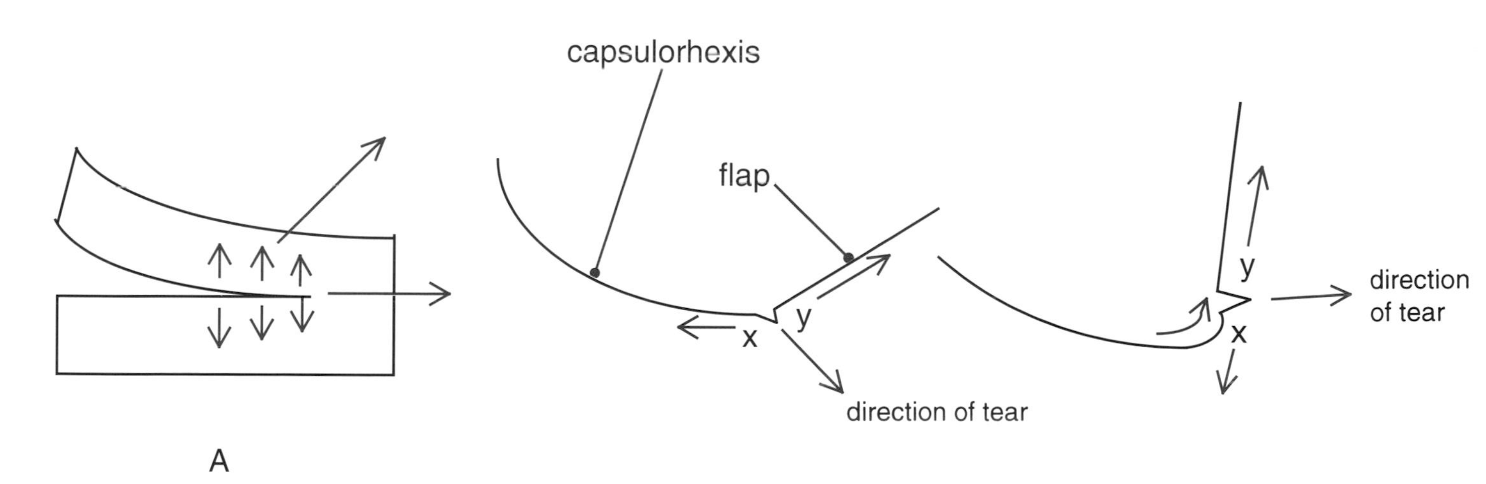

Figure 5-4-3 **Figure 5-4-4** **Figure 5-4-5**

Figure 5-4

Maintaining Chamber Depth

A shallow anterior chamber usually indicates that vitreous pressure is greater than anterior chamber pressure, resulting in the anterior displacement of the lens with zonular stress as shown in Figure 5-5-1. This stress acts on the site of a capsulorhexis tear at point x in a ripping configuration that will tend to peripherally extend the tear, sometimes even with just maintaining a grip at point y without any pulling (Figure 5-5-2). You can use viscoelastic to counteract the vitreous pressure and relieve stress on the zonules as in Figure 5-5-3; for this reason some surgeons like to perform the entire capsulorhexis with a cystotome on a viscoelastic syringe in order to readily compensate for any decrease in anterior chamber depth. Surgeons who prefer using capsulorhexis forceps should have viscoelastic readily available for injection through the side-port paracentesis incision in case of shallowing of the anterior chamber.

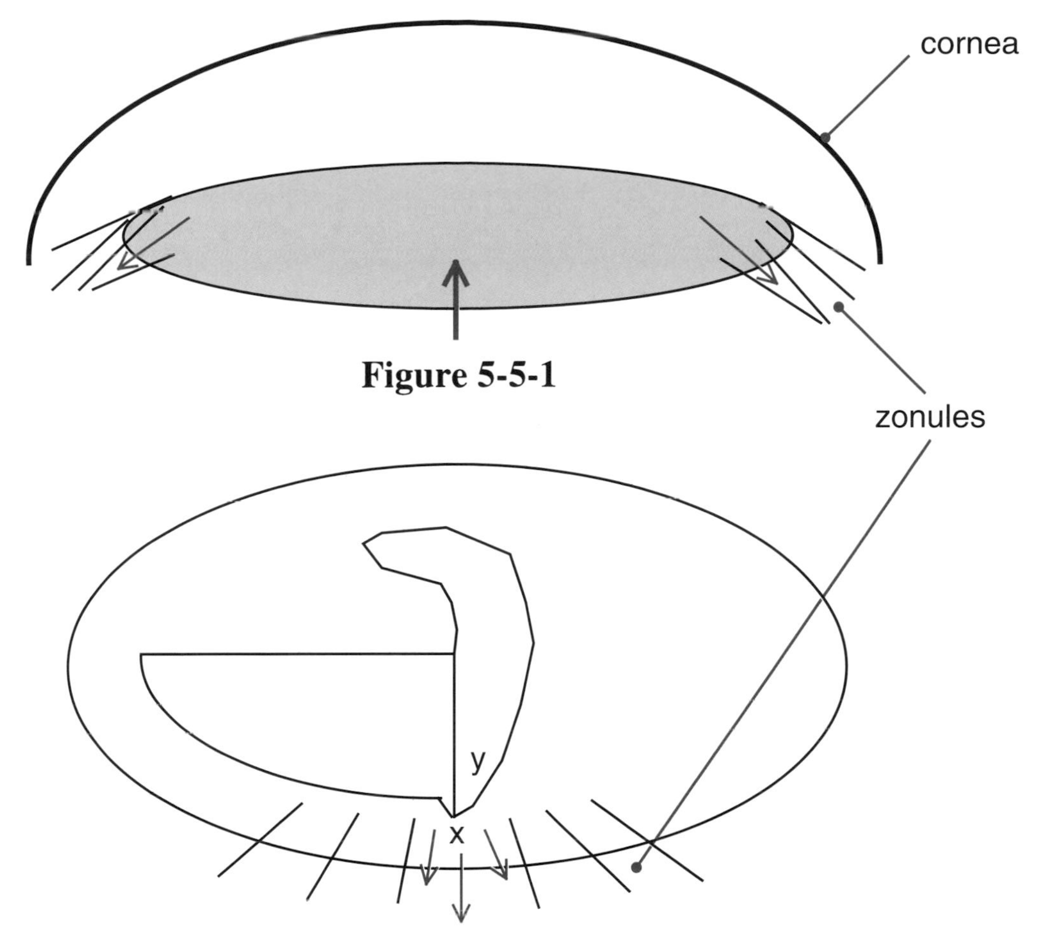

Figure 5-5-1

Figure 5-5-2

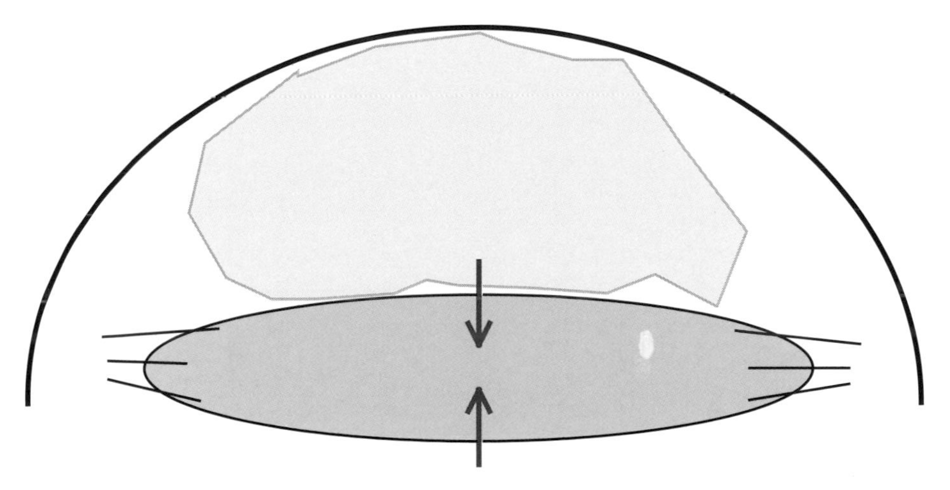

Figure 5-5-3

Figure 5-5

Combining Techniques

Figure 5-6-1 shows a capsulorhexis proceeding smoothly using a shearing technique; note the smooth mirror-image symmetry around point a. In Figure 5-6-2, a relative shallowing of the anterior chamber contributed to the peripheral extension of the tear. Point b is spear-/bullet-shaped instead of smoothly round. Attempting to correct the problem by abruptly changing direction with a shear technique (red arrow) will almost certainly produce more peripheral extension. The better option in this case is to convert to a ripping technique by engaging and pulling as indicated by the blue dot and arrow; viscoelastic is used to reinflate the chamber prior to executing the ripping maneuver. Once a desired configuration is again obtained, you can convert back to a shear technique as illustrated in Figure 5-6-3.

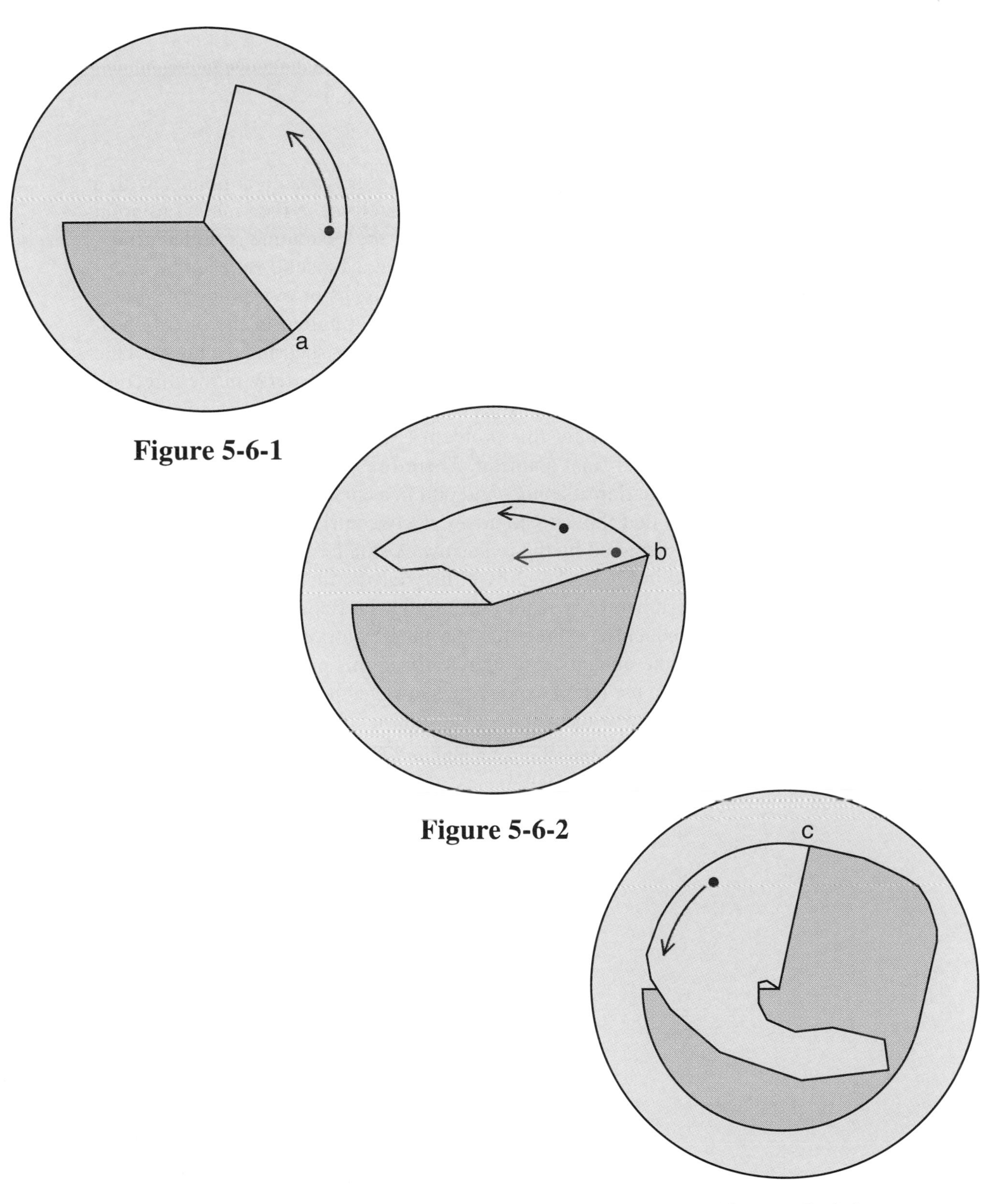

Figure 5-6-1

Figure 5-6-2

Figure 5-6-3

Figure 5-6

Capsulorhexis Initiation 1

One way to begin the capsulorhexis is by puncturing the capsule at point 1 with a side-cutting cystotome on a viscoelastic syringe. The cystotome is then moved to point 4, cleanly incising the capsule as it is moved. At point 4, the cystotome is pulled downward (blue arrow) to shear the capsule at this point so that a capsular flap can be created and rolled over as shown. The flap is engaged with forceps or cystotome at point y (originally the posterior surface of the anterior capsule) and pulled in the direction of the curvilinear green arrow to continue the capsulorhexis with a shearing technique. One problem with this technique is that the initial flap rarely shears exactly in the direction of the blue arrow as shown in Figure 5-7-1. It usually extends somewhat peripherally as shown in Figure 5-7-2. The remedy for this problem is to simply allow for it; point 4 should be central to your desired final diameter. Therefore, when given the configuration in Figure 5-7-2, engage the flap at point y and pull in a curvilinear fashion as depicted by the green arrow. Note that this curved arrow is concentric to the desired path of the capsulorhexis, which is depicted by the red arrow. A smaller diameter capsulorhexis could have been obtained in Figure 5-7-2 by either starting the flap closer to point 3 (thus allowing for some peripheral extension) or pulling the flap more centrally rather than concentrically to consequently redirect the tear more centrally (see Figure 5-3-4).

Note that point 1 is in the optical center; any error in this positioning should be to the right of center. If you err to the left of center (eg, starting at point 2), the resultant flap radius will be constrained such that the resultant capsulorhexis will be eccentric and too small. This error is of course easily rectified by making appropriate relaxing incisions to extend the flap radius to or beyond the center.

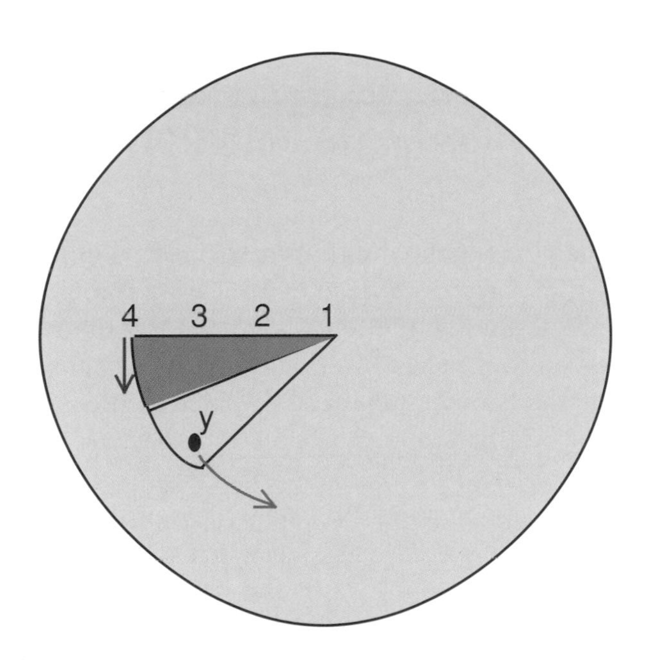

Figure 5-7-1

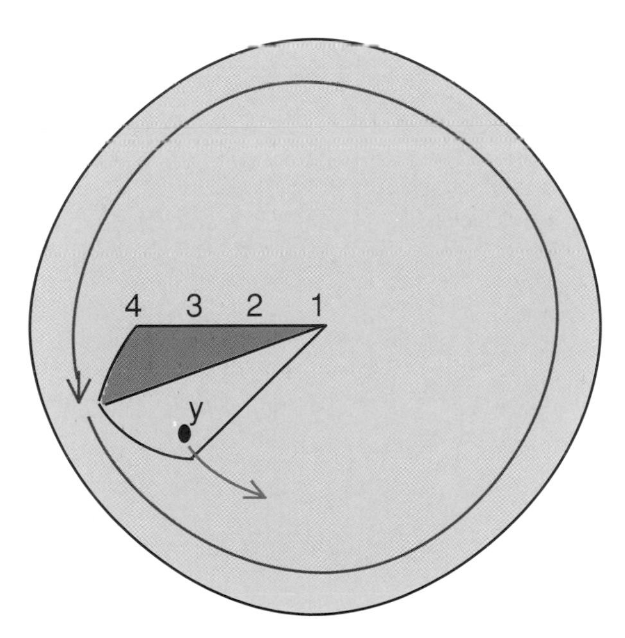

Figure 5-7-2

Figure 5-7

Capsulorhexis Initiation 2

Figure 5-8-1 illustrates the potential pitfalls associated with pulling the capsule at a point central to point 4 (blue arrow). Instead of a shearing force directed in the direction of the blue arrow right at point 4, the force is instead transmitted along the edge of the capsule (green arrows) to both ends of the incision, with consequent potential for peripheral extension of the incision at either end by ripping forces as shown by the red arrows. Extension at point 4 is particularly troublesome because if it extends into the zonules, recovery becomes difficult; conversion to a can-opener capsulotomy is often required in these cases. Extension at point 1 is usually less problematic. In fact, the possible extension at point 1 shown in Figure 5-8-2 can be used to begin the capsulorhexis by clockwise rotation of the flap as outlined by the red arrow. In general, however, if you wish to shear the capsule at point 4 to begin a flap, the most control can be achieved by pulling the capsule right at point 4 rather than more centrally.

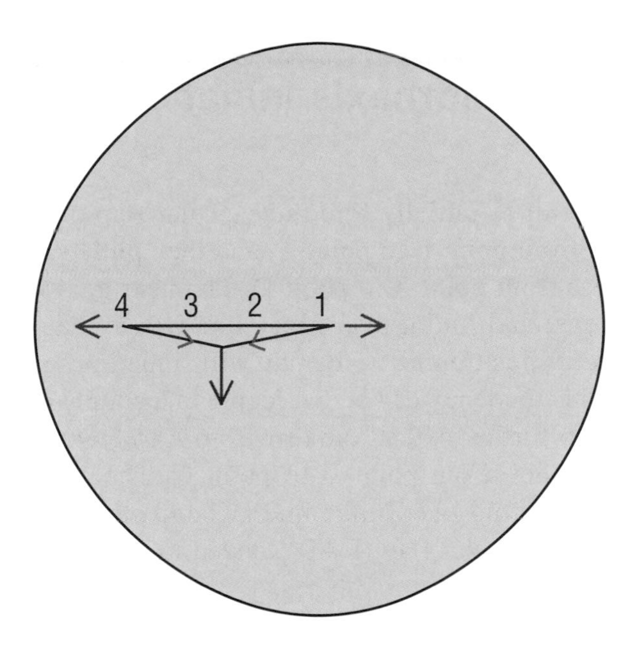

Figure 5-8-1

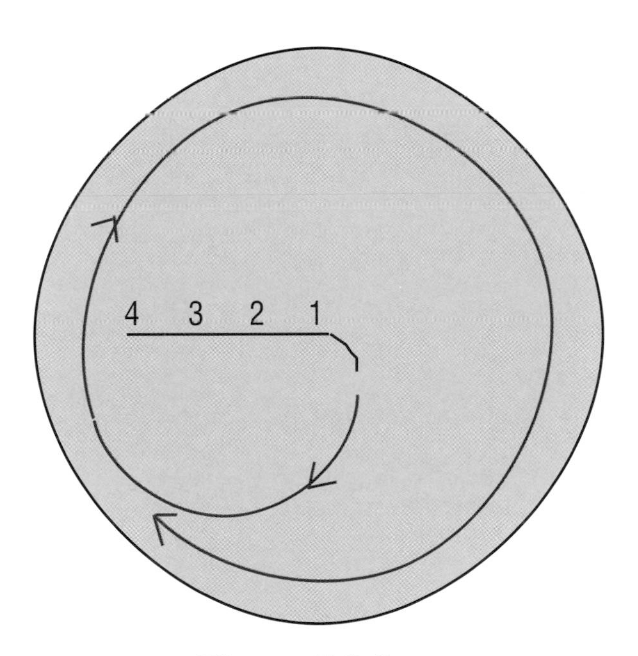

Figure 5-8-2

Figure 5-8

Capsulorhexis Initiation 3

Sometimes it is difficult to initially fold the capsular flap over. In Figure 5-9, the capsule has been incised from point B to point A, and then pulled downward at point A to create the shearing tear from point A to point D. The next goal is to engage the flap (with cystotome or forceps) and fold it over hinge line DB so that point A will overlie point E. However, after thus positioning it, the flap will sometimes spontaneously return to its original position. This tendency can be overcome in a couple of ways. More shearing force can be applied to further extend the tear from A to beyond D. Alternatively, a relaxing incision can be made from point B to point C. The resultant U-shaped flap (CBAD) will usually readily fold over hinge line DC and stabilize in the folded position, whereas the original triangular flap (BAD) tended to return to its in vivo position because of constraint at point B.

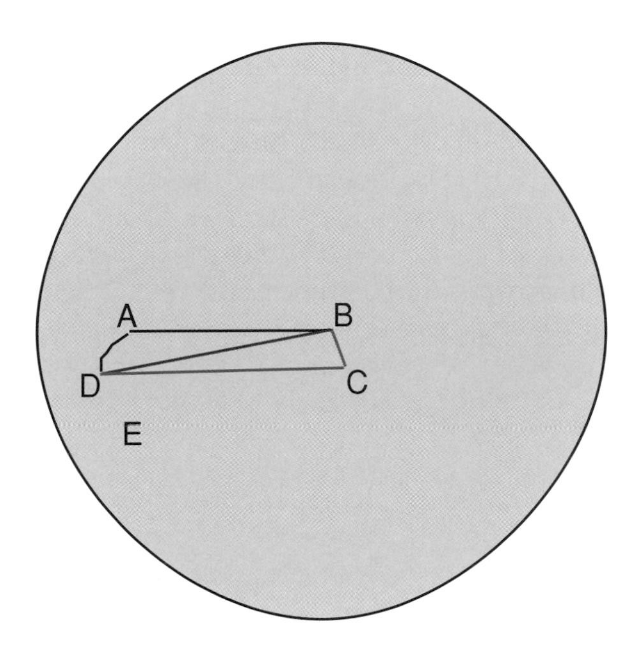

Figure 5-9

Capsulorhexis Initiation 4

An alternate method for beginning the capsulorhexis is shown in Figure 5-10-1. The capsule has been incised at point A; the ensuing triangular flap is grasped at point B and drawn in the direction of the red arrow. Shearing forces are acting roughly equally at points C and D, resulting in a capsule strip with parallel sides. In Figure 5-10-2, the pulling motion has changed to a curvilinear direction (red arrow), which results in the strip changing direction by curving from F to G with point E acting as a central pivot point; the lines EF and EG are radii of curvature for this portion of the tear. At this point, HG can be used as a radius of curvature instead of EG; this has been performed in Figure 5-10-3 where HI and HG (from Figure 5-10-2) serve as new radii of curvature. Notice how the curvilinear red arrow in 5-10-3 reflects this larger radius of curvature relative to the more tightly curved arrow in 5-10-2; these arrows represent the direction that the flap was pulled with either a cystotome or forceps to control the direction of the tear.

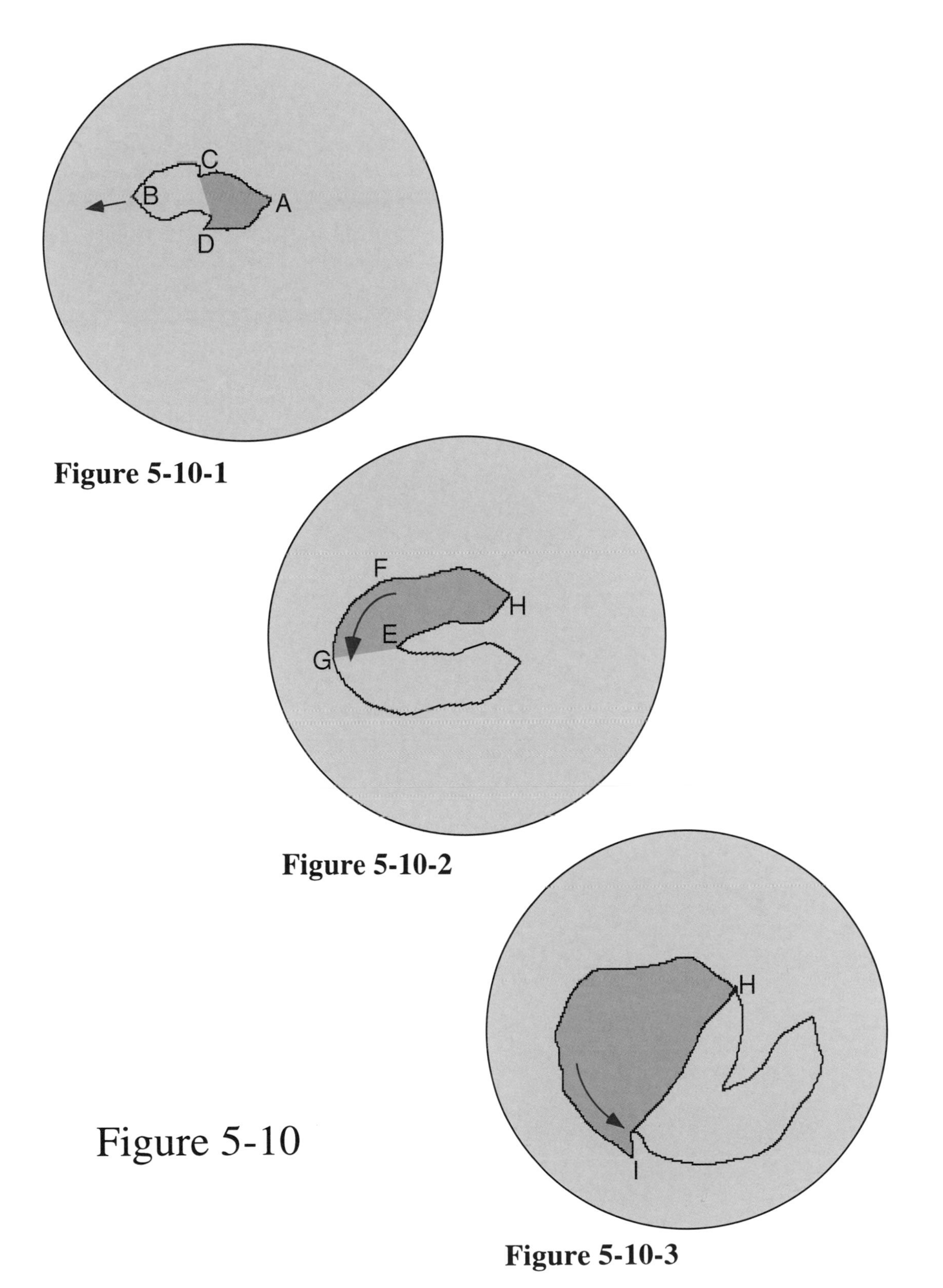

Figure 5-10-1

Figure 5-10-2

Figure 5-10

Figure 5-10-3

Anterior Cortical Opacities

Dense anterior cortical opacities can block the red reflex and interfere with visualization of the capsulorhexis. However, even though the point of tearing is obscured in Figure 5-11, its location can be extrapolated (green lines) from the adjacent visible capsulorhexis, the flap edge, and the line formed as the flap folds over on the intact capsule. Note that if the flap edge were visualized along the red line (b) instead of the black line (a), you could infer that the tearing point was too peripheral (d) and take appropriate measures, such as redirecting the flap more centrally or even converting to a ripping technique.

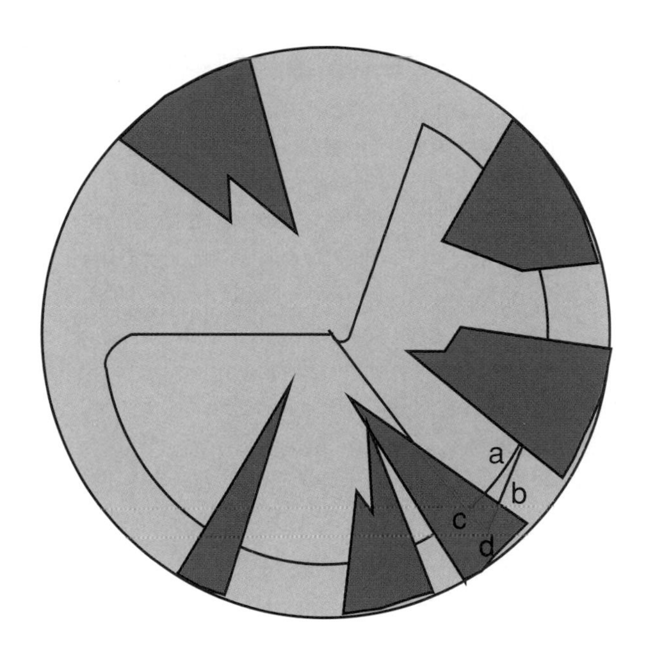

Figure 5-11

Capsulorhexis Enlargement

Figure 5-12-1 illustrates a borderline pupil; it was just large enough to allow a minimal capsulorhexis and subsequent phacoemulsification. However, forcing an implant through an insufficiently large capsulorhexis can cause a break in the continuous tear and/or (even more likely) cause zonular stress or rupture. Furthermore, a small capsulorhexis has the risk of scarring down to a visually compromising diameter. The opening can be enlarged by first inflating the capsular bag with viscoelastic to provide a safety margin for the posterior capsule. The anterior capsule is then incised with Vannas or Grieshaber scissors as shown in Figure 5-12-2. Note the exposure provided by a Lester, Seibel, or other angled instrument with a rounded tip inserted through the side-port incision. The flap is then grasped with capsule forceps and directed in a shearing manner as shown to enlarge the capsulotomy by removing a continuous strip. The Lester hook is repositioned as necessary to maintain exposure.

Another rationale might say to implant the lens in the bag prior to the enlargement. This course of action would not only stress the small capsulotomy and zonules as stated above, but it would also compromise the controllability of the enlargement by having extraneous forces acting on the tear via haptic tension on the bag. Another rationale might say to do this procedure prior to phaco to ensure maximum protection for the posterior capsule. However, the resultant prostaglandin release from the iris manipulation may result in pupillary contracture which would compromise the safety of phacoemulsification. Another option would be to stretch the pupil or to use Grieshaber or other iris retraction hooks and/or sphincterotomies to enlarge and maintain the pupil during the whole procedure. However, the pupil size may not be the only limitation. If cortical (see Figure 5-11) or other medial opacities interfere with the red reflex, it is often better to err on the side of making a smaller continuous tear capsulorhexis rather than risking a peripheral extension due to poor visualization. Then, after phaco and IA are complete and the red reflex is enhanced, you can use the same capsulorhexis enlargement method as in Figure 5-12-3.

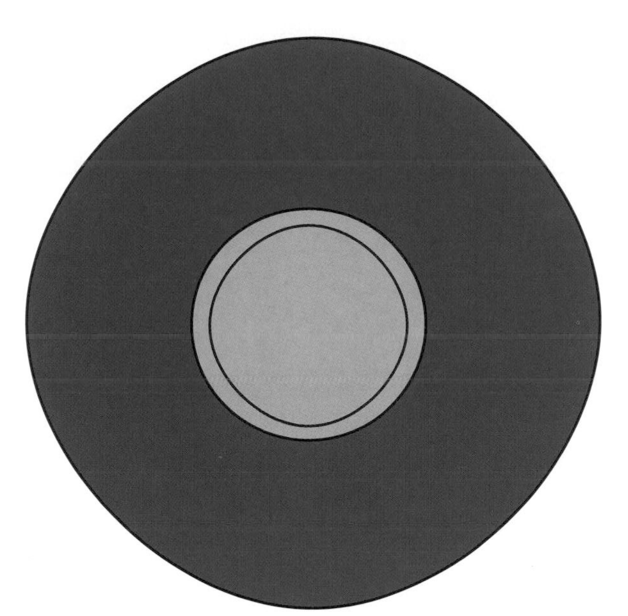

Figure 5-12-1

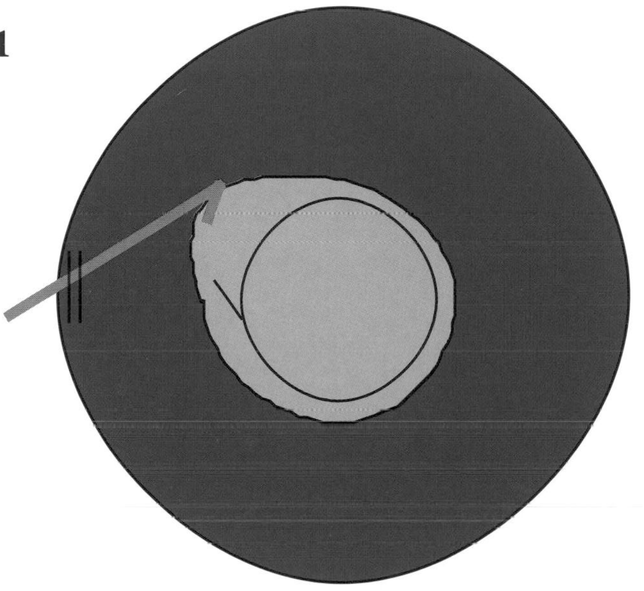

Figure 5-12-2

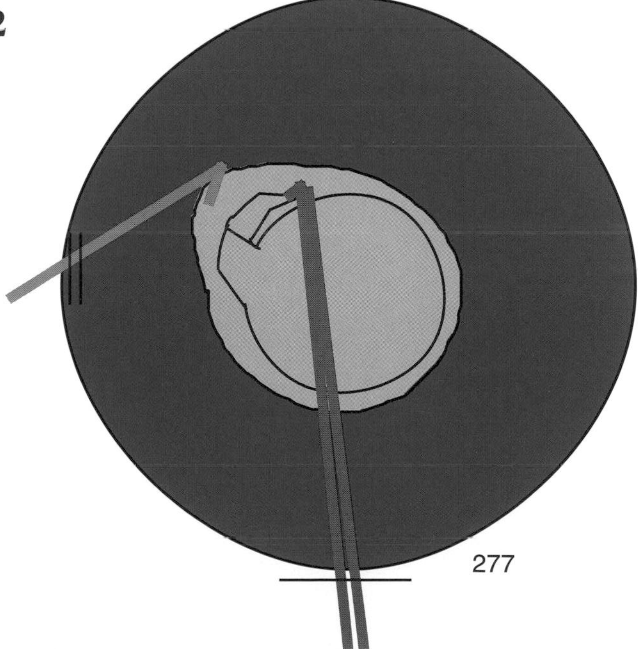

Figure 5-12-3

Figure 5-12

APPENDICES

Appendix A: Implied Surface Area in Units of mm Hg

The force required to suspend a column of mercury (Hg) of height (h), where volume of a cylinder = $\Pi r^2 h$ and density = ρ, is:

$$\mathbf{F = mass \cdot acceleration}$$

$$\mathbf{F = (density \cdot volume) \cdot g, \text{ where } g = gravitational\ acceleration}$$

$$\mathbf{F = \rho \cdot \Pi r^2 h \cdot g}$$

$$\mathbf{Pressure = \frac{force}{area}, \text{ and } area = \Pi r^2}$$

$$\mathbf{P = \frac{\rho \Pi r^2 hg}{\Pi r^2} = \rho hg}$$

So, P is a linear function of the column height (ie, mm of Hg). Also, note in the last line of the derivation that the units of surface area (Πr^2) in the numerator and denominator cancel each other out such that the final unit of mm Hg has the surface area implied but not expressed. Therefore, when calculating the force for a given pressure and surface area, it is more convenient to convert mm Hg to PSI (pounds per square inch), as seen in Appendix B.

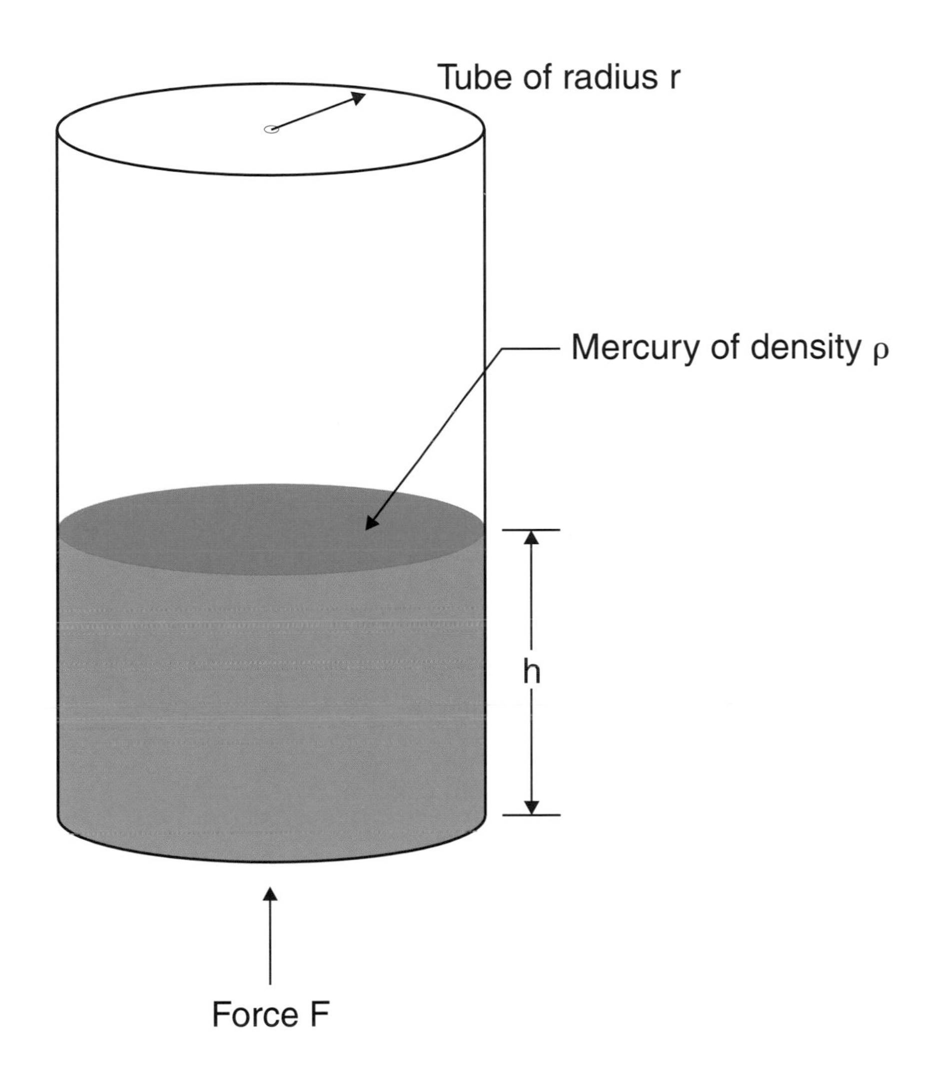
Tube of radius r
Mercury of density ρ
h
Force F

Appendix B: Aspiration Port Surface Area Derivation

The formula for the surface area of a circle is $\Pi r^2 = \Pi rr$, where r = radius of the needle's internal diameter (I.D.). The formula for the surface area of an oval is $\Pi r(r_l)$, where r is the short radius of the oval (same value as the radius of a circular cross-section of the needle) and r_l is the long radius of the oval. Since r_l is always greater than r, $r(r_l)$ will always be greater than r(r), and it follows that the oval cross-section of a beveled needle's aspiration port will have larger surface area than the circular cross-section of a 0° tip's aspiration port (see Figure 1-48). A standard phaco needle has an I.D. of 0.9mm = .035 inches. To compute r_l, the total length of the oval (diameter) is computed with trigonometric function as shown, such that:

$$\cos 45^\circ = \frac{b}{c}, \text{ where } \cos 45^\circ = .707 \text{ and } b = .035''$$

$$.707 = \frac{.035''}{c}$$

$$c = \frac{.035''}{.707} = .050'' = \text{long diameter of oval}$$

$$r_l = \text{long radius of oval} = \frac{\text{long diameter of oval}}{2} = \frac{.050''}{2} = .025''$$

$$r = \text{short radius of oval} = \text{radius of } 0^\circ \text{ tip} = \frac{.035''}{2} = .018''$$

$$\text{area of } 0^\circ \text{ tip} = \Pi r^2 = \Pi(.018'')^2 = .0010 \text{ sq. inch}$$

$$\text{area of } 45^\circ \text{ tip} = \Pi(r)(r_l) = \Pi(.018'')(.025'') = .0014 \text{ sq. inch}$$

to convert mm Hg to PSI use

$$\frac{14.7 \text{ PSI (atmospheric pressure at sea level)}}{760\text{mm Hg (atmospheric pressure at sea level)}} = \frac{.019 \text{ PSI}}{1\text{mm Hg}}$$

$$\text{so, for pump vacuum of 100mm Hg} = 100\text{mm Hg} \bullet \frac{.019 \text{ PSI}}{\text{mm Hg}} = 1.9 \text{ PSI}$$

$$\text{holding force of vacuum for } 0^\circ \text{ tip} = \frac{1.9 \text{ lbs.}}{\text{sq. inch}} \bullet .0010 \text{ sq. inch} = .0019 \text{ lbs.}$$

$$\text{holding force of vacuum for } 45^\circ \text{ tip} = \frac{1.9 \text{ lbs.}}{\text{sq. inch}} \bullet .0014 \text{ sq. inch} = .0027 \text{ lbs.}$$

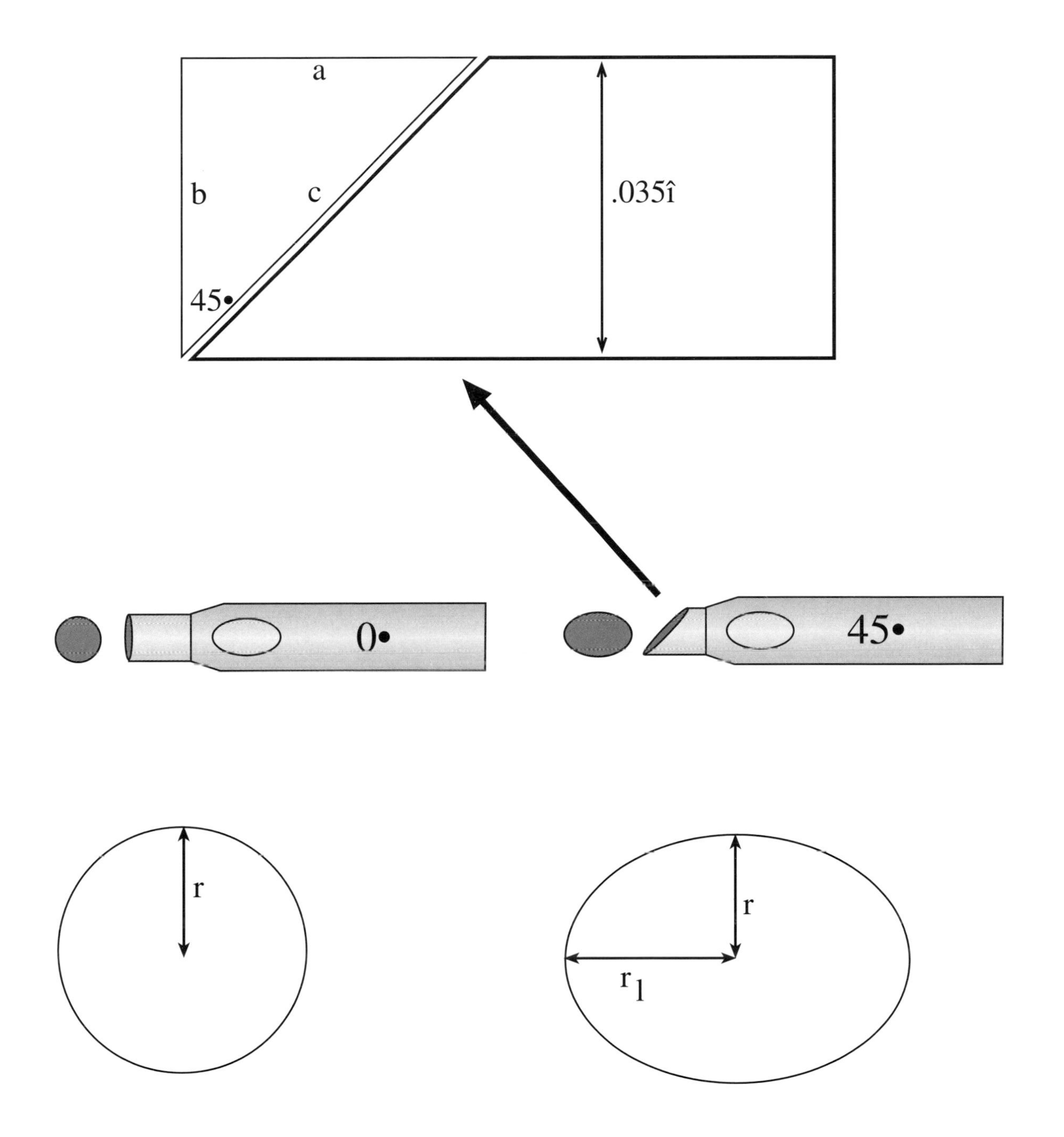
a
b
c
45•
.035î
0•
45•
r
r
r_1

Appendix C: Summary of Pressure Terminology

As defined in Appendix A, pressure is the force per unit area. Any pressure above the absolute vacuum of outer space is a positive value. However, pressures are often expressed as a pressure differential relative to atmospheric pressure at sea level, in which case pressures above atmospheric are expressed as positive numbers and pressures less than atmospheric are expressed as negative numbers. Pressures less than atmospheric are also often expressed as units of (relative) vacuum, which are by convention positive numbers. For example:

200mm Hg vacuum = -200mm Hg pressure

Both of the above values refer to a pressure that is 200mm Hg below ambient atmospheric pressure (see accompanying figure).

Atmospheric pressure is defined as 760mm Hg or 14.7 PSI at sea level. If a Goldmann Applanation Tonometer produces a reading of 20mm Hg, this then represents the positive pressure above atmospheric pressure, such that the eye's actual hydrostatic pressure is 760 + 20 = 780mm Hg. Similarly, a phaco pump which produces a holding force at the occluded tip of 100mm Hg vacuum (or equivalently -100mm Hg pressure) has an actual internal tip pressure of 760 - 100 = 660mm Hg. Therefore, it can be seen that the numbers used in phaco surgery, as well as ophthalmology in general, represent a pressure differential as opposed to an actual pressure. Moreover, a relative pressure differential or vacuum can exist between two pressures even if neither pressure is below atmospheric pressure (see Figure 1-9-1, as well as the discussion with Figure 1-37).

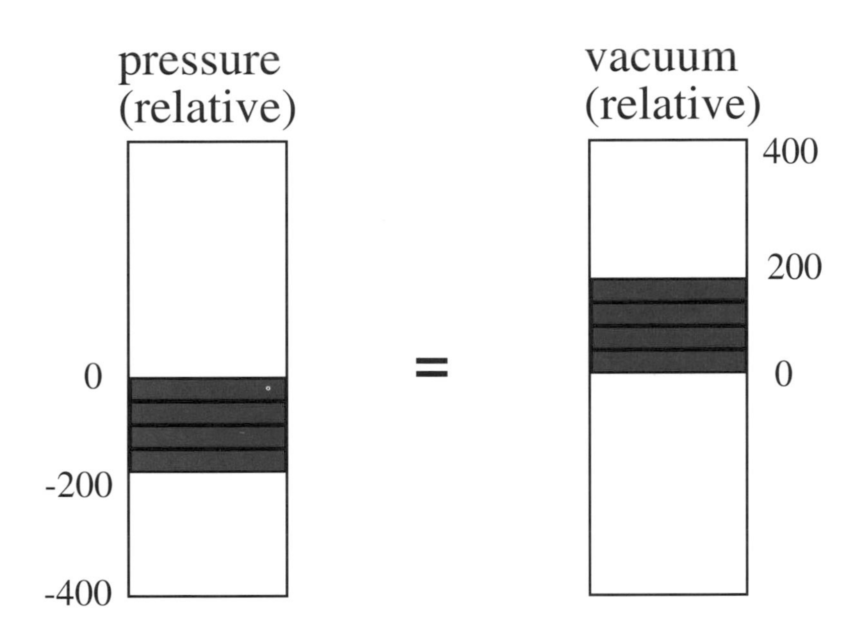

Zero (on meter) = atmospheric pressure
actual atmospheric pressure = 760mm Hg

Note: The irrigating bottle yields an IOP of 11mm Hg (above atmospheric pressure) for every 15cm (6 inches) of elevation above the eye. This relationship is accurate for hydrostatic pressures in pedal position 1; the IOP decreases in pedal positions 2 and 3 in proportion to the pump strength and to the degree of aspiration port occlusion (see Figures 1-10 and 1-35b).

Bibliography

Chip and Flip. Fine IH. *Video Journal of Ophthalmology*. 1991;VII(4).

Divide and Conquer. Gimbel HV. *Phacoemulsification*. ISBN 1-56283-004-X. *Video Journal of Ophthalmology*. 800-822-3100.

Four Quadrant Method. Shepherd JR. *Video Journal of Ophthalmology*. 1990;VI(2).

Kratz/Maloney Two-Handed Method. Maloney WF. *Video Journal of Ophthalmology*. 1987;III(4).

One-Handed Method. Allergan Medical Optics Department of Professional Education. *Small Incision Surgery with Richard Livernois, MD*. Irvine, Calif. Call for video 800-347-4500.

Osher RH. *The Mature Cataract and Its Sharp Edges: Fact or Fiction?* 1997 ASCRS Film Festival grand prize winner.

Phaco Chop. Nagahara K. *Video Journal of Ophthalmology*. 1993;IX(3).

Stop and Chop. Koch P. *Mastering Phacoemulsification*. Thorofare, NJ: SLACK Incorporated; 1993.

Index